Lecture Notes in Artificial Intelligence 7885

Subseries of Lecture Notes in Computer Science

LNAI Series Editors

Randy Goebel
University of Alberta, Edmonton, Canada
Yuzuru Tanaka
Hokkaido University, Sapporo, Japan
Wolfgang Wahlster
DFKI and Saarland University, Saarbrücken, Germany

LNAI Founding Series Editor

Joerg Siekmann
DFKI and Saarland University, Saarbrücken, Germany

W0234385

Niels Peek   Roque Marín Morales
Mor Peleg (Eds.)

Artificial Intelligence in Medicine

14th Conference on Artificial Intelligence
in Medicine, AIME 2013
Murcia, Spain, May 29 – June 1, 2013
Proceedings

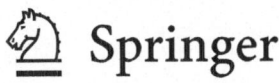 Springer

Series Editors

Randy Goebel, University of Alberta, Edmonton, Canada
Jörg Siekmann, University of Saarland, Saarbrücken, Germany
Wolfgang Wahlster, DFKI and University of Saarland, Saarbrücken, Germany

Volume Editors

Niels Peek
University of Amsterdam, Dept. of Medical Informatics
Meibergdreef 9, 1105 AZ Amsterdam, The Netherlands
E-mail: n.b.peek@amc.uva.nl

Roque Marín Morales
University of Murcia, Dept. of Information Engineering and Communications
Campus de Espinardo, 30100 Espinardo (Murcia), Spain
E-mail: roquemm@um.es

Mor Peleg
University of Haifa, Dept. of Information Systems
Rabin Bldg., 31905 Haifa, Israel
E-mail: morpeleg@is.haifa.ac.il

ISSN 0302-9743   e-ISSN 1611-3349
ISBN 978-3-642-38325-0   e-ISBN 978-3-642-38326-7
DOI 10.1007/978-3-642-38326-7
Springer Heidelberg Dordrecht London New York

Library of Congress Control Number: 2013937754

CR Subject Classification (1998): I.2, J.3, H.2.8, I.5, H.4, I.4, G.3

LNCS Sublibrary: SL 7 – Artificial Intelligence

Typesetting: Camera-ready by author, data conversion by Scientific Publishing Services, Chennai, India

Printed on acid-free paper

Springer is part of Springer Science+Business Media (www.springer.com)

Preface

The European Society for Artificial Intelligence in Medicine (AIME) was established in 1986 following a very successful workshop held in Pavia, Italy, the year before. The principal aims are to foster fundamental and applied research in the application of artificial intelligence (AI) techniques to medical care and medical research, and to provide a forum at biennial conferences for discussing any progress made. For this reason the main activity of the society was the organization of a series of biennial conferences, held in Marseilles, France (1987), London, UK (1989), Maastricht, The Netherlands (1991), Munich, Germany (1993), Pavia, Italy (1995), Grenoble, France (1997), Aalborg, Denmark (1999), Cascais, Portugal (2001), Protaras, Cyprus (2003), Aberdeen, UK (2005), Amsterdam, The Netherlands (2007), Verona, Italy (2009), and Bled, Slovenia (2011). This volume contains the proceedings of AIME 2013, the 14th Conference on Articial Intelligence in Medicine, held in Murcia, Spain, May 29-June 1, 2013.

The AIME 2013 goals were to present and consolidate the international state of the art of AI in biomedical research from the perspectives of theory, methodology, systems, and applications. A specific focus for the AIME 2013 conference was the role of AI in telemedicine and eHealth systems. The conference included two invited lectures, full and short papers, tutorials, workshops, and a doctoral consortium.

In the conference announcement, authors were solicited to submit original contributions regarding the development of theory, methods, systems, and applications for solving problems in the biomedical field, including AI approaches in biomedical informatics, molecular medicine, and healthcare organizational aspects. Authors of papers addressing theory were requested to describe the properties of novel AI models potentially useful for solving biomedical problems. Authors of papers addressing theory and methods were asked to describe the development or the extension of AI methods, to address the assumptions and limitations of the proposed techniques and to discuss their novelty with respect to the state of the art. Authors of papers addressing systems and applications were asked to describe the development, implementation, or evaluation of new AI-inspired tools and systems in the biomedical field. They were asked to link their work to underlying theory, and either analyze the potential benefits to solve biomedical problems or present empirical evidence of benefits in clinical practice.

AIME 2013 received 96 abstract submissions, 82 thereof were eventually submitted as complete papers. Submissions came from 25 different countries, including eight outside Europe. All papers were carefully peer-reviewed by experts from the Program Committee with the support of additional reviewers. Each submission was reviewed by at least two and in most cases three reviewers. The reviewers judged the overall quality of the submitted papers, together with their relevance to the AIME conference, technical correctness, novelty with respect to state of the art, scholarship and quality of presentation. In addition, the reviewers provided detailed written comments on each paper, and stated their confidence in the subject area.

A small committee consisting of the AIME 2013 Scientific Chair, Niels Peek, the Scientific Co-chair and Organizing Committee Chair, Roque Marin, and the AIME 2011 Scientific Chair, Mor Peleg, made the final decisions regarding the AIME 2013 scientific program. This process started with a virtual meeting held on February 14, 2013, using three-part video conferencing. In subsequent days short discussions followed. The process ended with a short visit of the Scientific Chair to Murcia.

As a result, 18 long papers (with an acceptance rate of about 27%) and 26 short papers were accepted. Each long paper was presented in a 25-minute oral presentation during the conference. Each short paper was presented in a 5-minute presentation and by a poster. The papers were organized according to their topics in the following main themes: (1) Decision Support, Guidelines and Protocols; (2) Semantic Technology I; (3) Bioinformatics; (4) Machine Learning; (5) Probabilistic Modelling and Reasoning; (6) Image and Signal Processing; (7) Semantic Technology II; (8) Temporal Data Visualization and Analysis; and (9) Natural Language Processing.

AIME 2013 had the privilege of hosting two invited speakers: Dominik Aronsky, from the Vanderbilt University Medical Center, USA, and Hermie Hermens, from the University of Twente, The Netherlands. Dominik Aronsky showed how an integrated information infrastructure with computer-based decision support can help care providers to deliver high-quality patient care, optimize operational activities, and facilitate clinical and informatics research studies in an emergency care setting. Hermie Hermens discussed historical and current trends in the field of telemedicine, and the challenges of adding intelligence to telemedicine systems.

The fifth Doctoral Consortium for the AIME series of conferences was organized this time by Nada Lavrač from the Jožef Stefan Institute in Llubljana, Slovenia. The Doctoral Consortium provided an opportunity for seven PhD students to present their preliminary work and to discuss their plans and preliminary results. A scientific panel consisting of Ameen Abu-Hanna, Steen Andreassen, Riccardo Bellazzi, Carlo Combi, Michel Dojat, Nada Lavrac, Peter Lucas, Roque Marin, Niels Peek, Silvana Quaglini, and Yuval Shahar discussed the contents of the students doctoral theses.

A significant number of full-day workshops were organized after the AIME 2013 main conference: the workshop entitled Knowledge Representation for Health Care and Process-Oriented Information Systems in Healthcare (KR4HC 2013 / ProHealth 2013), chaired by David Riaño (Universitat Rovira i Virgili, Spain) and Annette ten Teije (Vrije Universiteit Amsterdam, The Netherlands); the workshop Agents Applied in Health Care, chaired by Antonio Moreno (Universitat Rovira i Virgili, Spain); and the workshop Artificial Intelligence for Medical Data Streams, chaired by Pedro Pereira (University of Porto, Portugal). Moreover, three interactive tutorials were organized prior to the AIME 2013 main conference: An Introduction to Agent-Based Modeling, by John H. Holmes (University of Pennsylvania, USA); Bayesian Networks in Computational Neuroscience, by Pedro Larrañaga and Concha Bielza (Universidad Politécnica de Madrid, Spain); and Evaluating Prognostic Models in Medicine, by Ameen Abu-Hanna and Niels Peek (University of Amsterdam, The Netherlands).

We would like to thank everyone who contributed to AIME 2013. First of all we would like to thank the authors of the papers submitted and the members of the Program Committee together with the additional reviewers. Thanks are also due to the invited speakers as well as to the organizers of the workshops and the tutorial and doctoral consortium. Final thanks go to the Organizing Committee, who managed all the work making this conference possible. The free EasyChair conference Web system (http://www.easychair.org/) was an important tool supporting us in the management of submissions, reviews, selection of accepted papers, and preparation of the overall material for the final proceedings. We would like to thank the University of Murcia and the Campus Mare Nostrum, which hosted and sponsored the conference; the Fundación Séneca (Agence for Science and Technology of the Region of Murcia), who sponsored the conference through the Program for Mobility, Cooperation and Internationalization Jiménez de la Espada (Ref.18676/OC/12); and the Spanish Society of Artificial Intelligence (AEPIA), who provided a grant for young researchers. Finally, we thank the Springer team for helping us in the final preparation of this LNCS book.

March 2013   Niels Peek
                                                       Roque Marín Morales
                                                            Mor Peleg

Organization

Scientific Chair

Niels Peek

Program Committee

Raza Abidi, Canada

Ameen Abu-Hanna,
  The Netherlands
Klaus-Peter Adlassnig, Austria
Steen Andreassen, Denmark
Pedro Barahona, Portugal
Riccardo Bellazzi, Italy
Isabelle Bichindaritz, USA
Carlo Combi, Italy

Amar Das, USA
Michel Dojat, France
Henrik Eriksson, Sweden
Paulo Félix, Spain
Catherine Garbay, France
Adela Grando, UK
Femida Gwadry-Sridhar, Canada
Milos Hauskrecht, USA
Reinhold Haux, Germany
John Holmes, USA
Arjen Hommersom,
  The Netherlands
Werner Horn, Austria
Val Jones, The Netherlands
Katharina Kaiser, Austria
Elpida Keravnou, Cyprus
Pedro Larrañaga, Spain
Nada Lavrač, Slovenia
  (Doctoral Consortium Chair)
Xiaohui Liu, UK
Peter Lucas, The Netherlands
Mar Marcos, Spain

Roque Marín Morales, Spain
  (Local Organizing Committee Chair)

Michael Marscholleck, Germany
Carolyn McGregor, Canada
Paola Mello, Italy
Silvia Miksch, Austria
Stefania Montani, Italy
Barbara Oliboni, Italy
Niels Peek, The Netherlands (Scientic
  Program Committee Chair)
Mor Peleg, Israel
Christian Popow, Austria
Silvana Quaglini, Italy
Stephen Rees, Denmark
David Riaño, Spain
Lucia Sacchi, Italy
Abdul Sattar, Australia
Rainer Schmidt, Germany
Brigitte Seroussi, France
Yuval Shahar, Israel

Costas Spyropoulos, Greece
Annette ten Teije, The Netherlands
Paolo Terenziani, Italy
Samson Tu, USA
Allan Tucker, UK
Frank van Harmelen, The Netherlands

Alfredo Vellido, Spain
Dongwen Wang, USA
Blaz Zupan, Slovenia
Pierre Zweigenbaum, France

Local Organizing Committee

Manuel Campos
Jesualdo Fernandez
Jose Juarez Herrero (Co-chair)
Antonio Gomariz
Eduardo Lupiani

Roque Marín Morales (Chair)
Jose Palma
Guido Sciavicco
Rafael Valencia

Additional Reviewers

Álvarez, Miguel
Amizadeh, Saeed
Barbarini, Nicola
Batal, Iyad
Bottrighi, Alessio
Bragaglia, Stefano
Cariñena, Purificación
Chesani, Federico
Dentler, Kathrin
Hoffmann, Stephan
Khanna, Sankalp
Konstantopoulos, Stasinos
Koukourikos, Antonis
Krithara, Anastasia
Lammarsch, Tim
Lappenschaar, Martijn
López-Vallverdú, Joan Albert

Martínez-Salvador, Begoña
Messai, Nizar
Milian, Krystina
Minard, Anne-Lyse
Petasis, Georgios
Petridis, Sergios
Portet, François
Pozzani, Gabriele
Presedo, Jesús
Riguzzi, Fabrizio
Rind, Alexander
Sottara, Davide
Teijeiro, Tomás
Torres-Sospedra, Joaquín
Valizadegan, Hamed
Velikova, Marina

Doctoral Consortium Committee

Ameen Abu-Hanna, The Netherlands
Steen Andreassen, Denmark
Riccardo Bellazzi, Italy
Carlo Combi, Italy
Michel Dojat, France
Nada Lavrač, Slovenia (Chair)

Peter Lucas, The Netherlands
Roque Marín Morales, Spain
Niels Peek, The Netherlands
Silvana Quaglini, Italy
Yuval Shahar, Israel

Workshops

Knowledge Representation for Health Care and Process-Oriented Information Systems in Healthcare (KR4HC 2013/ProHealth 2013)

Co-chairs:

Richard Lenz	University of Erlangen-Nuremberg, Germany
Silvia Miksch	Vienna University of Technology, Austria
Mor Peleg	University of Haifa, Israel
Manfred Reichert	University of Ulm, Germany
David Riaño	Universitat Rovira i Virgili, Tarragona, Spain
Annette ten Teije	Vrije Universiteit, Amsterdam, The Netherlands

Agents Applied in Health Care

Co-chairs:

Antonio Moreno	Universitat Rovira i Virgili, Tarragona, Spain
Ulises Cortés	Technical University of Catalonia, Barcelona, Spain
Magí Lluch-Ariet	Barcelona Digital, Spain
Helena Lindgren	University of Umea, Sweden
Michael Schumacher	University of Applied Sciences Western Switzerland, Sierre, Switzerland
David Isern	Universitat Rovira i Virgili, Tarragona, Spain

Artificial Intelligence for Medical Data Streams

Co-chairs:

Pedro Pereira Rodrigues	University of Porto, Portugal
Mykola Pechenizkiy	Eindhoven University of Technology, The Netherlands
João Gama	University of Porto, Portugal
Mohamed Medhat Gaber	University of Portsmouth, UK
Carolyn McGregor	University of Ontario Institute of Technology, Canada

Tutorials

Introduction to Agent-Based Modeling

John H. Holmes	University of Pennsylvania, USA

Bayesian Networks in Computational Neuroscience

Pedro Larrañaga and Concha Bielza	Universidad Politécnica de Madrid, Spain

Evaluating Prognostic Models in Medicine

Ameen Abu-Hanna and
    Niels Peek   University of Amsterdam, The Netherlands

Computer-Based Decision Support in the Emergency Department

Dominik Aronsky[1]

[1] Dept. of Biomedical Informatics & Emergency Medicine, Eskind Biomedical Library, Vanderbilt University, Nashville, TN, USA

Abstract. The Emergency Department is a fast-paced, information intensive environment that can benefit from improved information management. The presentation will discuss how an integrated information system infrastructure can support providers to deliver high-quality patient care, optimize operational activities, and facilitate clinical and informatics research studies in an emergency care setting. Illustrative examples will include improvement of pneumonia-care processes, implementation of asthma guidelines, and forecasting Emergency Department overcrowding.

Towards Intelligent Telemedicine Services

Hermie Hermens[1,2]

[1] Telemedicine Group, Roessingh Research and Development, Enschede,
The Netherlands
[2] Telemedicine Group, University of Twente, Enschede, The Netherlands

Abstract. Telemedicine is an area of innovation in the delivery of health care services, which is expected to have a great impact by making health care more efficient and cost effective, and by supporting independent living and self-management. Especially these last two are crucial as the number of people with chronic conditions who need long term care increases while our limited health service resources become more and more stretched.

Telemedicine has gone through a number of cycles of evolution. In the 80's it was demonstrated that remote consultation was possible and clinically valid; later the feasibility of remote detection of critical events such as seizures was established. More recently larger scale studies (e.g. Clear, Myotel, HelloDoc) showed that clinical outcomes are comparable to conventional care and that by replacing parts of the current care process by telemedicine solutions, cost effective results can be obtained.

Telemedicine is now challenged to enter the phase of mature solutions and large scale deployment. One of the main obstacles to reaching this goal is the lack of intelligence in current systems. Clinicians need to be supported by intelligent decision support systems and patients need to be coached to support their ambitions to be independent and to change their adverse behavior, hence intelligent, safe supporting environments need to be created.

Examples of ongoing research in these directions will be presented which illustrate the integration of clinical practice guidelines into decision support systems (Mobiguide); smart activity coaching (IS-Active); and monitoring of patient behavior at home (Carebox).

Table of Contents

1. Decision Support, Guidelines and Protocols

2. Semantic Technology I

3. Bioinformatics

4. Machine Learning

5. Probabilistic Modelling and Reasoning

6. Image and Signal Processing

7. Semantic Technology II

8. Temporal Data Visualization and Analysis

9. Natural Language Processing

From Decision to Shared-Decision: Introducing Patients' Preferences in Clinical Decision Analysis - A Case Study in Thromboembolic Risk Prevention

Lucia Sacchi[1,*], Carla Rognoni[1,2], Stefania Rubrichi[1], Silvia Panzarasa[1], and Silvana Quaglini[1]

[1] Dipartimento di Ingegneria Industriale e dell'Informazione,
University of Pavia, Pavia, Italy
{lucia.sacchi,stefania.rubrichi,carla.rognoni,
silvia.panzarasa,silvana.quaglini}@unipv.it
[2] Centre for Research on Health and Social Care Management (CERGAS),
Bocconi University, Milan, Italy

Abstract. In the context of the EU project MobiGuide, the development of a patient-centric decision support system based on clinical guidelines is the main focus. The project is addressed to patients with chronic illnesses, including atrial fibrillation (AF). In this paper we describe a shared-decision model framework to address those situations, described in the guideline, where the lack of hard evidence makes it important for the care provider to share the decision with the patient and/or his relatives. To illustrate this subject we focus on an important subject tackled in the AF guideline: thromboembolic risk prevention. We introduce a utility model and a cost model to collect patient's preferences. On the basis of these preferences and of literature data, a decision model is implemented to compare different therapeutic options. The development of this framework increases the involvement of patients in the process of care focusing on the centrality of individual subjects.

Keywords: Decision Trees, Patient Preferences, QALYs, Atrial Fibrillation.

1   Introduction

Taking into account patients' preferences is nowadays an essential requirement in health decision-making [1,2]. As a matter of fact, patients increasingly want their personal perspectives to be considered in the process of care. Besides genetic-based personalized care, which is another way of viewing personalized medicine, our attention is focused on addressing individual attitudes, considering patient's perception of his health status, personal context, job-related requirements and economic conditions.

Clinical decision analysis refers to the process of exploiting a decision model to evaluate situations that imply the choice between two or more alternatives [3]. Such alternatives might regard for example choosing between two pharmacological treatments, between a surgical intervention and a drug, etc. As a matter of fact, even in an evidence-based setting where directions are summarized into a clinical practice

N. Peek, R. Marín Morales, and M. Peleg (Eds.): AIME 2013, LNAI 7885, pp. 1–10, 2013.
© Springer-Verlag Berlin Heidelberg 2013

guideline (CPG), there might exist situations, highlighted by the guideline itself, where it is important for the care provider to involve the patient in the decision. The process during which the patient and his care provider reach a clinical decision together is known as *shared decision* [4] and its main goal is to take into account both the available scientific evidence and the patient's perception of the consequences of different options [5].

The key point to turn a clinical decision into a shared decision is the introduction of patients' preferences in the analysis. In particular, we introduce a web-based framework that can be used by physicians to first elicit patient preferences and consequently run a decision model, using (also) values directly derived from the patient under observation. The concept of preference in this paper refers to both a patient's perception of the health states he is experiencing or he might experience as a consequence of the therapeutic choice, and to the economic impact such choices might have from his viewpoint. To take into account all this information, we have developed a utility model and a cost model. Such models are coupled to a theoretical decision model framework to solve the decision task. The final decision will thus account for patient-specific parameters, which might be different from population parameters derived from the literature.

The framework was developed in the context of the MobiGuide project (http://www.mobiguide-project.eu/). MobiGuide is a European funded project carried on by a consortium of 13 partners from several countries in Europe (Italy, Israel, The Netherlands, Spain, and Austria). It is aimed at developing a knowledge-based patient guidance system based on computer-interpretable guidelines (CIGs) and designed for the management of chronic illnesses, including Atrial Fibrillation (AF). The main components of the MobiGuide System are a Decision Support System (DSS), devoted to the representation and execution of CIGs, and a Body Area Network (BAN), including a network of sensors and a smartphone, to support telemonitoring of the patient. The data collected by the system are stored in a Patient Health Record (PHR). Among all the challenging objectives of the project, one involves the identification in the CPG of those recommendations where the lack of hard evidence requires a shared decision. Once those recommendations are identified, a suitable framework is set up to allow the physician managing the shared decision process. To illustrate the proposed framework, in this paper we focus on the AF Guideline [6] and in particular on a recommendation regarding the therapeutic management of antithrombotic risk for patients belonging to a specific risk category. In the following we will first introduce some theoretical bases and we will then present the proposed models and the implemented interfaces for thromboembolic risk prevention in AF.

2   Methods

Building the shared-decision framework involved using different methodologies and technologies for (i) dealing with the collection of patients' preferences and (ii) developing and running decision-theoretic models. The first issue included the design of a utility model and a cost model, and resulted into an interface that requires an active participation of the patient and the physician (or better the psychologist) to collect the most relevant patient-specific variables. The second issue is related to computational formalisms for decision making: even though other formalisms, such as influence diagrams or decision tables are available, we chose to use the decision tree formalism, because it allows easier knowledge elicitation from the doctors. Once fed with parameters suitably elicited from the patient and/or taken from the literature, the model automatically runs relying on a specific commercial software tool.

Moreover, we rely on a relational database to store both the tree characteristics necessary for the user interaction (i.e. the represented health states and some numerical parameters) and the tree results. Results are stored together with data about the interaction session, such as the identity of patient and physicians participating to the encounter, and their opinion on the usefulness of such interaction. All these data will be used for a future evaluation of the framework.

2.1   Collecting Patient's Preferences – Values, Utilities and Costs

The ultimate goal of a decision process is to select one out of several *decision options*, which are the possible treatment alternatives, object of the analysis. During the course of the analyzed disease, a patient may experience a set of different *health states*. Starting from a specific decision option and moving through the health states, the model leads to the determination of a specific *outcome*. The probability of occurrence of each health state and of transition between states is highly dependent on the treatment option selected. Intuitively, different subjects may perceive differently the quality of life related to health states. Moreover, one patient might consider the economic impact of a specific treatment more relevant for the choice with respect to another subject. For this reason, it is very important to tailor the decision process on the single patient, taking into account this variety of aspects. This moves the perspective of the clinical decision process towards a shared decision model, where the physician, during a face-to-face encounter with the patient, elicits his preferences related to different future scenarios.

From the observations above, it is clear that it is important to measure the quality of life the patient associates to specific conditions. Quality-Adjusted Life Years (QALYs) [7] is one of the most known and used indicators combining in a single value the life expectancy and the subjective perception of the health states considering physical, mental and social aspects. Given a time span T divided into n time intervals t_i, i=1 .. n, each one spent in a particular health state s_i, QALYs are defined as $\Sigma_{i=1,n}$ $(t_i u_i)$, where u_i is the *utility coefficient* (UC) for s_i. To define QALYs, we thus need to characterize each health state by a UC, ranging from 0 (death) to 1 (perfect health). Literature and web provide UCs for several health states (e.g. [8,9]). Such coefficients can be also conveniently elicited from the single patient, according to the physician/psychologist judgment about the patient's capability of understanding the elicitation methods that we will briefly describe below. Note that UCs are related to health states, so if different decision options lead to the same states, UCs are only elicited once. In addition, periodical reassessment of UCs may be necessary, as patients' perception of health states may change in time.

The Utility Model

The MobiGuide framework for shared decision is provided with the three classical methods for eliciting values and utilities: rating scale (RS), standard gamble (SG) and time trade-off (TTO). In the RS method, the patient is asked to rate all the states represented in the decision model on a scale ranging for example from 0 to 100. While not suitable for QALY calculation [10], these values, rescaled to 0-1, represent a patient-specific ranking of the states, useful for further consistency check.

The TTO method was specifically developed for use in health care [11]. To elicit utility for a specific health state, the subject is asked to compare two different scenarios: 1) to stay in that specific state for a time t (computed as the life expectancy of an individual with that chronic condition) until death or 2) to live an healthy life for a time $x < t$. During elicitation, time x is varied until the patient is indifferent between the two alternatives and the UC for the examined state is computed as the ratio x/t.

In the SG approach [12], the subject is offered two alternatives. Alternative 1 is a treatment that, if successful, might enable the patient to live in perfect health for the rest of his life. Such treatment, though, carries a certain risk of death r (think for example to a surgical intervention). Alternative 2 is that the subject lives all his life in the specific chronic state under analysis. During the face-to-face encounter the value for r is varied until the patient is indifferent between the two alternatives, and the UC is computed as $1-r$.

The Cost Model

Besides quantifying the patient's perception of different health states, it is also useful to involve him in the quantification of a cost model. In this model we consider the so-called "out-of-pocket" costs, which are the costs directly burdening the patient and causing an economic impact on his activities. While in the utility model the patient gives his opinion about the health states, for the cost model the patient is asked to provide information needed for quantifying the costs related to the clinical paths that are generated as a consequence of the different decision options. We have considered three categories of costs: (a) Costs related to the visits the patient has to undergo during his treatment; (b) Costs related to domiciliary care the patient may be in need of and (c) Home adaptation costs. As regards point (a), the value for the costs of the visits directly imputed to a patient depends on the position of the patient with respect to the national healthcare service, as some patients in Italy can have the visits costs totally covered. Besides the specific visits costs, we also took into account non-healthcare resources that are:

- The cost of the travel to the medical center where the visit is performed: this is a patient-specific value that depends on the distance the patient has to travel, the transportation   facility, etc.;
- The cost of the meals that the patient might have to pay for during the visit day;
- Patient's productivity loss, in case the patient is self-employed or retired;
- The cost related to an assistant possibly needed by the patient to reach the visit location: the model takes into account the cost for his/her travel and meals. In addition, it is possible to quantify the assistant's time in terms of productivity loss or salary.

The inclusion of costs related to domiciliary care is based on the fact that, after some specific events (such as for example a stroke) the patient might need domiciliary assistance. This is quantified by the salary given to the assistant in the case he/she is a professional employed by the patient. In case the assistant is a member of the patient's family, the cost is quantified in terms of productivity loss.

Assistance to the patient after a specific health event may also imply some home adaptation to manage the impairments the patients may experience after the event. These costs are assessed based on the results presented in [13], where the authors present an analysis of the overall social costs of stroke in Italy in terms of direct costs and productivity losses.

Since several cost components are related to the specific patient's context, the quantification holds as long as the context remains the same.

2.2   The Decision Models

As mentioned, in MobiGuide we have used Decision Trees (DT) [3]. DTs are one of the most used formalisms in the analysis of the logical structure and timing of clinical decision. They connect the alternative decision options to their expected effects and the final outcomes of each possible scenario. This is done following a formalism based on the combination of nodes and branches.

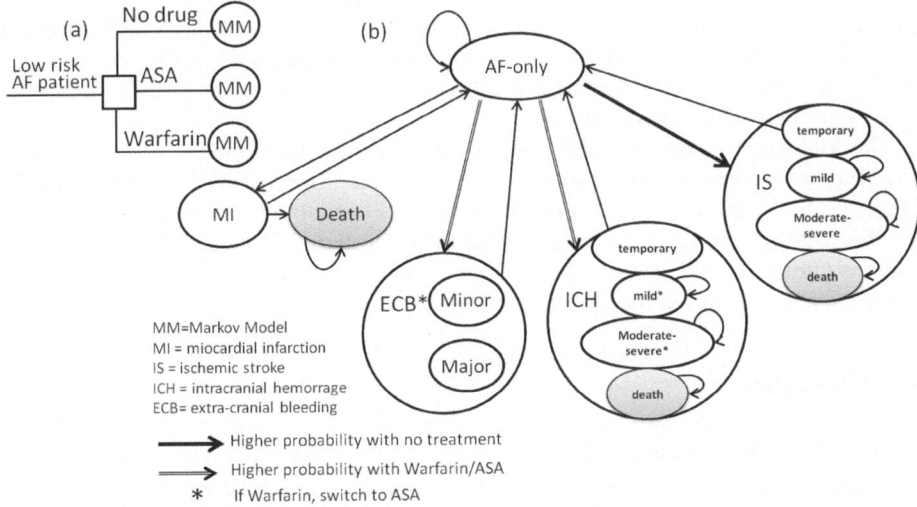

Fig. 1. (a) The initial part of the decision tree. Nodes labeled with "MM" are the starting point of the (simplified) Markov process represented in (b), where different line types indicate a trade-off between decreasing the risk of stroke and decreasing the risk of bleeding.

Figure 1 shows a scratch of a DT structure. It refers to the DT used for choosing the antithrombotic prophylaxis (note that, while the utility and the cost models presented so far are generic, i.e. they can be used for any type of shared decision, for every specific decision problem a specific decision-theoretic model must be implemented).

In a DT there are decision nodes, chance nodes and terminal nodes. Decision nodes are the starting points for the alternative options the study is considering. In the example shown in Figure 1, the decision node is the one labeled as "low risk AF patient", i.e. a patient eligible for that DT. Chance nodes symbolize an uncertain event, with a finite number of possible outcomes, which must be exhaustive and mutually exclusive. Each outcome is associated with its occurrence probability. A terminal node identifies the end of a path. It is associated with a *payoff* value, characteristic of that path, i.e. an outcome that the decision maker wants to maximize (e.g. QALYs) or minimize (e.g. cost). If events recur over time, and transitions among states must be represented, a Markov Model (MM) [14] is combined into the DT.

Running or solving a decision tree means calculating the expected values of the payoffs for all the possible decision options, by weighting the values at the end of the paths with their probability of occurrence. After a tree is run, the decision node shows, for each strategy, these expected values. The solution suggested by the model is the one optimizing the payoff. In case of multiple, competing payoffs, the results of the tree cannot be used as direct suggestions, but they just represent quantitative values useful to reason about. For example, suppose Option 1 gives better results in terms of QALYs than Option 2, which instead gives less out-of-pocket costs. In this case, the final choice could depend on the financial status of the patient.

In our framework, DTs are initially fed with probabilities and UCs found in the literature, and can be used as they are, when physicians judge that the patient is not able to provide additional, more personalized information. For the most frequent case, though, when the patient is able to provide his own preferences and context details, DTs can be personalized with patient's preferences and patient's profile features collected and stored through the above-illustrated generic models. As a result, decision-options are ranked on a personalized basis.

The MobiGuide trees are built using the commercial tool TreeAge (TreeAge Software Inc, www.treeage.com). Moreover, we have developed a web interface using the TreeAge Pro Interactive Tool, to make the models available also to the end users less familiar with the modeling technique. The physician will thus be able to browse probabilities, utilities, and costs, and to adjust values according to his knowledge if needed. Then he will run the decision tree and see the results.

3   Results

In this section we present the implementation of the proposed framework for shared decisions. To illustrate the specific developed decision model, we consider a recommendation included in the AF guideline on the management of thromboembolic risk:

*For primary prevention of thromboembolism in patients with nonvalvular AF who have just 1 of the following validated risk factors, **antithrombotic therapy with either aspirin or a vitamin K antagonist is reasonable**, based upon an assessment of the risk of bleeding complications, ability to safely sustain adjusted chronic anticoagulation, and **patient preferences**: age greater than or equal to 75 y (especially in female patients), hypertension, HF, impaired LV function, or diabetes mellitus*

This recommendation involves first of all the choice whether to treat or not, and in case of treatment, the choice between two drug options, namely acetyl salicylic acid (ASA) or oral anticoagulant therapy (OAT) with vitamin K antagonists such as warfarin. Thus, this is a case where the CPG recommendation itself suggests considering patient's preferences in the decision process.

3.1   The Decision Tree for Managing Antithrombotic Risk

In this paper we used an adapted version of a DT combined with MMs to compare the clinical pathways of an AF patient who may undergo the aforementioned treatment strategies for stroke prevention, or who takes no drug therapy at all [15]. During the Markov process, individuals move among health states that recur over time according to transition probabilities, which also may vary on time.

As shown in the diagram presented in Figure 1 (b), the health states implemented in the model are: AF-only, ischemic stroke (IS, which can be temporary, mild, moderate-severe, fatal), intracranial hemorrhage (ICH, which also can be temporary, mild, moderate-severe, fatal), myocardial infarction (MI), extra-cranial bleeding (minor and major), combined events and death. As outcomes, we have considered life years, QALYs, and costs. Figure 1 (b) shows a simplified representation of the implemented MM: the patient enters the process in the AF-only state. During the course of the disease, he can experience events such as MI, IS, ICH, and extra cranial bleedings. Temporary IS or ICH are events that cause only a transient disability and after which the patient recovers and goes back to the AF-only state. A patient experiencing more severe events, such as a mild/moderate-severe IS or ICH, is often subject to permanent impairment. The occurrence of these events depends on the different transition probabilities that are related both to the treatment and to the patient's risk for stroke, calculated on the basis of $CHADS_2$ score [16]. The administration of warfarin or ASA decreases the probability of occurrence of IS, but increases the probability of ICH and extra-cranial bleedings. On the other hand, the choice of not prescribing any therapy increases the probability of IS while limiting the occurrence of ICH and extra-cranial bleedings. If, while undergoing therapy with warfarin, a patient in the AF-only state experiences an ICH or a major extra-cranial bleeding, OAT therapy is interrupted and replaced by ASA, to decrease the probability of further bleedings.

In order to make the decision analysis a *shared* decision, we have implemented a user interface to allow the doctor to elicit from the patient his UCs for each health state, as described in the following section.

3.2   The Utility Coefficients and Costs Elicitation Interface

The utility model is implemented through an interface to be used during face-to-face encounters between patients and physicians. Through this interface, the physician is able to interact with the patient to elicit values and UCs using all the methods presented in Section 2.1. The interface has been designed to give the patient the best possible understanding of the questions he has to answer. Consider for example the interface for the SG method. As previously explained, with this method the patient is asked to reason about a risky procedure potentially able to heal him. Since showing only the numeric value of the risk is not very intuitive for the patient, we have added a graphical representation that, for each value of the risk, turns into red a random set of yellow smileys corresponding to this percentage.

In the developed framework, we give the physician the possibility of evaluating UCs with both the described methods (SG and TTO). In this case, the final UC is calculated as the average value, which can also be a weighted average, according to the physician's confidence on one or the other method for that specific patient.

Besides utilities, costs are the other aspect that tailors the framework to the specific patient. On the basis of the cost model, a questionnaire has been designed to ask the patient the necessary personal data for cost calculation. The part of the questionnaire related to the cost for anticoagulant treatment monitoring is reported in Figure 2.

MobiGuide   INR Control Visit Costs Questionnaire

Productivity loss

Q1 **Employment?**
   ☐ Retired ☐ Self-employed ☐ Other

Q2 **Do you need any assistance to reach the visit location?**
   ☐ Yes, a family member/friend
   ☐ Yes, a caregiver
   ☐ No

Travel

Thinking of the suggested INR center:

Q4 **How would you travel to the visit location?**
   (Please check all the boxes that apply)
   ☐ Car/Motorbike

Q4.1.1 How many kilometers would you have to cover by car/motorbike? .... km

Q4.1.2 Do you know your car/motorbike features?
   Brand and model: ....
   Fuel type:
      ☐ Fuel
      ☐ Diesel

☐ Train/Intercity bus
Q4.2.1 How many kilometers would you cover by train/intercity bus? .... Km
☐ City Bus
☐ On foot

Meals

Please, fill in this section just in case of "INR medical report in loco"

☐ **INR medical report via fax/email**
☐ **INR medical report in loco**

Q5 Usually, the INR examination results are available after a few hours (early in the afternoon).
In this case, I prefer to:
   ☐ wait for the report at the medical centre

Q5.1.1 If you have lunch there, how much   do you think it will cost, approximately?
   ....
   ☐ go home and return later

☐ **INR medical report elsewhere (e.g. general practitioner)**

Fig. 2. A portion of the questionnaire for valuing the cost model. INR is a laboratory test required to monitor anticoagulant therapy effects, and it must be done in general every 15 days.

3.3   Showing Decision Analysis Results

Results are presented in the interface as shown in Figure 3. The expected values for all the defined payoffs for each decision option are listed. The most common case is that the most expensive option is also the most effective from the health outcomes point of view. As well, it may happen that an option shows higher life expectancy but lower QALY than another one. These are the situations that require the patient to reason with his doctor about the best choice.

Expected Values			
Payoff	Warfarin	ASA	No therapy
Life Years	22 years 3 months	22 years 1 months	21 years 1 months
QALYs	15 years 12 months	15 years 10 months	15 years 0 months
Patient Costs	10154 €	3179 €	3041 €

Fig. 3. Example of the results provided by running the decision tree for a specific patient: expected values of the payoffs (rows) for the possible therapeutic options (columns)

4   Conclusions and Future Developments

In this paper we have presented the design and implementation choices underlying the definition of a shared decision framework to be used by physicians and patients to introduce patient preferences and run a patient-specific clinical decision model. We believe that such a framework might be of help to improve patients' empowerment, increasing their involvement in the process of care focusing on the centrality of the individual instead of considering populations or cohorts.

The novelty of our work relies in the possibility of fully personalizing and deploying decision trees on the web. This represents a possible future exploitation of the MobiGuide project results, putting the basis for a repository of web-interactive tools for medical decision making.

The very next step will include system usability tests. As a matter of fact, the current interface is the result of a set of iterations performed together with physicians involved in MobiGuide. Further usability tests with external users are thus required to check additional system characteristics.

Acknowledgments. This work is supported by the EU funded MobiGuide project (FP7 287811). We are grateful to all the MobiGuide team, and in particular to Prof. Mor Peleg, Prof. Yuval Shahar, and Dr. Carlo Napolitano, for fruitful discussion on the shared-decision topic. We would also like to thank Dr. Lucio Liberato and Dr. Monia Marchetti for their help with the DT model.

References

1. Llewellyn-Thomas, H.A., Crump, T.: Decision Support for Patients: Values Clarification and Preference Elicitation. Med. Care Res. Rev. (2012) (Epub ahead of print)
2. Hack, T.F., Degner, L.F., Watson, P., Sinha, L.: Do patients benefit from participating in medical decision making? Longitudinal follow-up of women with breast cancer. Psychooncology 15(1), 9–19 (2006)
3. Weinstein, M.C., Fineberg, H.V.: Clinical Decision Analysis. Saunders, Philadelphia (1980)
4. Charles, C., Gafni, A., Whelan, T.: Shared decision- making in the medical encounter: What does it mean? Social Science Medicine 44, 681–692 (1997)

5. Stacey, D., Murray, M.A., Légaré, F., Sandy, D., Menard, P., O'Connor, A.: Decision coaching to support shared decision making: A framework, evidence, and implications for nursing practice, education, and policy. Worldviews Evid. Based Nurs. 5(1), 25–35 (2008)
6. American College of Cardiology Foundation/American Heart Association Task Force: 2011 ACCF/AHA/HRS focused updates incorporated into the ACC/AHA/ESC 2006 guidelines for the management of patients with atrial fibrillation: A report of the American College of Cardiology Foundation/American Heart Association Task Force on practice guidelines. Circulation 123(10), e269–e367 (2011)
7. Soares, M.O.: Is the QALY blind, deaf and dumb to equity? NICE's considerations over equity. Br. Med. Bull. 101, 17–31 (2012)
8. Bell, C.M., Chapman, R.H., Stone, P.W., Sandberg, E.A., Neumann, P.J.: An off-the-shelf help list: A comprehensive catalog of preference scores from published cost-utility analyses. Med. Decis. Making 21(4), 288–294 (2001)
9. CEA Registry website, https://research.tufts-nemc.org/cear4/ (last access March 13, 2013)
10. Bleichrodt, H., Johannesson, M.: An Experimental Test of a Theoretical Foundation for Rating-scale Valuations. Med. Decis. Making 17, 208–216 (1997)
11. Torrance, G.W., Thomas, W.H., Sackett, D.L.: A utility maximization model for evaluation of health care programs. Health Services Res. 7, 118–133 (1972)
12. Von Neumann, J., Morgenstern, O.: Theory of Games and Economic behavior. Princeton University Press (1944)
13. Gerzeli, S., Tarricone, R., Zolo, P., Colangelo, I., Busca, M.R., Gandolfo, C.: The economic burden of stroke in Italy. The EcLIPSE Study: Economic Longitudinal Incidence-based Project for Stroke Evaluation. Neurol. Sci. 26(2), 72–80 (2005)
14. Sonnenberg, F.A., Beck, J.R.: Markov models in medical decision making: A practical guide. Med. Decis. Making 13(4), 322–338 (1993)
15. Liberato, N.L., Rognoni, C., Marchetti, M., Quaglini, S.: Cost-effectiveness of new oral anticoagulants for stroke prophylaxis in atrial fibrillation. To appear on: Internal and Emergency Medicine (2012)
16. Lip, G.Y.H.: Stroke in atrial fibrillation: Epidemiology and thromboprophylaxis. J. Thromb Haemost 9 (suppl. 1), 344–351 (2011)

Model-Based Combination of Treatments for the Management of Chronic Comorbid Patients

David Riaño[1] and Antoni Collado[2]

[1] Research Group on Artificial Intelligence
Universitat Rovira i Virgili, Tarragona, Spain
david.riano@urv.net
[2] SAGESSA Group, Reus, Spain
acollado@grupsagessa.com

Abstract. The prevalence of chronic diseases is growing year after year. This implies that health care systems must deal with an increasing number of patients with several simultaneous pathologies (i.e., comorbid patients), which involves interventions combining primary, specialist, and hospital cares. Clinical practice guidelines provide evidence-based information on these interventions, but only on individual pathologies. This sets up the urgent need of developing ways of merging multiple single-disease interventions to provide professional assistance to comorbid patients. Here, we propose an integrated care model formalizing the treatment of chronic comorbid patients across primary, specialist and hospital cares. The model establishes the baseline of a divide-and-conquer approach to the complex task of multiple therapy combination that was tested on the comorbidity of hypertension and chronic heart failure.

Keywords: Computerized Clinical Practice Guidelines, Clinical Decision Support Systems, Health Care Modeling, Therapy Combination.

1 Introduction

Chronic diseases are prevalent health conditions that affect large sections of the population and burden National Health Systems worldwide. Their management uses to involve primary care GPs, specialists, and hospital interventions, and their treatments use to be described in clinical practice guidelines. Such guidelines are conceived to deal with a single disease [3] as they refer to other guidelines when a secondary disease is observed. So, in order to manage comorbid patients, health care professionals have to work with several guidelines simultaneously.

This problem has been addressed with several AI technologies. Some of these technologies propose the unification of treatments as an alignment of common actions [1], the use of GLINDA [4], the generalization of the intersecting patient conditions addressed by the guidelines to be merged [5], or the supervised unification of automatically customized guidelines [7]. In spite of these interesting advances, these approaches have not completely solved the problem of easy combination of multiple treatments, in part because of the complexity of this task.

N. Peek, R. Marín Morales, and M. Peleg (Eds.): AIME 2013, LNAI 7885, pp. 11–16, 2013.
© Springer-Verlag Berlin Heidelberg 2013

Other approaches such as automated drug interaction alerts [2] or computerized physician order entry systems (CPOE) [8] provide useful detection of drug interactions but still limited support to suggest equivalent treatments that solve unwanted interactions. Some experimental systems such as [6] use predefined rules to solve clinical interactions for the management of comorbid patients.

Here, we propose a *divide and conquer* strategy that contributes to simplify the task of combining multiple treatments, and therefore to ease the implementation of computer intelligent systems to automate such sort of combinations. The process followed was to analyze the guidelines of five chronic diseases, and to detect a generic model representing GP-specialist-hospital interventions for the long term treatment of chronic comorbid patients.

In section 2, we discuss the method and describe the generic model found. In section 3, we use this model to construct concrete multi-pathology treatments. In section 4, we summarize the conclusions and future work.

2   Methods

This work is founded on the analysis of five clinical practice guidelines corresponding to hypertension [9] (HT), diabetes mellitus [10], chronic heart failure [11] (HF), ischaemic heart disease [12], and hypercholesterolemia [13]. They were analyzed by a senior GP who concluded with a treatment model for each one of the diseases. After this, a software & knowledge engineer formalized the models and proposed a generic treatment model encompassing all the disease models. The engineering process was clinically supervised and validated by the GP.

2.1   The Underlying Generic Treatment Model

Figure 1 shows the modular description of the generic treatment model that we found for the management of chronic patients involving primary, specialist, and hospital cares. It is composed of decisions and treatments. Decisions are used to orientate the treatment in one direction or another. For example, if an urgent treatment is needed or not. In the model, we distinguish three sorts of decisions: *seriousness* of the current patient condition, with values mild, serious, and very serious taking different meanings depending on the considered disease; *evolution* or change in the patient condition, with values improves, keeps, and worsens meaning a decrement, stable, or increment of seriousness, respectively, and *acuteness* or whether the patient requires a referral to a hospital.

Treatments in the model represent clinical interventions either as sets of actions (action blocks) or treatment tables (table blocks). **Action Blocks** describe sets of clinical actions. For example, ANALYSIS OF SERIOUSNESS (I) is a set of tests to detect the seriousness of a case in primary care, ADDITIONAL ANALYSES are optional tests upon confirmation that the patient does not require acute treatment, TREATMENT (EMERGENCY) are the immediate actions before a transferral to a hospital, and PREPARE REFERRAL TO EMERGENCY the actions to prepare the patient for a transfer to the hospital. **Table Blocks** are matrices

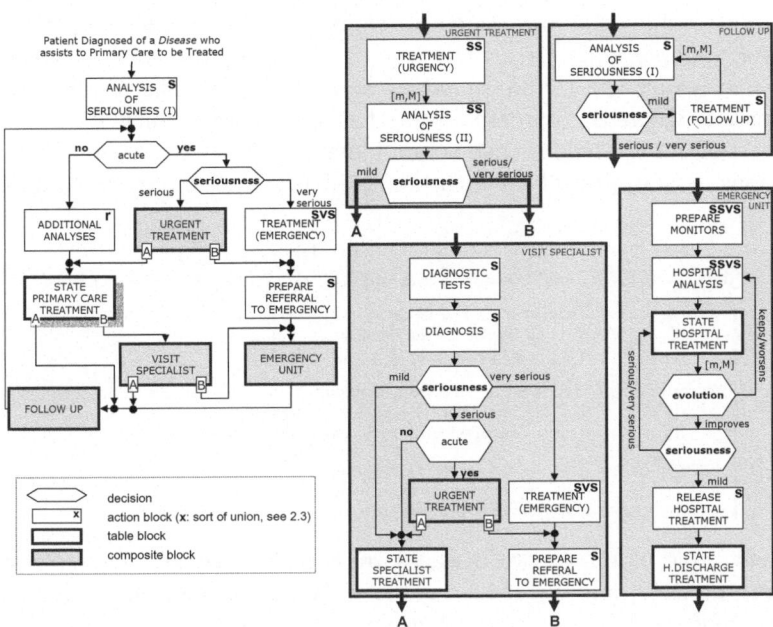

Fig. 1. Modular description of the Generic Treatment Model

T that, for a current treatment t and symptoms s of the patient, a treatment $T(t, s)$ is recommended. Related to the treatment a $[min,max]$ time interval can be given informing about the recommended time for the next visit, and the place p for this visit (*i.e.*, primary care, specialists, or hospital). Both, *min-max* values can be undefined, representing *now* and *infinite*, respectively.

With this model we can automate the process of merging treatments for several chronic diseases by pairwise combination ($\oplus$ operator) of equivalent blocks.

2.2 The $\oplus$ Operator for Merging Treatments

For time intervals, $[t_1, t_2] \oplus [t'_1, t'_2] = [\min\{t_1, t'_1\}, \min\{t_2, t'_2\}]$. For the acute condition of two diseases $acute_1 \oplus acute_1 = or\{acute_1, acute_2\}$ (*i.e.*, a comorbid case is considered acute if some morbidity is acute). For patient *evolution*, $improves_1 \oplus improves_2 = and\{improves_1, improves_2\}$ (*i.e.*, comorbidity improves if all diseases improve, otherwise the patient is considered to keep or worsen). For *seriousness*, $\oplus$ is as it follows:

seriousness condition ($i = 1, 2$)	$\oplus$ combination
(serious$_i$, very-serious$_i$)	($or_i\{$serious$_i\}$, $or_i\{$very-serious$_i\}$)
(mild$_i$, serious/very-serious$_i$)	($and_i\{$mild$_i\}$, $or_i\{$serious/very-serious$_i\}$)
(mild$_i$, *otherwise*, very-serious$_i$)	($and_i\{$mild$\}$, *otherwise*, $or_i\{$very-serious$_i\}$)

In order to combine sets of actions S_i, we provide five implementations of the $\oplus$ operator: *simple union* (s), *recall union* (r), *mild-serious union* (ss), *serious-very-serious union* (svs), and *simplified serious-very-serious union* (ssvs). See equations 2-5, where S_i^p represents the set of actions preceding S_i.

The sort of union used for each action block is indicated in figure 1. Unwanted interactions in $S_{1 \oplus 2}$ are solved with the rule-based system described in [6].

$$S_{1 \oplus 2} = \{d_1 : s : s \in S_1 - S_2\} \cup \{d_2 : s : s \in S_2 - S_1\} \cup \{d_1, d_2 : s : s \in S_1 \cap S_2\} \tag{1}$$

$$S_{1 \oplus 2} = \{d_1 : s : s \in S_1 - (S_2 \cup S_2^p)\} \cup \{d_2 : s : s \in S_2 - (S_1 \cup S_1^p)\} \cup \{d_1, d_2 : s : s \in (S_2 \cap S_1) - (S_1^p \cup S_2^p)\} \tag{2}$$

$$S_{1 \oplus 2} = \begin{cases} union(S_1, S_2) & \text{if } d_1 \text{ and } d_2 \text{ are } \texttt{serious} \\ d_1 : S_1 & \text{if } d_1 \text{ is } \texttt{serious} \text{ and } d_2 \text{ is } \texttt{mild} \\ d_2 : S_2 & \text{if } d_1 \text{ is } \texttt{mild} \text{ and } d_2 \text{ is } \texttt{serious} \end{cases} \tag{3}$$

$$S_{1 \oplus 2} = \begin{cases} union(S_1, S_2) & \text{if } d_1 \text{ and } d_2 \text{ are } \texttt{very-serious} \\ d_1 : S_1 & \text{if } d_1 \text{ is } \texttt{very serious} \text{ and } d_2 \text{ is } \texttt{serious} \\ d_2 : S_2 & \text{if } d_1 \text{ is } \texttt{serious} \text{ and } d_2 \text{ is } \texttt{very serious} \end{cases} \tag{4}$$

$$S_{1 \oplus 2} = \begin{cases} union(S_1, S_2) & \text{if } d_1 \text{ and } d_2 \text{ are } \texttt{very-serious} \\ d_1 : S_1 & \text{if } d_1 \text{ is } \texttt{very serious} \text{ and } d_2 \text{ is not } \texttt{very-serious} \\ d_2 : S_2 & \text{if } d_2 \text{ is } \texttt{very serious} \text{ and } d_1 \text{ is not } \texttt{very-serious} \end{cases} \tag{5}$$

Equivalent table blocks of two diseases are combined by storing the respective treatment tables T_1 and T_2 inside the block. When a comorbid patient p arrives with a current treatment t, both tables are applied to obtain the treatments for each disease. The resulting comorbid treatment is calculated as $T_{1 \oplus 2} = \cup_i \{d_i : t : t \in T_i(t, p)\}$. The system in [6] is applied to solve the conflicts in $T_{1 \oplus 2}$.

3   Combining Hypertension and Heart Failure Treatments

The guidelines [9,11] were used to fill in all the blocks in figure 1. Then, the tools described in the previous section were used to obtain a combined treatment for the comorbidity. The result was validated by a senior GP.

Decision Elements. *Seriousness* of HT is mild when there is not a risk of target organ damage (TOD) and the blood pressure is normal (BP<140/90), serious when not TOD but BP≥140/90, and very serious when TOD. For HF, mild stands for functional class I/II (FC I/II), serious for FC III, and very serious for FC IV. For HT an *acute* patient condition is when BP increases above 140/90, and there is an increment of symptoms (i.e., headache, dyspnea, breast pain, or dizziness). For HF, a patient condition is *acute* when there is an increment of FC that reaches level III or IV.

Action Blocks. Some of the action blocks obtained are shown in columns HT and HF of table 1, together with their $\oplus$-combination in column HT+HF.

Table Blocks. Table blocks in figure 1 were also obtained after the analysis of [9,11]. When two blocks are combined, their tables are stored for later combined use. Some interesting results showed the GP testing the system that the tool was able to detect and solve common treatment conflicts. For example, for a patient with BP≤120/80 and FC I, the STATE PRIMARY CARE HT table recommended [9] the prescription of one drug, among which calcium channel blockers (CCB) such as diltiazem are possible. On the other hand, the STATE

Table 1. Some action blocks for HT, HF, and comorbidity

action block	HT	⊕	HF	=	HT+HF
ANALYSIS OF SERIOUSNESS (I)	Check Medical Record Measure BP Anamnaesis	⊕	Check Medical Record Physical Examination EKG	=	HT,HF: Check Medical Record HT: Measure BP HT: Anamnaesis HF: Physical Examination HF: EKG
ADDITIONAL ANALYSES	General Analytics EKG	⊕	Torax RX General Analytics	=	HT, HF: General Analytics HF: Torax RX
TREATMENT (EMERGENCY) and TREATMENT (URGENCY)	Calm patient down Anxiety=>Diazepam 5-10mg/sl Captopril 25mg/sl/30min 1-3 times Opt=>Captopril 5-10mg/mouth	⊕	Diuretic full dose/intravenous	=	HT: Calm patient down HT: Anxiety=>Diazepam 5-10mg/sl HT: Captopril 25mg/sl/30min 1-3 times HT: Opt=>Captopril 5-10mg/mouth HF: Diuretic fd/iv
PREPARE REFERRAL TO EMERGENCY	Intravenous Supine Position Oxygen	⊕	Intravenous Supine Position Oxygen	=	HT, HF: Intravenous HT, HF: Supine Position HT, HF: Oxygen

PRIMARY CARE HF table recommended [11] an ACE inhibitor (e.g. enalapril) and a β-blocker (e.g., atenolol), but the system detected an unwanted interaction in the combined treatment that was solved after automatic removal of the CCB.

4 Conclusions

The combination of treatments for chronic comorbid patients has been implemented with a fully automated process which uses a divide and conquer strategy that models treatment in primary, specialist, and hospital cares as the interaction of a fixed number of decision and treatment blocks. Treatment combination is the result of pairwise combination of blocks of the same sort in the model.

References

1. Abidi, S.R., Abidi, S.S.R.: Towards the Merging of Multiple Clinical Protocols and Guidelines via Ontology-Driven Modeling. In: Combi, C., Shahar, Y., Abu-Hanna, A. (eds.) AIME 2009. LNCS, vol. 5651, pp. 81–85. Springer, Heidelberg (2009)
2. Ammenwerth, E., Schnell-Inderst, P., Machan, C., Siebert, U.: The Effect of Electronic Prescribing on Medication Errors and Adverse Drug Events: A Systematic Review. JAMIA 15(5), 585–600 (2008)
3. Boyd, C.M., Darer, J., et al.: Clinical Practice Guidelines and Quality of Care for Older Patients with Multiple Comorbid Diseases. JAMIA 294(6), 716–724 (2005)
4. GuiLine Interaction Detection Architecture (Glinda) project (March 2013), http://glinda-project.stanford.edu
5. Isern, D., Moreno, A., Sánchez, D., Hajnal, A., Pedone, G., Varga, L.Z.: Agent-based execution of personalised home care treatments. Appl. Intell. 34(2), 155–180 (2012)
6. López-Vallverdú, J.A., Riaño, D., Collado, A.: Rule-based combination of comorbid treatments for chronic diseases applied to hypertension, diabetes mellitus and heart failure. In: Lenz, R., Miksch, S., Peleg, M., Reichert, M., Riaño, D., ten Teije, A. (eds.) ProHealth 2012/KR4HC 2012. LNCS (LNAI), vol. 7738, pp. 30–41. Springer, Heidelberg (2013)
7. Riaño, D., Real, F., et al.: An ontology-based personalization of health-care knowledge to support clinical decisions for chronically ill patients. JBI 45, 429–446 (2012)
8. Schedlbauer, A., et al.: What Evidence Supports the Use of Computerized Alerts and Prompts to Improve Clinicians' Prescribing Behavior? JAMIA 16, 531–538 (2009)

9. 7th Report on Prevention, Detection, Evaluation, and Treatment of High Blood Pressure. US Dept. Health Human Services (2003)
10. Guia de maneig de la diabetes (March 2013) (in Catalan), www.grupsagessa.com/documents/menupai/pai_diabetis-catala.pdf
11. Dickstein, K., et al.: ESC Guidelines for the diagnosis and treatment of acute and chronic heart failure 2008. European Heart Journal 29, 2388–2442 (2008)
12. Unstable angina and NSTEMI (March 2013), http://www.nice.org.uk/guidance/CG94
13. Guia de maneig de la hipercolesterolèmia (March 2013) (in Catalan), www.grupsagessa.com/documents/menupai/pai_hipercolesterolemia-catala.pdf

Using Constraint Logic Programming to Implement Iterative Actions and Numerical Measures during Mitigation of Concurrently Applied Clinical Practice Guidelines

Martin Michalowski[1], Szymon Wilk[2], Wojtek Michalowski[3], Di Lin[4], Ken Farion[5], and Subhra Mohapatra[3]

[1] Adventium Labs, Minneapolis MN, USA
martin.michalowski@adventiumlabs.com
[2] Poznan University of Technology, Poznan, Poland
[3] University of Ottawa, Ottawa ON, Canada
[4] McGill University, Montreal, PQ, Canada
[5] Children's Hospital of Eastern Ontario, Ottawa ON, Canada

Abstract. There is a pressing need in clinical practice to mitigate (identify and address) adverse interactions that occur when a comorbid patient is managed according to multiple concurrently applied disease-specific clinical practice guidelines (CPGs). In our previous work we described an automatic algorithm for mitigating pairs of CPGs. The algorithm constructs logical models of processed CPGs and employs constraint logic programming to solve them. However, the original algorithm was unable to handle two important issues frequently occurring in CPGs – iterative actions forming a cycle and numerical measurements. Dealing with these two issues in practice relies on a physician's knowledge and the manual analysis of CPGs. Yet for guidelines to be considered stand-alone and an easy to use clinical decision support tool this process needs to be automated. In this paper we take an additional step towards building such a tool by extending the original mitigation algorithm to handle cycles and numerical measurements present in CPGs.

Keywords: Clinical Decision Support Systems, Computerized Clinical Practice Guidelines, Constraint Logic Programming, Comorbidity.

1 Introduction

Developing CPGs that explicitly address all potential comorbid diseases is not only difficult, but also impractical, and there is a need for formal methods that would allow combining several disease-specific CPGs in order to customize them to a patient [1]. Studies show that the lack of such methods is one of the obstacles in the adoption of CPGs in clinical practice and the development of these methods has been identified as one of the "grand challenges" for clinical decision support [2]. Our previous research [3] responded to the above challenge by proposing an automatic mitigation algorithm that verifies if pairs of CPGs can

N. Peek, R. Marín Morales, and M. Peleg (Eds.): AIME 2013, LNAI 7885, pp. 17–22, 2013.

be applied simultaneously to a patient with comorbid diseases. We described the novel use of a *constraint logic programming* (CLP) model to represent guidelines. We also explained how to codify domain knowledge associated with using these guidelines, and presented an algorithm that manipulates and solves the CLP model to propose a combined therapy for comorbid patient. The mitigation algorithm was originally developed under a number of assumptions, two of them being no iterative actions that may produce a cycle and the use of only binary action variables (i.e., variables associated with actions prescribed by a CPG). This paper revises the mitigation algorithm to relax these two assumptions.

2   Motivating Clinical Scenario

Consider an elderly male patient complaining of palpitations, shortness of breath and a syncopal episode. At the time of presentation he was not in any distress but had a rapid irregular pulse. A 12-lead ECG was done and revealed an irregular, wide complex tachycardia consistent with atrial fibrillation (AF) in the setting of Wolff-Parkinsons-White (WPW) syndrome. The attending physician concluded that the patient has a chronic condition (WPW) and an acute disease (AF).

When treating a patient for both AF and WPW there is an interplay between medications, specifically oral flecainide prescribed for WPW, and IV flecainide or amiodarone prescribed for AF. Overdosing the patient leads to a level of the drug in the blood that results in toxicity. Therefore dosages of flecainide need to be expressed in terms of exact, patient-specific (numerical) values that are revised during the management process. Additionally, the CPG for WPW contains a treatment cycle that adjusts flecainide dosages. Thus, handling both iterative actions manifesting as a cycle and the dosage of flecainide is essential to developing a combined therapy for this patient. While AF and WPW serve as the motivating clinical example, the described issues are common across many other pairs of diseases.

3   Extended Mitigation Algorithm

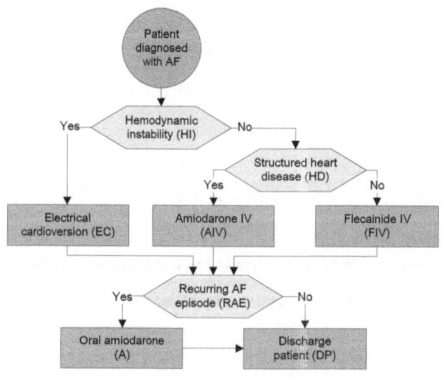

Fig. 1. AG_{AF}

Our mitigation algorithm (presented in detail in [3]) checks for possible adverse interactions between CPGs, addresses identified interactions and finally finds a combined therapy consisting of individual therapies derived from both CPGs. It accepts as input two CPGs given as actionable graphs and available patient information represented as a set of variable-value pairs. An actionable graph is a directed acyclic graph with context, action and decision nodes corresponding to context, decision and action steps that appear in most formal CPG representations [4] and it can be obtained automatically from these representation [5]. An AG that represents CPG for AF (AG_{AF}) is given in Fig. 1.

The mitigation algorithm consists of three main phases: preparation, mitigating direct interactions, and mitigating indirect interactions. The extensions to handle iterative actions and numerical values, described below, affect the preparation phase of the algorithm where logical representations of actionable graphs are constructed.

Handling cycles requires a new step in the preparation phase, where a cyclic actionable graph is transformed into an acyclic one by expanding the cycle. The two key issues with cycles are: (1) they pose a problem when transforming an actionable graph into a logical model because a unique variable is needed for each action (and actions in cycles occur multiple times), and (2) often there is no clear definition of the number of iterations or a stopping condition. Based on consultations with medical experts we developed a two-step *expand* procedure (Figure 2) to remove a cycle by estimating the number of iterations (extracted directly from a CPG in the easy case or approximated using expert knowledge in the complex case) and expanding the identified cycle.

Require: $AG_i, Stop_i$
$Cycle_i \leftarrow identify\_cycle(AG_i)$
$MaxIter_i \leftarrow check\_conditions(Cycle_i, Stop_i)$
$ForwardPath_i \leftarrow create\_path(Cycle_i)$
$AG_i^{exp} \leftarrow replace\_cycle(AG_i, ForwardPath_i, MaxIter_i)$
return AG_i^{exp}

Fig. 2. The *expand* procedure

The procedure begins by identifying the cycle in the actionable graph (AG_i) using a path-based strong component algorithm [6]. Note that the identification step assumes a single cycle only (handling multiple cycles could be done by using a recursive invocation of the *expand* procedure with AG_i). The procedure then uses the identified cycle and a stopping condition ($Stop_i$) to determine the maximum number of iterations ($MaxIter_i$). We establish the stopping condition according to expert's opinion, evidence, or patient information.

Next, we create a forward path ($ForwardPath_i$) to resolve the cycle. A forward path starts with the first node identified in the original cycle and includes the remaining cycle nodes. Finally, we create a revised actionable graph where the cycle is replaced by a set of connected forward paths, the number of these paths is equal to the maximum number of iterations. The updated actionable graph (AG_i^{exp}) is then used to create a logical model. We note that even in simple cases where the number of iterations is known, invoking the *expand* procedure is still necessary to introduce new variables needed to expand the cycle.

Numerical variables need special attention when creating logical models and they affect how action and decision variables are used. In the case of action variables, numerical variables add support for actions that are more complex than "go/no go" flags. For example, where previously a variable representing the administration of flecainide was represented by a binary variable $F := true/false$, introducing a numerical variable $DF := [0\ldots500]$ enables considering administration of a medication and an associated dosage (medication is administered if its dosage is greater than 0). Numerical variables also allow for algebraic expressions that define conditions and they enable the computation of values for these variables. Whereas, previously considered logical models only allowed expressions such as $\neg(A \wedge F)$, after introducing this extension these models can include expressions such as $\neg(A \wedge DF \geq DF0) \wedge (DF = DF1 + DF2 + DF3 + \ldots)$.

4   Evaluation

To evaluate the extended mitigation algorithm, we use an instance of the clinical scenario described in Section 2. We apply interaction operators to represent external domain knowledge that describes indirect interactions between the maximum safe oral dosage of flecainide ($DF_{safe}(P) = 200mg$, coming from the guideline for WPW, where P indicates the level of plasma in blood) and oral dosage of amiodarone or IV flecainide. A revision operator is included that reduces the dosage of flecainide from the maximum safe level to 75% of this safety threshold (a revision developed after consulting with medical experts). We remove iterative actions from AG_{WPW} by invoking the *expand* procedure, resulting in AG_{WPW}^{exp} given in Fig. 3 (please note only AG_{AF} is given in Fig. 1 due to space limitations).

Consider a patient, who has not been stabilized within the first three rounds of flecainide therapy (variables $WS0 = WS1 = WS2 = n$), has hemodynamic instability ($HI=y$), and who has a reoccurrence of AF ($RAE = y$). Given the logical model and an initial assignment of values to variables as defined by the above patient information, the extended mitigation algorithm

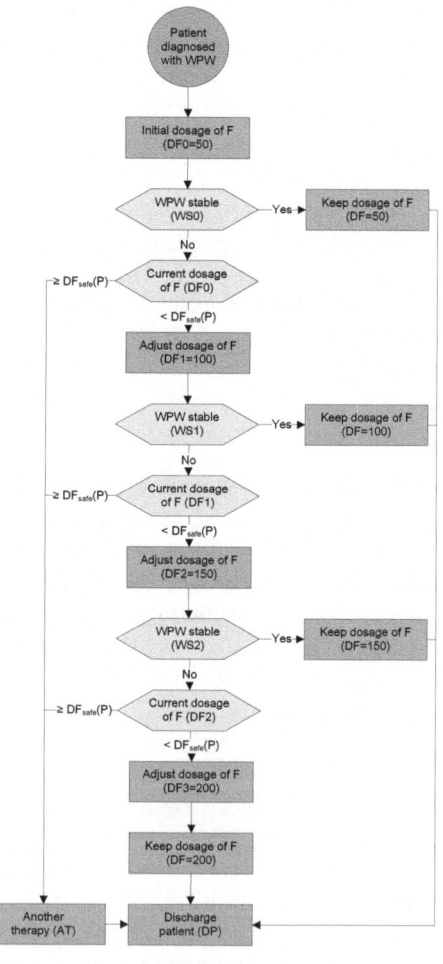

Fig. 3. AG_{WPW}^{exp}

invokes a CLP solver (we use the ECL^iPS^e system [7]) . No direct adverse interactions are detected so the model is augmented with the interaction operators described above and the solver is again invoked. This time, an adverse indirect interaction is detected, corresponding to interplay between the dosage of flecainide and oral amiodarone. The extended mitigation algorithm proceeds to resolve this interaction by invoking the revision operator that lowers the dosage of flecainide from $DF_{safe}(P)$ by 25% (given P = 0.7, it translates to lowering from 200mg to 150mg). The revised model is passed to ECL^iPS^e and the solver produces the following solution: [*WS0 = n, WS1 = n, WS2 = n, DF0 = 50, DF1 = 100, DF2 = 150, DF3 = 200, DF= 150, HI = y, EC = true, RAE = y, PD = true*] that represents a combined therapy. In layman's terms this solution indicates that the dosage of flecainide is set to 150mg ($DF = 150$) as indicated by the revision operator, the patient undergoes electrical cardioversion ($EC = true$) and is discharged ($PD = true$). For instances with no found solution, we return the possible source of infeasibility to the physician who can use this information to determine the correct next steps given the patient information.

5   Discussion

In this paper we presented extensions to our mitigation algorithm. These extensions allow for numerical variables and add support for algebraic expressions and conditions. We introduced the *expand* procedure to identify and expand cycles, thus enabling the mitigation algorithm to operate on guidelines with complex relationships. This is an important step towards our goal of creating a comprehensive alerting system for physicians that will support the concurrent application of multiple CPGs. The extended mitigation algorithm is currently being incorporated into a mobile clinical decision support system to create a proof-of-concept application for evaluation in a clinical scenario. Further, we are working on a formal theory for representing and mitigating CPGs that will enable us to operationalize the application across a broad range of clinical scenarios.

References

[1] Fox, J., Glasspool, D., Patkar, V., Austin, M., Black, L., South, M., Robertson, D., Vincent, C.: Delivering clinical decision support services: There is nothing as practical as a good theory. J. Biomed. Inform. 43, 831–843 (2010)
[2] Sittig, D., Wright, A., Osheroff, J., Middleton, B., Teich, J., Ash, J., Campbell, E., Bates, D.: Grand challenges in clinical decision support. J. Biomed. Inform. 41, 387–392 (2008)
[3] Wilk, S., Michalowski, W., Michalowski, M., Farion, K., Hing, M., Mohapatra, S.: Mitigation of adverse interactions in pairs of clinical practice guidelines using constraint logic programming. Journal of Biomedical Informatics 46(2), 341–353 (2013)
[4] Isern, D., Moreno, A.: Computer-based execution of clinical guidelines: A review. Int. J. Med. Inform. 77, 787–808 (2008)

[5] Hing, M., Michalowski, M., Wilk, S., Michalowski, W., Farion, K.: Identifying inconsistencies in multiple clinical practice guidelines for a patient with·co-morbidity. In: Proceedings of KEDDH 2010, pp. 447–452 (2010)
[6] Tarjan, R.: Depth-first search and linear graph algorithms. SIAM J. Comput. 1(2), 146–160 (1972)
[7] The ECLiPSe Constraint Programming System, http://www.eclipseclp.org

A Multi-agent Planning Approach for the Generation of Personalized Treatment Plans of Comorbid Patients*

Inmaculada Sánchez-Garzón[1], Juan Fdez-Olivares[1], Eva Onaindía[2],
Gonzalo Milla[1], Jaume Jordán[2], and Pablo Castejón[2]

[1] Department of Computer Science and AI, Universidad de Granada, Spain
[2] Department of Computer Science, Universitat Politècnica de València, Spain

Abstract. This work addresses the generation of a personalized treatment plan from multiple clinical guidelines, for a patient with multiple diseases (comorbid patient), as a multi-agent cooperative planning process that provides support to collaborative medical decision-making. The proposal is based on a multi-agent planning architecture in which each agent is capable of (1) planning a personalized treatment from a temporal Hierarchical Task Network (HTN) representation of a single-disease guideline, and (2) coordinating with other planning agents by both sharing disease specific knowledge, and resolving the eventual conflicts that may arise when conciliating different guidelines by merging single-disease treatment plans. The architecture follows a life cycle that starting from a common specification of the main high-level steps of a treatment for a given comorbid patient, results in a detailed treatment plan without harmful interactions among the single-disease personalized treatments.

Keywords: multi-agent planning, comorbidity, guideline conciliation.

1 Introduction

The generation of personalized treatment plans for patients with a single disease is a widely studied problem in the field of AI in Medicine. Most of the proposed approaches implement sophisticated problem solving processes that (1) take as input a knowledge base containing a Computer Interpretable Guideline (CIG[1]); and (2) adapt the activities of the formal guideline, from patient-focused clinical data, in order to generate a personalized treatment to be performed at the point of care. Although these approaches provide decision support in order for the clinical staff to efficiently follow the guidance provided by CPGs, they either have neglected or do not have deeply addressed the problem of planning personalized treatments for comorbid patients (i.e., patients with multiple and simultaneous diseases [3]). This is mainly due to the fact that a CPG gathers

---

* Work partially supported by projects P08-TIC-3572 and TIN2011-27652-C03-03/01.
[1] Clinical Practice Guideline (CPG) represented in a formal language.

N. Peek, R. Marín Morales, and M. Peleg (Eds.): AIME 2013, LNAI 7885, pp. 23–27, 2013.
© Springer-Verlag Berlin Heidelberg 2013

the clinical evidence for a concrete disease, and rarely considers patients with multiple diseases in clinical trials [8].

However, the problem of tailoring a treatment plan for a comorbid patient requires to conciliate the activities recommended by several single-disease CPGs. In this scenario, new problem solving capabilities are needed in order to detect and resolve eventual interactions (or conflicts) between different clinical knowledge sources. These interactions may be of different types, like conflicts between recommended medications of different diseases (drug-drug interactions), adverse effects on other diseases when treating the target disease (drug-disease interactions), inefficient scheduling of activities or even contradictory/redundant recommendations [3]. Regarding this problem, different perspectives have been proposed as [7], [2] or [6]. However, the use of multi-agent techniques appears to be a very suitable approach, since agents can encapsulate the expertise and skills of a specialist (or team of specialists). The strength of these techniques has been exploited in projects like GLINDA [1].

Some other features can be identified in this new scenario: (1) The medical expertise is distributed among different CPGs; (2) There is a common task that consists of the design of a personalized treatment plan, without harmful interactions, for a comorbid patient; (3) It has to be accomplished by at least two clinicians or by one clinician consulting at least two different knowledge sources and; (4) Each specialist has both disease-specific problem solving and cooperation capabilities that can exploit to carry out a collaborative medical decision-making process. These features fulfill the main requirements of a cooperative distributed problem solving process. Moreover, the generation of a personalized treatment plan from multiple CPGs, for a comorbid patient, can be addressed as a multi-agent cooperative planning process. Concretely this work presents a multi-agent planning architecture in which each agent is capable of (1) *planning* a personalized treatment for a given patient, from a temporal Hierarchical Task Network (HTN) representation of a single-disease guideline, and (2) *coordinating* with other planning agents by both sharing their local, disease-specific recommendations, and resolving the eventual conflicts that may arise when conciliating their single-disease plans. Thus, the architecture follows a life cycle that starting from a common specification of the main high-level steps of the treatment for a given patient, it will result in a personalized plan without harmful interactions.

2 Multi-agent Planning Architecture

Figure 1(a) shows the proposed Multi-Agent Planning (MAP[2]) architecture that is composed of an *Initiator Agent* and several *Planning Agents*. A planning agent can be seen as the representation of a clinical specialist capable of (1) planning a personalized, single-disease care plan (*HTN planner* module); (2) coordinating with other specialists, by sharing its single-disease recommendations and experience (*Coordinator* module) and (3) detecting and resolving conflicts between its recommendations and those of others (*Conflict Solver* module).

---

[2] MAP is the combination of multi-agent techniques and planning techniques [9].

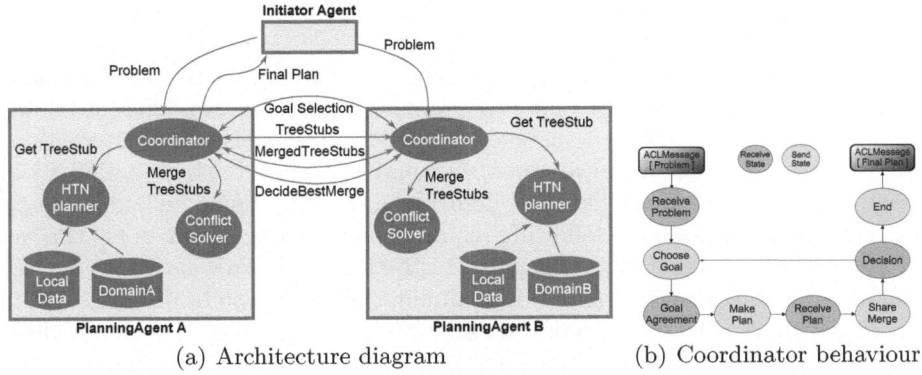

(a) Architecture diagram   (b) Coordinator behaviour

Fig. 1. Multi-Agent Planning approach

The mission of the *Initiator Agent* is to send the global problem to the *Planning Agents*. A global problem may be defined by a starting time point and a list with the high-level steps of the care plan. For instance, the following code shows a problem denoting that the phases of diagnosis, treatment and follow-up have to be designed for the patient $?p$ starting from a specific date: $((\$start == "2012/12/21")(Diagnosis\ ?p)(Treatment\ ?p)(FollowUp\ ?p))$.

Note that the process of designing a treatment plan for a comorbid patient is a cooperative planning process that iterates over the high-level tasks of the global problem and for each task a joint treatment plan is obtained. Such joint plan is generated by a merging process developed by the *Conflict Solver* module in which single-disease treatments (automatically generated by *HTN planners*) are combined in order to detect and solve eventual interactions. Next subsections briefly describe the different modules of a *Planning Agent*.

2.1 HTN Planner : Single-Disease Treatment Planning

The HTN planner takes as inputs a *planning domain* (i.e., a hierarchy of tasks representing compound and primitive activities) and a *planning problem*. A planning domain encodes a single-disease CPG based on HPDL, a temporal HTN planning language as expressive as standard CIGs languages [5]. HPDL provides support to represent time-annotated guidelines and it is capable of representing decisions, different execution flows and iterative task decomposition schemas. A planning problem represents the set of goals to be achieved during the planning process (e.g., $(Treatment\ ?p)$) as well as the initial state, which is encoded in the block *Local Data* of Figure 1(a). Local Data contains information about patients (e.g., demographic and clinical data), drug medication patterns (e.g., dose, frequency, administration mode) as well as interactions (e.g., drug-drug interactions, drug-disease interactions). As result, the HTN planner[3] generates a *TreeStub* composed of a personalized, single-disease plan (with time-annotated primitive actions) and the rules of the planning domain applied to generate it.

---

[3] For more information about the planning process, please see our previous work [4,5].

2.2   Conflict Solver : Plan Merging Strategy

This module develops a plan merging process by combining the planning domains of two *TreeStubs*. This means that every conflict solver uses two different knowledge sources[4] for generating a merged, conflict-free treatment plan. Interactions are avoided by means of the *preconditions* and *effects* (expressed in HPDL) of the primitive actions of the planning domain. In this way, before including a new action to the joint plan, the following requirements must be satisfied: (1) this action is not contraindicated for the patient, (2) this action does not generate any drug-drug or drug-disease conflict. In planning time, such conditions are checked by comparing the clinical data of the patient (e.g., list of prescribed drugs, diagnosed diseases and contraindicated actions) with the knowledge extracted from CPGs (e.g., interactions between drug-drug and drug-disease). Note that this data are encoded in the Local Data block. Moreover, after adding an action to the plan, its effects are applied updating the clinical data of the patient.

2.3   Coordinator : Multi-agent Planning Cooperation

Figure 1(b) shows a finite state machine model of the behaviour of the *Coordinator* module. There are two different kind of states: (1) *receive*, where the agent waits for an *ACLMessage*[5]. from other agents, and (2) *send*, where the agent performs some actions and sends an *ACLMessage* to other agents.

In the first state (*Receive Problem*), the coordinator receives the global problem. Then, after choosing a specific task-goal of the problem and sending it to the other agent (*Choose Goal*), it waits for the reception of the other agent's goal (*Goal Agreement*). When both agents agree on the goal to solve, each one calls to its HTN planner to generate a local plan (*Make Plan*), as explained before. Then, the planner returns a *TreeStub*, which is send to the other agent. In the next state (*Receive Plan*), the coordinator receives the *TreeStub* from the other agent and then, a merging process is performed by the conflict solver in order to combine the just received *TreeStub* with its local plan (*Share Merge*). Then, agents share their merged treatments and select the best one as the final global plan. The coordinator also analyses if the planning process has finished (*End*), in which case it sends the final global plan in an *ACLMessage* to the initiator agent. Otherwise, it selects the next task-goal to achieve (*Choose Goal*).

Finally, the best plan is selected according to an utility function that may incorporate different clinical criteria: (1) *Efficiency* from the institutional point of view, by optimizing the used resources (e.g., lower cost of drugs) or the temporal cost (e.g., lower duration of treatment); (2) *Complexity* from the patient point of view, by quantifying the complexity of the medication regimen (as proposed in [3]) and selecting the easiest one. In fact, for elderly people, it is preferable a medication regimen with few drugs and few different dosage schedules.

---

[4] More clinical knowledge than the used previously by the HTN planner.

[5] A message whose content is based of the standard FIPA ACL (Agent Communication Language) http://www.fipa.org/specs/fipa00061/.

3   Conclusions and Future Work

The proposed multi-agent planning architecture provides support for the generation of treatment plans for comorbid patients by carrying out a cooperative planning process that, starting from a high-level description of the main steps of a care plan, results in an interaction-free, personalized treatment plan. Such plan is generated and merged from multiple clinical guidelines (represented as HTN domains), in a collaborative process based on both the sharing of local treatments (obtained by different temporal HTN planners) and the selection of the best proposal according to some clinical criteria (efficiency or complexity).

By means of a previous experimental evaluation, some *simulated* CPGs were represented and some preliminary results were obtained, which support this work. We are presently engaged in a detailed experimentation with real CPGs of the most prevalent diseases in comorbid patients, since our research group has already experience in the representation of real clinical knowledge in HPDL [4]. Furthermore, we intend to work on both a more collaborative plan merging approach with clinicians and on argumentation techniques to reach agreements.

References

1. GLINDA: GuideLine INteraction Detection Architecture,
   http://glinda-project.stanford.edu/
2. Abidi, S.R.: A conceptual framework for ontology based automating and merging of clinical pathways of comorbidities. In: Riaño, D. (ed.) K4HelP 2008. LNCS, vol. 5626, pp. 55–66. Springer, Heidelberg (2009)
3. Boyd, C.M., Darer, J., Boult, C., Fried, L.P., Boult, L., Wu, A.W.: Clinical practice guidelines and quality of care for older patients with multiple comorbid diseases: Implications for pay for performance. JAMA 294(10), 716–724 (2005)
4. Fdez-Olivares, J., Castillo, L., Cózar, J., García Pérez, O.: Supporting clinical processes and decisions by hierarchical planning and scheduling. Comput. Intell. 27(1), 103–122 (2011)
5. González-Ferrer, A., ten Teije, A., Fdez-Olivares, J., Milian, K.: Automated generation of patient-tailored electronic care pathways by translating computer-interpretable guidelines into hierarchical task networks. Artif. Intell. Med. (2012) (in Press)
6. Hing, M.M., Michalowski, M., Wilk, S., Michalowski, W., Farion, K.: Identifying inconsistencies in multiple clinical practice guidelines for a patient with co-morbidity. In: IEEE International Conference on BIBM Wkshp., pp. 447–452 (2010)
7. Lozano, E., Marcos, M., Martínez-Salvador, B., Alonso, A., Alonso, J.R.: Experiences in the development of electronic care plans for the management of comorbidities. In: Riaño, D., ten Teije, A., Miksch, S., Peleg, M. (eds.) KR4HC 2009. LNCS, vol. 5943, pp. 113–123. Springer, Heidelberg (2010)
8. Lugtenberg, M., Burgers, J.S., Clancy, C., Westert, G.P., Schneider, E.C.: Current guidelines have limited applicability to patients with comorbid conditions: A systematic analysis of evidence-based guidelines. PLoS ONE 6(10), e25987 (2011)
9. de Weerdt, M., Clement, B.: Introduction to planning in multiagent systems. Multiagent and Grid Systems 5(4), 345–355 (2009)

Merging Disease-Specific Clinical Guidelines to Handle Comorbidities in a Clinical Decision Support Setting

Borna Jafarpour and Syed Sibte Raza Abidi

Computer Science Department, Dalhousie University, Halifax, Canada
{borna,sraza}@cs.dal.ca

Abstract. From a clinical decision support perspective the treatment of co-morbid diseases is a challenge since it demands the coordination between the disease-specific therapeutic plans of the co-morbid diseases. Although clinical guidelines provide clinical recommendations, they focus on a single disease and for comorbid disease management there is a requirement to have multiple concurrently active clinical guidelines. Merging computerized clinical practice guidelines (CPG) related to comorbidities and using them in clinical decision support systems is a potential solution to manage comorbidities in a clinical decision support system. We have developed a CPG merging framework to merge computerized CPG. The central aspect of our framework is a merge representation ontology that captures the merging criteria to achieve the merging of multiple CPG whilst satisfying medical, workflow, institutional and temporal constraints. We have used our framework successfully to create therapy plans for patients treated for Atrial Fibrillation and Chronic Heart Failure comorbidity.

Keywords: Practice Guideline, OWL, SWRL, Comorbidity, Execution Engine.

1 Introduction

The treatment of co-morbid diseases—i.e. the simultaneous presentation of multiple medical conditions in a patient—is a challenge since it demands the coordination between the disease-specific therapeutic plans of the co-morbid diseases. Typically the diagnostic and therapeutic plans for single diseases are presented as Clinical Practice Guidelines (CPG). However, CPG do not give a detailed account of strategies and recommendations to handle comorbid conditions [2].

From a clinical decision support perspective, the concurrent use of multiple CPG covering the comorbid diseases is not an optimal solution as it leads to unnecessary duplication of tasks, resources and even conflicts around treatment options. One solution to handle comorbid conditions in a clinical decision support environment is to systematically merge the independent CPG of the comorbid conditions to generate a mutually consistent comorbid CPG. Merging CPG is defined by Abidi [2] as: "Merging multiple CPG is the process of merging the knowledge which is encapsulated in them into a unified CPG that can be used to treat the patients for their co-morbidities while the integrity and pragmatics of the medical knowledge is kept intact".

In this paper, we present a semantic web based framework to dynamically integrate/merge two or more disease-specific CPG to generate a clinically pragmatic and

N. Peek, R. Marín Morales, and M. Peleg (Eds.): AIME 2013, LNAI 7885, pp. 28–32, 2013.

clinically safe comorbid CPG. The tenets of our framework are as follows: (a) To computerize paper based CPG we use an existing OWL-based CPG ontology that models clinical tasks, diagnostic concepts, and therapeutic decisions [2]; (b) To represent the CPG merge criteria, we have developed an OWL-based Merge Representation Ontology (MRO) that captures the potential merge points between two or more CPG as per the judgment of a domain expert; and (c) To achieve CPG merging, we have augmented an already existing OWL-based execution engine [4] by OWL axioms and SWRL rules which calculate the effect of each CPG on others based on the merge criteria. The input to our merging execution engine is two or more computerized CPG and an instantiation of the MRO which encompasses the merge criteria and the output is the recommendations based on the individual CPG and the merge criteria. Fig. 1 shows the system level architecture of our CPG merging framework.

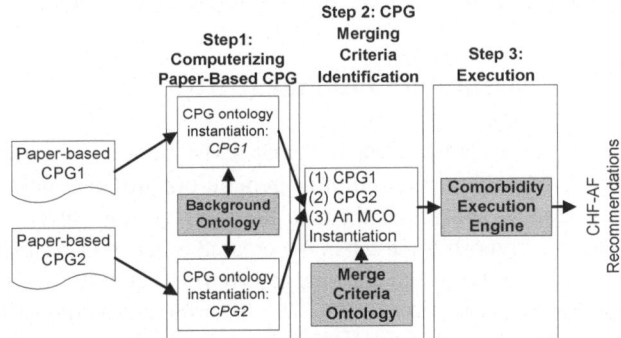

Fig. 1. System level architecture of our CPG merging framework

Our contributions are twofold: (1) An expressive ontology-based language for capturing comorbidity merge criteria between the computerized CPG; and (2) A merging execution engine capable of dynamically merging several CPG during their execution.

2   Related Work

Computerized CPG related to comorbidities can be merged either before or during the execution [5]. These two approaches are called (a) Pre-Execution Level and (b) Execution Level merging respectively.

In the pre-execution level merging, several CPG computerized in the same CPG representation can be manually or automatically merged. Two examples of manual merging of CHF related comorbidities have been performed in [2] and [6]. In these approaches, the identical tasks have been identified and reused in the unified merged CPG. Computerized CPG can also be merged in the pre-execution level automatically using specialized algorithms. In the approach introduced by Riano et al. in [3], CPG are broken into several state-action structures and then merged into a conflict-free unified CPG. We believe this is not a safe solution as it rearranges individual CPG. Hing et al. [1] have proposed a CPG merging approach based on constraint logic programming where they perform modifications on CPG based on mitigation operators to remove the adverse interactions and contradicting states. We believe that none of the pre-execution level merging approaches is practical as they merge the CPG by making assumptions about the execution paths and their starting times. However, the merged CPG cannot be used for treatment of comorbid patient if these assumptions do not hold true during execution.

Merging at the execution level is accomplished by dynamically merging several CPG based on the execution flow and patients' information. It is the most challenging approach and hence has been pursued the least. The only research in this area suggests the use of SWRL rules to map common tasks across multiple CPG in order to achieve CPG merging [5] however not enough detail for an implementation exists.

Literature review concludes that CPG merging, especially at the execution level, is a challenging problem that needs innovative solution approaches for modeling the merge criteria and dynamically merging several computerized CPG.

3   Merge Representation Ontology (MRO)

In order to identify the merge criteria that may exist between the tasks of two or more comorbidity CPG, we interviewed three general practitioners with experience in treating comorbid patients and asked them to list the merging criteria that they may consider while treating comorbid patients. We created a list of criteria and developed an OWL-Lite ontology to represent the merge criteria. The MRO is instantiated to capture the merge points between two CPG. We describe below the MRO, properties are listed in italics and classes are both italicized and Capitalized.

The *Constraint* class represents the potential merging points between two or more tasks from different CPG. Properties *hasTask1*, *hasTask2* with the domain of *Constraint* and range of *Task* are used to indicate the merged tasks. *Task* class represents the medical task in our CPG ontology. Merging constraints can be categorized under three types represented by the following subclasses of the *Constraints* class: *WorkflowConstraint*, *InstitutionalConstraint* and *MedicalConstraint*. *WorkflowConstraint*: This class represents the constraint that affects how the workflow structures of the CPG are interpreted for comorbid patient. A workflow constraint may indicate that tasks indicated by properties *hasTask1* and *hasTask2* (1) are identical, (2) should be executed simultaneously, (3) have a sequential constraint between them or (4) can be combined into a new and more effective task. For instance the following instantiation of the MRO expresses that tasks treatment_with_beta_blockers_and_ACEI from the CHF CPG and the task anticoagulation_with_Warfarin from the AF CPG should be executed simultaneously during the treatment of CHF-AF patients.

```
MRO:simacconst1   a MRO:SimultaneousActionConstraint;
  MRO:hasTask1 chf:treatment_with_beta_blockers_and_ACEI;
  MRO:hasTask2 af:anticoagulation_with_Warfarin;
  MRO:task1CanWait "7"^^xsd:int. #7 days
```

Property *task1CanWait* is used to indicate that if task1is about to be executed while the other CPG has not reached task2, task1 can wait for 7 days in the pending state until the behind CPG catches up so that both of the tasks can be executed simultaneously. *InstitutionalConstraint* is used to capture institutional constraints that may affect merging two CPG at a specific institute. These constraints may indicate, for instance, that two tasks cannot be executed in the same location or at the same time due to institutional policies or resource limitations. *MedicalConstraint* class may express the circumstances under which re-using the result of the previously executed tasks is possible or two tasks from different CPG may be conflicting. More details of this ontology are skipped due to the space limitation.

4   Comorbidity Execution Engine

Existing CPG execution engines work based on the concept of task state transition systems. These engines are designed to execute only one CPG rather than several comorbidity CPG. Merging constraints may change the way CPG are executed by affecting the state transition of the tasks. Hence, in order to successfully execute several merged CPG related to a comorbidity we need to model (a) Tasks' state transition and (b) the effect of constraints on tasks' state transitions.

We augment an existing OWL-based CPG execution engine which models tasks states and their transitions in an ontology using OWL axioms and SWRL rules. We add a set of OWL axioms and SWRL rules to the CPG execution engine which can be used by an OWL reasoner to find the effect of the constraints on the tasks' state transitions. Each type of constraint has its own special effect on execution of the merged CPG by triggering state transitions in tasks. For instance, if two tasks are merged by *SimultaneousActionConstraint*, it will force the task ahead (t1) to go to the pending state in order to wait for the behind CPG to reach the merging point (t2). The following rule written in SWRL implements the desired behavior:

```
SimultaneousActionConstraint(?const), has-
Task1(?const,?t1), StartedTask(?t1), has-
Task2(?const,?t2), InactiveTask(?t2)→ PendingTask(?t1)
```

Reasoning on this rule will help the execution engine infer that t1 should go to the pending state. In this way the effect of the merging constraints on the tasks' state will be taken into consideration during dynamic merging of several CPG. Using similar rules, when the behind t2 becomes started, this constraint will cause the t1 to go to started state as well so they both can be executed simultaneously. All other constraints have similar rules that make the necessary state transitions. These state transitions are caused by constraints will help the OWL-based execution engine to dynamically merge several CPG according to merge criteria.

5   Evaluation

Our evaluation shows that our ontology is consistent, in OWL-Lite and as a result decidable. Completeness evaluations also show that our ontology can capture all of the interactions and merges indentified in the related literature on merging computerized CPG. Moreover, we have found several new possible merging constraints such as simultaneous action constraint that have not been reported in the existing literature. The usefulness of these new merging constraints is yet to be fully evaluated in merging complex comorbidity CPG. To evaluate the efficacy of the MRO, we experimented with the merging of CPG for CHF and AF. We were able to express the merge criteria in a more detailed and precise manner compared to [2]. For instance, an unaccounted simultaneous constraint were found and modeled in MRO. We also used our CPG merging execution engine to execute CHF and AF CPG along with the instantiation of MRO. Domain expert believe that dynamically merging these two CPG enhances the relevance and timing of the recommendation as it does not make any assumptions about the execution flow of the CPG before execution and the decisions are made when the relevant information is available.

Acknowledgements. This research project is sponsored by a research grant from Green Shield, Canada.

References

1. Hing, M.M., Michalowski, M., Wilk, S., Michalowski, W., Farion, K.: Identifying Inconsistencies in Multiple Clinical Practice Guidelines for a Patient with Co-Morbidity. In: 2010 IEEE International Conference on Bioinformatics and Biomedicine Workshops (BIBMW), pp. 447–452. IEEE Press (2010)
2. Abidi, S.R.: A Knowledge Management Framework to Develop, Model, Align and Operationalize Clinical Pathways to Provide Decision Support for Comorbid Diseases, PhD dissertation, Dalhousie University, Halifax, Canada (2010)
3. Real, F., Riaño, D.: Automatic Combination of Formal Intervention Plans Using SDA* representation model. In: Riaño, D. (ed.) K4CARE 2007. LNCS (LNAI), vol. 4924, pp. 75–86. Springer, Heidelberg (2008)
4. Jafarpour, B., Abidi, S.R., Abidi, S.S.R.: Exploiting OWL reasoning services to execute ontologically-modeled clinical practice guidelines. In: Peleg, M., Lavrač, N., Combi, C. (eds.) AIME 2011. LNCS (LNAI), vol. 6747, pp. 307–311. Springer, Heidelberg (2011)
5. Abidi, S.R.: A conceptual framework for ontology based automating and merging of clinical pathways of comorbidities. In: Riaño, D. (ed.) K4HelP 2008. LNCS, vol. 5626, pp. 55–66. Springer, Heidelberg (2009)
6. Lozano, E., Marcos, M., Martínez-Salvador, B., Alonso, A., Alonso, J.R.: Experiences in the Development of Electronic Care Plans for the Management of Comorbidities. In: Riaño, D., ten Teije, A., Miksch, S., Peleg, M. (eds.) KR4HC 2009. LNCS, vol. 5943, pp. 113–123. Springer, Heidelberg (2010)

Multiparty Argumentation Game for Consensual Expansion Applied to Evidence Based Medicine

Stefano Bromuri[1] and Maxime Morge[2]

[1] Institute of Business Information Systems
University of Applied Sciences Western Switzerland
Stefano.Bromuri@hevs.ch
[2] Laboratoire d'Informatique Fondamentale de Lille
Université Lille 1
Maxime.Morge@univ-lille1.fr

Abstract. Evidence based medicine (EBM) requires many different sources of knowledge when dealing with complex patients. Such a discipline inherently involves the issue of conflicts arising amongst arguments coming from different sources, such as guidelines, trials and clinical studies. In this paper we consider a set of agents with their own medical argumentation which exchange medical arguments to enrich their own knowledge and suggest a set of treatments resulting from the argumentation process.

1 Introduction

Evidence Based Medicine (EBM) involves the application of the best practice towards a treatment as supported by the scientific method [1]. One way used by medical doctors to implement EBM is to use medical guidelines in their clinical practice. However, contradictions happen between the different guidelines and clinical trials. Multi-Agent Systems can help EBM by combining existing medical guidelines. In Argumentation Theory, the positions (arguments) and the oppositions (attacks) are first-class citizens. In this paper, we adopt a dialectical approach of argumentation where the argumentation is the outcome of a dispute process [2,3,4]. Agents play a game to decide the best treatment to be applied to a patient and highlight where the conflicts are. In [5] we focused on formalizing the argumentation game while the significance of this paper resides in its application for EBM. In particular, we evaluate our approach with a case study involving a patient affected by hypertension, dyslipidemia and cardiovascular complications.

2 Background

In order to represent evidence, here we adopt the abstract approach to argumentation proposed in [2]. Medical arguments are viewed as abstract entities supporting claims about treatments to be proposed for a patient. The fact that an argument is challenged by another captures the notion of conflict in the treatments.

N. Peek, R. Marín Morales, and M. Peleg (Eds.): AIME 2013, LNAI 7885, pp. 33–37, 2013.

Definition 1 *(AF). An Argumentation Framework is a couple $AF = \langle A, R \rangle$ where A is a finite set of arguments, $R \subseteq A \times A$ is a binary relation called* attack relation.

Contrary to [6], arguments are atomic entities representing the drugs to be used in a treatment for a patient, while attacks represent conflicts amongst the drugs related to the particular patient status. For example, for a dyslipidemic patient that has a history of myocardial infarction, n-3 fatty acids (N3FA) and statins are arguments and N3FA attack statins due to the patient's history.

An argumentation framework does not allow to model missing information. That is the reason why [7] introduce the *Partial Argumentation Framework (PAF)* representing the fact that an argument attacks (or not) a second argument can be ignored.

Definition 2 *(PAF). A partial argumentation framework is a triplet $PAF = \langle A, R, I \rangle$ where: $\langle A, R \rangle$ is the underlying AF as defined in Def. 1, $I \subseteq A \times A$ is the* ignorance relation *which verifies that $R \cap I = \emptyset$. We call* non-attack relation $N = (A \times A) \setminus (R \cup I)$.

To capture the heterogeneous viewpoints related to medical guidelines, trials and meta analysis, we consider a set of agents, each of them having its own arguments and conflicts. The agents aim at expanding their argumentation based on a consensus.

Formally, we consider here a profile of n argumentation frameworks $S = \langle AF_1, \ldots, AF_n \rangle$. Our goal is to expand this vector in a profile of partial argumentation frameworks $P = \langle PAF_1, \ldots, PAF_n \rangle$ where each PAF_i expands the corresponding AF_i with S by taking account the arguments, the attacks and the non-attacks from the other AFs in S. For this purpose, we focus on the consensual expansion proposed by [7]. In order to expand an AF_i on a PAF_i, we consider all the arguments and only the consensual attacks.

Definition 3 (Consensual Expansion). *Let $S = \langle AF_1, \ldots, AF_n \rangle$ be a profile of n argumentation frameworks $AF_i = \langle A_i, R_i \rangle$ with $1 \leq i \leq n$. Let $conf(S) = (\bigcup_i R_i) \cap (\bigcup_i N_i)$ be the set of non-consensual attacks. The consensual expansion of AF_i with S is a partial argumentation framework $PAF_i = \langle A'_i, R'_i, I'_i \rangle$ where: $A'_i = \bigcup_i A_i$, $R'_i = R_i \cup ((\bigcup_{j \neq i} R_j) \setminus conf(S))$ and $I'_i = conf(S) \setminus (A_i \times A_i)$. Then, $N'_i = (A'_i \times A'_i) \setminus (R'_i \cup I'_i)$.*

The arguments in the consensual expansion (A'_i) are all the arguments from the initial profile. A new attack is added (R'_i) if it is consensual, i.e. if all agents which initially consider these arguments agree on this conflict. An attack is ignored (I'_i) if it is not consensual $(conf(S))$ and if it was not considered *a priori* $(A_i \times A_i)$.

3 Proposal

We adopt an individual-oriented approach where the consensual expansion emerges from the interactions between the agents. Our proposal consists of a multiparty argumentation game, where more than two agents play and observe moves on a gameboard. At the end of the game, each agent builds its *PAF* with the arguments and the conflicts recorded on the gameboard.

Definition 4 *(gb). The gameboard is an objective representation of the game with a triplet $gb = \langle AM, RM, DM \rangle$ where: AM is the record list of argument moves, RM is the record list of attack moves and DM is the record list of denial moves.*

Agents perceive the gameboard and can act on it by adding arguments, attacks and non-attacks. These moves are evaluated via an artifact which records the dialogue history. Each utterance of a move is interpreted by the artifact for updating the gameboard in order to build the common partial argumentation framework.

Definition 5 (AF_{gb}). *We call common partial argumentation framework $PAF_{gb} = \langle A_{gb}, R_{gb}, D_{gb} \rangle$, the argumentation framework defined such that: A_{gb} is the set of arguments in the argument moves from AM, R_{gb} is the set attacks in the attack moves from RM and D_{gb} is the set of ignorances in the denial moves from DM.*

We aim at defining the game such that the rational rules of utterances and the rules of the game leads to a common partial argumentation framework $PAF_{gb} = \langle A_{gb}, R_{gb}, D_{gb} \rangle$.

The game we propose is a n-players simultaneous game based on the gameboard. Our argumentation game is subdivided into two subgames. The first one, the **argument game**, aims at collecting the agents' arguments. The second game, the **attack game**, collects all the consensual and non-consensual attacks. The argument (resp. attack) game ends when all the players withdraw, i.e. when they have no more arguments (resp. attacks) to push forward. Agents communicate by playing moves. The content of the moves depends on the subgame.

Argument Game. Agents can submit new arguments. A move is well-formed iff it contains an argument ($m = \langle i, assert(a) \rangle$ with $1 \leq i \leq n$ and $a \in \bigcup_i A_i$).

Attack Game. Agents can add or rectract attacks. A move is well-formed iff it contains an attack ($m = \langle i, assert(a,b) \rangle$ with $1 \leq i \leq n$ and $a,b \in A_{gb}$) or a non-attack ($m = \langle i, j, deny(a,b) \rangle$ with $1 \leq i, j \leq n$, $a,b \in A_{gb}$ and there is a move $m = \langle j, assert(a,b) \rangle$ in AM). Contrary to the attack moves, the non-attack moves are replying moves.

Rational Rules. Each player i can check the legality of moves and submit it if it is the case. During the argument game (resp. the attack game), an agent submits a move based on the rational rule (1) (resp. (2)):

$$ag_i \text{ utters} \begin{cases} m = \langle i, assert(a) \rangle \\ \quad \text{if } \exists a \in A_i \land a \notin A_{gb} \quad (1) \\ m = \langle i, withdraw \rangle \text{ else} \end{cases} \qquad ag_i \text{ utters} \begin{cases} m = \langle i, assert(a,b) \rangle \text{ if} \\ \quad \exists (a,b) \in R_i \land (a,b) \notin D_{gb} \\ m = \langle i, j, deny(a,b) \rangle \text{ if} \quad (2) \\ \quad \exists (a,b) \in N_i \land (a,b) \notin D_{gb} \\ m = \langle i, withdraw \rangle \text{ else} \end{cases}$$

The game is regulated by a scheduler which gives the token to agents in a fair way. Here we assume that agents are honest. At the end of the game, each player expands its argumentation framework with the arguments, the attacks and the denials reported in the common partial argumentation framework:

Definition 6 (Game Expansion). *Let $S = \langle AF_1, \ldots, AF_n \rangle$ be a profile of n argumentation frameworks and $AF_i = \langle A_i, R_i \rangle$ be one of them. The expansion of AF_i with $PAF_{gb} = \langle A_{gb}, R_{gb}, D_{gb} \rangle$ is the partial argumentation framework $PAF_i = \langle A_i'', R_i'', I_i'' \rangle$ defined such that: $A_i'' = A_{gb}$, $R_i'' = R_i \cup R_{gb}$, $I_i'' = D_{gb} \setminus (A_i \times A_i)$.*

Contrary to [7], agents do not need to know the arguments and the attacks of all the other agents but only the outcome of the game. As demonstrated in [5], the common partial argumentation framework allows to expand the individual argumentation frameworks in a consensual manner.

4   Usecase

We use our argumentation game to compare the results of different clinical trials, when a doctor is called to make a decision about a 55 years old patient who is affected by chronic hypertension, dyslipidemia and has coexistent cardiovascular complications. The problem for the medical doctor that has to decide about such a patient is to combine a set of drugs so that the probability of certain outcomes, such as myocardial infarction or kindey failure, are minimized.

We used the meta-analysis in [8,9,10], which compare different treatments for dyslipidemia, hypertension and cardiovascular complications: Statins, N3FA (n-3 fatty acid), Resins, Angiotensin-converting enzyme (ACE) and Diet. Fig. 1 compares the risk for the treatments. For instance, the risks due to cardiac mortality are less with N3FA rather than Resins (a_4). The other risks of mortality are equivalent for these two treatments (a_9). We consider five agents. Each of them is associated with an Argumentation Framework. The first evaluates cardiac mortality (AF_1), the second focuses on other mortality (AF_2), the third considers myocardial infarction (AF_3), the fourth focuses on stroke (AF_4) and the last one is interested in kidney outcome. The profile of the corresponding argumentation frameworks is in Fig. 1.

Treatments are represented by arguments: Statins (S), N3FA (N), Resins (R), ACE (A) and Diet (D). Each pairwise comparison is captured by an attack when there is an evidence for the benefit of one treatment over another one. The output of our argumentation game is represented in bottom of Fig. 1. Finally, our system allows to conclude that introducing N3FA, statins and ACE inhibitors is the treatment which has the lower risk. The clinical trials lead to the same conclusion. Resins, would be a good drug to

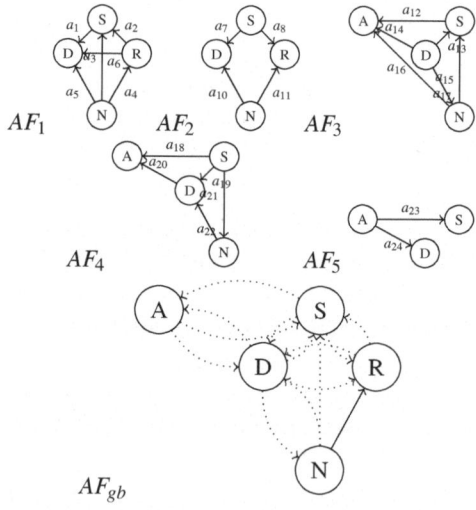

Id	Treatment	Comparison	Treatment	Indicator
a_1	Statins		Diet	card. mort.
a_2	Statins	<	Resins	card. mort.
a_3	Statins	<	N3FA	card. mort.
a_4	Resins	<	N3FA	card. mort.
a_5	Diet	<	N3FA	card. mort.
a_6	Diet	<	Resins	card. mort.
a_7	Statins	>	Diet	other mort.
a_8	Statins	>	Resins	other mort.
a_9	Statins	=	N3FA	other mort.
a_{10}	N3FA	>	Diet	other mort.
a_{11}	N3FA	>	Resins	other mort.
a_{12}	Statins	>	ACE	Myocardial
a_{13}	Statins	<	Diet	Myocardial
a_{14}	ACE	<	Diet	Myocardial
a_{15}	N3FA	>	Statins	Myocardial
a_{16}	N3FA	>	ACE	Myocardial
a_{17}	N3FA	<	Diet	Myocardial
a_{18}	Statins	>	ACE	Stroke
a_{19}	Statins	>	Diet	Stroke
a_{20}	ACE	<	Diet	Stroke
a_{21}	N3FA	<	Statins	Stroke
a_{22}	N3FA	>	Diet	Stroke
a_{23}	Statins	<	ACE	kidney out.
a_{24}	ACE	>	Diet	kidney out.

Fig. 1. Comparison of treatments (at left), the profile of argumentation frameworks (at top right) and the output (at bottom right)

deal with dyslipidemia, but the trials indicate that resins rise the probability of mortality for other causes, so, as a first choice, Statins are more indicated. In the case that the dyslipidemia worsens then the doctor will have to decide if the risk of cardiovascular complications justify the introduction of a combined therapy, but this case is outside the scope of this paper.

5   Conclusion

In this paper, we have considered a set of agents, each of them is equipped with its own argumentation framework. We have formalized a multiparty argumentation game, where more than two agents play and observe moves on a gameboard. In our individual-oriented approach, the building of the consensual expansions emerges from the interactions between the agents. Furthermore, our model is explanatory since it renders intelligible the conflicts between the agents which appear during the process, i.e. the contradiction in the medical guidelines.

Acknowledgement. This work was supported by the FP7 287841 COMMODITY12 project and a grant from Lille 1 University.

References

1. Timmermans, S., Mauck, A.: The promises and pitfalls of evidence-based medicine. Health Aff. (Millwood) 24(1), 18–28 (2005)
2. Dung, P.: On the acceptability of arguments and its fundamental role in nonmonotonic reasoning, logic programming and n-person games. Artif. Intell. 77, 321–357 (1995)
3. Prakken, H.: Formal systems for persuasion dialogue. KER 21, 163–188 (2006)
4. Bonzon, E., Maudet, N.: On the outcomes of multiparty persuasion. In: Proc. of AAMAS, IFAAMAS, pp. 47–54 (2011)
5. Bromuri, S., Morge, M.: Multiparty argumentation game for consensual expansion. In: Proc. of ICAART, pp. 160–165. INSTICC Press (2013)
6. Hunter, A., Williams, M.: Aggregating evidence about the positive and negative effects of treatments. Artif. Intell. Med. 56, 173–190 (2012)
7. Coste-Marquis, S., Devred, S., Konieczny, S., Lagasquie-Schiex, M.C., Marquis, P.: On the merging of Dung's argumentation systems. Artif. Intell. 171, 730–753 (2007)
8. Studer, M., Briel, M., Leimenstoll, B., Glass, T.R., Bucher, H.C.: Effect of different antilipidemic agents and diets on mortality: A systematic review. Arch. Intern. Med. 165(7), 725–730 (2005)
9. Bucher, H.C., Hengstler, P., Schindler, C., Meier, G.: N-3 polyunsaturated fatty acids in coronary heart disease: A meta-analysis of randomized controlled trials. Am. J. Med. 112(4), 298–304 (2002)
10. Larsson, S.C., Orsini, N.: Fish consumption and the risk of stroke: A dose-response meta-analysis. Stroke 42(12), 3621–3623 (2011)

Rule-Based Formalization of Eligibility Criteria for Clinical Trials

Zhisheng Huang, Annette ten Teije, and Frank van Harmelen

Department of Computer Science,
VU University Amsterdam, The Netherlands
{huang,annette,Frank.van.Harmelen}@cs.vu.nl

Abstract. In this paper, we propose a rule-based formalization of eligibility criteria for clinical trials. The rule-based formalization is implemented by using the logic programming language Prolog. Compared with existing formalizations such as pattern-based and script-based languages, the rule-based formalization has the advantages of being declarative, expressive, reusable and easy to maintain. Our rule-based formalization is based on a general framework for eligibility criteria containing three types of knowledge: (1) trial-specific knowledge, (2) domain-specific knowledge and (3) common knowledge. This framework enables the reuse of several parts of the formalization of eligibility criteria. We have implemented the proposed rule-based formalization in SemanticCT, a semantically-enabled system for clinical trials, showing the feasibility of using our rule-based formalization of eligibility criteria for supporting patient recruitment in clinical trial systems.

1 Introduction

Clinical trials have played important roles in medical research and drug development, because they provide sets of tests which generate safety and efficacy data for health interventions. However, the work in clinical trials have been considered to be laborious, sometimes, exhausting, because many procedures in clinical trials, such as patient recruitment (i.e., finding eligible patients for a trial) and trial finding (i.e., finding suitable trials for a patient), usually require manually processes. The goal of the formalizations of eligibility criteria is to provide faster identification of patients for trials and automatic identification of clinical trials for patients. That requires the implementation of the advanced reasoning services for matching patient data with formalized eligibility criteria.

There have been several attempts to the formulizations of eligibility criteria for clinical trials, which include pattern-based formalization, semantic-annotation–based formalization, and script-based formalization [3]. Compared with existing formalizations, a rule-based formalization is expected to be efficient and effective, because of their declarative nature, their high expressiveness, their reusability and easy maintenance. We have implemented the proposed rule-based formulization in SemanticCT, a semantically-enabled system for clinical trials [5][1].

---

[1] http://wasp.cs.vu.nl/sct

N. Peek, R. Marín Morales, and M. Peleg (Eds.): AIME 2013, LNAI 7885, pp. 38–47, 2013.
© Springer-Verlag Berlin Heidelberg 2013

SemanticCT provides semantic integration of various data in clinical trials. The system is designed to be a semantically-enabled system for decision support in various settings of clinical trials. In this paper we will show that the rule-based formalization of eligibility criteria is an efficient approach to identifying eligible patients for clinical trials.

2   Motivation for Rules and Prolog

2.1   Rules

A rule-based formalization is expected to be an efficient and effective formalism to support automatic patient recruitment and trial feasibility testing, because of the following features:

Declarative. A rule-based formalization is a declarative language that expresses the logic of a computation without the need of exactly describing its control flow. That is significantly different from traditional programming languages, like Java, which use a procedural approach for the specification of control flow in the computation. A declarative formalization is more suitable for knowledge representation and reasoning because it needs no carefully design its computation (or reasoning) procedure. Thus, a rule-based formalization of eligibility criteria would provide a more convenient and efficient way for the automatic patient recruitments in clinical trials, compared with other procedural approaches, like the script-based formalization, which relies procedural scripts, and the pattern-based approach, which is based on SPARQL queries with regular expressions.

Easy Maintenance. Rule-based formalization provides an approach in which specified knowledge is easy to be understood for human users, because they are very close to human knowledge. It would not be too hard for human users to check the correctness of the specification of eligibility criteria if they are formalized as a set of rules. Furthermore, changing or revising a single rule would not make an effect on other part of the formalization significantly, because the meaning of the specification is usually represented in the specific rule. Thus, it is much easier for maintenance of knowledge, compared with procedural/scripting approaches of the formalization of eligibility criteria.

Reusability. In a rule-based formalization, a single rule (or a set of rules) is usually considered to be independent from other part of knowledge. Thus, it is much more convenient to re-use some rules of a formalized clinical trial for formalization of other trials. Furthermore, some rules which specify common knowledge, such as rules for temporal reasoning, and domain knowledge, and those that specify knowledge of diseases, can be designed to be a common library, which can be re-used for the formalization of other trials.

Expressiveness. Automatic patient recruitment usually involves comprehensive scenarios of deliberation and decision-making procedures. To facilitate those capabilities, it may require sophisticated data processing in workflows. An expressive rule-based language can support various functionalities of data processing. Thus, it provides the possibility to build workflows for various scenarios of medical applications.

2.2   Rule-Based Language Prolog

There exist various rule languages which can be used for the formalization of eligibility criteria. In the researches of artificial intelligence, logic programming languages, like Prolog, are well known and popular rule-based languages. Several rule-based languages, like SWRL[2] and RIF[3], have been proposed for the semantics-enable rule-based language. In biomedical domain, the Arden syntax[4] has been developed to formalize rule-like medical knowledge. However, compared with logic programming language Prolog, both SWRL, RIF and the Arden syntax have very limited functionalities for data processing.

In this paper, we will propose a rule-based formalization, which is based on the logic programming language Prolog. Prolog is a general purpose logic programming language associated with artificial intelligence. An example of Prolog rule

```
triple_negative(Patient):-
    er_negative(Patient), pr_negative(Patient), her2_negative(Patient).
```

means that a patient of breast cancer is triple negative if it is ER negative, PR negative, and HER2 negative.

3   Framework

3.1   Eligibility Criteria

Eligibility criteria consist of inclusion criteria, which state a set of conditions that must be met, and exclusion criteria, which state a set of conditions that must not be met, in order to participate in a clinical trial.

Take the example of the trial NCT00002720, the eligibility criteria are:

```
DISEASE CHARACTERISTICS:
  - Histologically proven stage I, invasive breast cancer
  - Hormone receptor status:
    - Estrogen receptor positive
    - Progesterone receptor positive or negative
PATIENT CHARACTERISTICS:
  Age: 65 to 80, Sex: Female, Menopausal status: Postmenopausal
  Other: - No serious disease that would preclude surgery
         - No other prior or concurrent malignancy except basal cell
           carcinoma or carcinoma in situ of the cervix
```

Those inclusion criteria (such as 'invasive breast cancer') and exclusion criteria (such as 'No serious disease that would preclude surgery') are trial specific. However, in order to check whether or not a required item (i.e., a criterion) has been met by a patient record, we need some domain knowledge to interpret

---

[2] http://www.w3.org/Submission/SWRL/

[3] http://www.w3.org/TR/rif-overview/

[4] http://www.hl7.org/special/Committees/arden/index.cfm

the requirement and make it directly checkable from patient data. For example, 'invasive breast cancer' can be defined as either 'invasive ductal carcinoma' or 'invasive lobular carcinoma' in the diagnosis. Furthermore, we need some knowledge, such as temporal reasoning knowledge, to deal with temporal aspects of criteria, and service interface knowledge, to get the corresponding patient data from the EHR or CMR servers.

3.2 Different Knowledge Levels

We can formalize the knowledge rules of the specification of eligibility criteria of clinical trials with respect to the following different re-usable knowledge types:

Trial-specific Knowledge. Trial-specific knowledge are those rules which specify the concrete details of the eligibility criteria of a specific clinical trial. Those criteria are different from one trial to another. This is the formalization of which specific inclusion criteria and exclusion criteria are required for a particular clinical trial. The formalization of the criteria themselves are part of the other levels of knowledge.

Domain-specific Knowledge. Those trial-specific rules above may involve some knowledge which is domain specific, but that domain knowledge is in principle trial independent. Such domain specific, but trial independent knowledge can be formalized in re-usable libraries. For example, for clinical trials of breast cancer, we formalize the knowledge of breast cancer in the knowledge bases of breast cancer, a domain-specific library of rules. An example of this type of knowledge is a patient of breast cancer is triple negative if the patient has estrogon receptor negative, progesterone receptor negative and protein HER2 negative status.

Common Knowledge. The specification of the eligibility criteria may involve some knowledge which is domain independent, like for example knowledge about temporal reasoning and the knowledge for manipulating semantic data and interacting with data servers, e.g. how to obtain the data from SPARQL endpoints. We formalize those knowledge in several rule libraries, which can again be reused across different applications.

4 Formalization

4.1 Formalization of Trial-Specific knowledge

For the specification of eligibility criteria, we usually formalize their inclusion criteria and exclusion criteria respectively.

Given a patient ID, we suppose that we can obtain its patient data through the common knowledge of the interface with SPARQL endpoints and its internal data storage. Thus, in order to check if a patient meets an inclusion criterion, we can check if its patient data meet the criterion. Furthermore, we would not expect to check all the criteria with respect to the patient data, because some of those required data may be missing in the patient data. We introduce a special predicate getNotYetCheckedItems to collect those criteria which have not yet been formalized for the trial.

The inclusion criteria in the trial NCT00002720 above can be formalized in the following:

```
meetInclusionCriteria(_PatientID, PatientData, CT, NotYetCheckedItems):-
                    CT = 'nct00002720',
                    breast_cancer_stage(PatientData, '1'),
                    invasive_breast_cancer(PatientData),
                    er_positive(PatientData),
                    known_pr_status(PatientData),
                    age_between(PatientData, 65, 80),
                    postmenopausal(PatientData),
                    getNotYetCheckedItems(CT, NotYetCheckedItems).
```

We formalize the criteria which have not been checked in a rule like this:

```
getNotYetCheckedItems('nct00002720', NotYetCheckedItems):-
Item1 = 'No serious disease that would preclude surgery',
Item2 = 'No other prior or concurrent malignancy except
  basal cell carcinoma or carcinoma in situ of the cervix',
NotYetCheckedItems = [Item1, Item2].
```

4.2   Formalization of Domain-Specific Knowledge

We consider patient data as a set of property-value pairs. A general format of patient data, called the PrologCMR format, is designed to be a list of property-value pairs, like this:

```
[gender:Gender, birthyear:BirthYear, menopause:Menopause,
diagnosis:Diagnosis, her2:HER2, er:ER, pr:PR, stage:Stage,...]
```

The values in the pairs of the Prolog CMR format can be a term (i.e., a string or a number) or a list with the PrologCMR format. Namely it allows for a tree-structured data. For example, we can merge the properties of hormone receptors in the list above into a property-value pair, like this: hermone_receptor_status: [her2:HER2, er:ER, pr:PR].

This general format of patient data is flexible enough to represent the data from different formats of CMRs, because we can design a CMR-specific interface to obtain the corresponding data via different data servers, which can be a SPARQL endpoint, internal data storage server, or a database server. Then, we can convert the patient data into the PrologCMR format. We introduce the general predicate getItem(PatientData, Property, Value) to get the value of the property from the patient data.

Several receptor status of breast cancer cells have been considered to be very important for the classification of breast cancer. Those important receptors are estrogen receptor (ER), progesterone receptor (PR), and Human Epidermal growth factor Receptor 2(HER2). These receptor status can be straightforward formalized as follows:

```
er_positive(PatientData):- getItem(PatientData, er, ER), ER = 'positive'.
er_negative(PatientData):- getItem(PatientData, er, ER), ER = 'negative'.
```

Similarly we can define the predicates for PR and HER2.

More complex criteria where real domain knowledge is involved for instance the triple-negative breast cancer status which means that a patient of breast cancer is triple negative if she is ER negative, PR negative, and HER2 negative. This can be formalized as follows:

```
triple_negative(PatientData):- er_negative(PatientData),
    pr_negative(PatientData), her2_negative(PatientData).
```

The menopausal status of a female patient is simply considered as a value of a property in the patient data. Actually in medical science, menopausal status is defined in terms of menstrual periods.

```
last_time(Patient, menstrual_period, LastMenstrucalPeriod):-
hasPatientData(Patient,PatientData), postmenopausal(PatientData),
    today(Today), at_least_earlier(LastMenstrucalPeriod, Today, 1, year).
```

The definitions of those temporal predicates (e.g. *at_least_earlier*) belong to the common knowledge level.

4.3   Formalization of Common Knowledge

Temporal Reasoning. The rules for formalizing temporal reasoning and others are not domain- specific, because that kind of knowledge can be used in different applications. For reasoning with breast cancer knowledge, we may need various temporal operators(i.e., predicates), like those "before", "after", "until", "today", "no less than 6 months before", "at least two weeks" etc. Such general temporal operators are well known from the AI literature [1]. Thus, they are designed to be separated libraries, which are different from the domain specific libraries.

To summerise the general framework has three knowledge types: (1) clinical trial specific knowledge, (2) domain-specific knowledge, and (3) common knowledge. The clinical trial specific knowledge specified the eligibility criteria in terms of predicates defined in the domain-specific level if they are domain dependent and in the common knowledge level if they are domain independent but common knowledge. The levels (2) and (3) are the reusable parts for the formalization of eligibility criteria whereas (1) use those re-usable parts in the formalization of a specific eligibility criteria.

5   Implementation and Feasibility Experiment

Implementation. SWI-Prolog[8] provides a powerful Semantic Web library, by which we can achieve semantic interoperability in the rule-based formulation efficiently and effectively. SWI-Prolog handles the semantic web RDF model and OWL data naturally. RDF and OWL provide stable models for knowledge representation with nice support for semantic interoperability.

The rule-based formulation of eligibility criteria of clinical trials is developed with the support of the following two semantic web libraries in SWI-Prolog:

Web-server and client library. This is the core semantic web package of SWI-Prolog. It provides an HTTP server and client, session handling, authorization, logging, etc, and libraries for generating HTML pages and JSON. Based on this library, we developed the interface with SPARQL endpoints to obtain semantic data for the rule-based formulation of eligibility criteria.

For example, the following rule in Prolog is designed to obtain the patient data for a SPARQL endpoint, which is located at the localhost with a port:

```
getPatientData(PatientID, PatientData):-
    get_sparql_query(patientdata, Query, PatientID),
    findall(Row, (sparql_query(Query, Row,[host('localhost'), port(8183),
            path('/sparql/')])), Answers),
    sparql_answer_to_list(patientdata(PatientID), Answers, PatientData).
```

Namely, given a patienID, the predicate 'getPatientData' would return the patient data from the corresponding SPARQL endpoint. We use the predicate get_sparql_query(patient, Query, PatientID) to get a system specific SPARQL query for the given patient ID. We use the built-in predicate sparql_query to obtain the result Answers from the SPARQL endpoint. We design a predicate sparql_answer_to_list to convert the answers from the SPARQL endpoint into the internal representation of the patient data (i.e., a Prolog list), so that the patient data can be processed further by the predicate getItem, as we have discussed in the section about the formalization of domain specific knowledge.

RDF storage and query library. SWI-Prolog provides powerful support for the storage and manipulation of semantic data, like loading and saving RDF data and querying them. This RDF library loads and saves XML/RDF and Turtle. It also provides simple RDFS and OWL support which is sufficient for the temporary internal storage of semantic data in the rule-based formulation of eligibility criteria.

Feasibility. SemanticCT[5] is a semantically enabled system for clinical trials. The goals of SemanticCT are not only to achieve interoperability by semantic integration of heterogeneous data in clinical trials, but also to facilitate automatic reasoning and data processing services for decision support systems in various settings of clinical trials.

SemanticCT is built on the top of the LarKC (Large Knowledge Collider) platform[6], a platform for scalable semantic data processing. We have implemented the rule-based formulization of eligibility criteria as a component of SemanticCT for the service of automatic identification of eligible patients for clinical trials.

Experiment design: An ideal experimental scenario would look as follows: (i) take realistic corpus of patient records for included and excluded patients for a given set of trials; (ii) formalize the inclusion and exclusion conditions for these trials; (iii) execute these formalized criteria on the data of included and excluded

---

[5] http://wasp.cs.vu.nl/sct
[6] http://www.larkc.eu

patients; and (iv) compare precision and recall of the automatically selected set of patients against the actual selections as given in the corpus.

Available data: A corpus of current and past clinical trials is readily available[7] but given the lack of a realistic collection of patient data for such trials, we limit ourselves in this paper to a *feasibility* study that shows how two important tasks can in principle be supported by the formalization and implementation that we discussed above. Our experiments concern a *patient recruitment* task (= finding patients that qualify for a given trial), and a *trial feasibility* task (= checking if a set of inclusion and exclusion criteria for a newly designed trial results in a sufficient number of recruitable patients).

For a small corpus of clinical trials in our experiments, we have picked up 10 clinical trials of breast cancer out of the 4665 NCT clinical trials (1,200,565 triples) and we formalized the eligibility criteria of those selected trials (the trial ID numbers are listed in the tables that follow).

For patient data, we generated a set of 10,000 plausible patient files created by our Knowledge-based Patient Data Generator[8]. This Knowledge-Based Patient Data Generator uses clinical and epidemiological background knowledge to generate a patient population that is both medically plausible, and that has a realistic statistical distribution. *Experiment 1: Patient Recruitment:* Some eligibility criteria cannot be checked automatically over the patient data, because they need additional input from patients, like the criteria 'Patients must be mentally competent to understand and give informed consent for the protocol'. Some eligibility criteria have not yet been checked, because their corresponding data have not yet been available in the existing patient data format, like the criteria 'Must have regular menstrual cycles (21-35 days)'.

Table 1. Checked Eligibility Criteria. IC:Inclusion Criteria, EC: Exclusion Criteria, NYC: Not Yet Checked Items.

Clinical Trial ID	Total Criteria	Checked Criteria	Total IC	Total EC	Checked IC	Checked EC	NYC IC	NYC EC	Checked Criteria Rate(%)
NCT00001250	22	15	11	11	7	8	4	3	68.18
NCT00001385	18	15	9	9	7	8	2	1	83.33
NCT00002720	10	7	9	1	7	0	2	1	70.00
NCT00002762	15	7	10	5	5	2	5	3	46.67
NCT00002934	26	10	20	6	9	1	11	5	38.46
NCT00003329	6	3	5	1	3	0	2	1	50.00
NCT00003654	18	11	1 0	8	9	2	1	6	61.11
NCT00005023	29	10	27	2	9	1	18	1	34.48
NCT00005079	18	11	10	8	7	4	3	4	61.11
NCT00005587	16	10	12	4	10	0	2	4	62.50

Table 1 reports on a (simulated) *patient recruitment scenario*, and summarizes how many criteria have been checked in the test. The table shows that we can check maximally 83.33% of the criteria, and minimally 34.48% of the

---

[7] e.g. clinicaltrial.gov

[8] http://wasp.cs.vu.nl/apdg

Table 2. Trial Feasibility

Clinical TrialID	T200 Founded	T200 Rate(%)	T300 Founded	T300 Rate(%)	T500 Founded	T500 Rate(%)	T750 Founded	T750 Rate (%)
NCT00001250	200	100	300	100	500	100.00	750	100
NCT00001385	200	100	300	100	500	100	750	100
NCT00002720	200	100	300	100	397	79.40	397	52.93
NCT00002762	200	100	241	80.33	241	48.20	241	32.13
NCT00002934	200	100	300	100	500	100	750	100
NCT00003329	200	100	300	100	500	100	750	100
NCT00003654	200	100	300	100	500	100	750	100
NCT00005023	200	100	300	100	500	100	501	66.80
NCT00005079	200	100	281	93.67	281	56.20	281	37.47
NCT00005587	200	100	300	100	500	100	750	100

criteria, based on the given patient data. *Experiment 2: Trial Feasibility* In this feasibility experiment, we use our system to automatically determine if a given target number of patients can be recruited for a trial: T200 stands for finding 200 candidate patients, and T500 stands for finding 500 candidate patients, from the total 10,000 patients. Table 2 shows the results of trial feasibility with different targets. For the lower target (e.g., T200), we can always find the targeted numbers of the candidate patients who meet the checked criteria. For the higher target (e.g., T750), we cannot find enough candidate patients for four trials. Furthermore, a lower percentage of checked items does not necessary lead to higher recruitment rate. For example, Trial 'NCT00002762' (with checked item rate 46.67) can find only 32.13 percent of the target. That means that some of checked criteria in this trial have low feasibility, and the limited number of the patient data also lead to the difficulties.

These experiments show that conditions of realistic trials can be formalized and implemented in such a way that, at least on our artificially generated but medically and statistically plausible patient data, both patient recruitment and trial feasibility can be supported.

6   Related Work, Discussion and Conclusion

[6] translates each free-text eligibility criterion into a machine executable statement using a derivation of the Arden Syntax. Clinical trial protocols were then structured as collections of these eligibility criteria using XML. In our work, we use a more expressive rule-based language and then structured the eligibility criteria as RDF. [2] presents a method entirely based on standard semantic web technologies and tools, that allows the automatic recruitment of a patient to available clinical trials. They use a domain specific ontology to represent data from patients' health records and use SWRL to verify the eligibility of patients to clinical trials. Although we propose an even more expressive language for modeling the eligibility criteria this is in the same spirit as our approach. Furthermore, we proposed a general framework for specifying the eligibility criteria in three

types of knowledge to facilitate reuse. The empirical analysis in [7] shows that the vast majority (85%) of trial criteria is of "significant semantic complexity". This justifies our choice for an expressive rule-based formalism. The paper also observes that temporal data play a role in 40% of all criteria, justifying our choice for a separate layer for this in our formalization.

For clinical trials, identifying eligible patients are mostly manually. Thus, it often results in low clinical trial enrolment. The formulation of eligibility criteria provides the possibility for faster identification of patients for clinical trials. Based on the rule-based formulation of eligibility criteria, we can achieve an efficient way for automatic identification of eligible patients whenever possible.

With the support of the Semantic Web library in the Prolog-based formalism, we can achieve the semantic interoperability among EHR and clinical trial systems, because the relevant can be exploited to allow more efficient patient enrolment in clinical trials. Semantic interoperability between EHR and CT systems enables us to provide solutions for patient recruitment that help avoid double data entry.

However, automatic patient recruitment for clinical trials would not be considered as a simple system of automatic checking with the criteria of patient data. In many application scenarios of patient recruitment, it should be considered to be one with a decision making system, which involves complex procedure and comprehensive processing over various data and workflows. It would be also beneficial if the formalism can accommodate and integrate with the clinical guidelines for specific diseases[4]. We leave it as one of the future work.

Acknowledgments. This work is partially supported by the European 7th framework programme EURECA Project(FP7-ICT-2011-7, Grant 288048).

References

1. Allen, J.F.: Maintaining knowledge about temporal intervals. Commun. ACM 26(11), 832–843 (1983)
2. Besana, P., Cuggia, M., Zekri, O., Bourde, A., Burgun, A.: Using semantic web technologies for clinical trial recruitment. In: Patel-Schneider, P.F., Pan, Y., Hitzler, P., Mika, P., Zhang, L., Pan, J.Z., Horrocks, I., Glimm, B. (eds.) ISWC 2010, Part II. LNCS, vol. 6497, pp. 34–49. Springer, Heidelberg (2010)
3. Bucur, A., ten Teije, A., van Harmelen, F., Tagni, G., Kondylakis, H., van Leeuwen, J., Schepper, K.D., Huang, Z.: Formalization of eligibility conditions of CT and a patient recruitment method, D6.1. Technical report, EURECA Project (2012)
4. de Clercq, P., Blom, J., Korsten, H., Hasman, A.: Approaches for creating computer-interpretable guidelines that facilitate decision support. Artif. Intell. Med. 1, 1–27 (2004)
5. Huang, Z., ten Teije, A., van Harmelen, F.: SemanticCT: A semantically enabled clinical trial system. Technical report, Vrije University Amsterdam (March 2013)
6. Ohno-Machado, L., Wang, S.J., Mar, P., Boxwala, A.A.: Decision support for clinical trial eligibility determination in breast cancer. In: Proc. AMIA Symp., pp. 340–344 (1999)
7. Ross, J., Tu, S., Carini, S., Sim, I.: Analysis of eligibility criteria complexity in clinical trials. AMIA Summits Transl. Sci. Proc. 2010, 46–50 (2010)
8. Wielemaker, J., Huang, Z., van der Meij, L.: SWI-Prolog and the web. Journal of Theory and Practice of Logic Programming 3, 363–392 (2008)

Characterizing Health-Related Information Needs of Domain Experts

Eya Znaidi[1], Lynda Tamine[1], Cecile Chouquet[2], and Chiraz Latiri[3]

[1] IRIT, University of Toulouse
[2] Institute of Mathematics, University of Toulouse
[3] Computer Sciences Department, Faculty of Sciences of Tunis

Abstract. In information retrieval literature, understanding the users'
intents behind the queries is critically important to gain a better insight
of how to select relevant results. While many studies investigated how
users in general carry out exploratory health searches in digital environments, a few focused on how are the queries formulated, specifically by
domain expert users. This study intends to fill this gap by studying 173
health expert queries issued from 3 medical information retrieval tasks
within 2 different evaluation compaigns. A statistical analysis has been
carried out to study both variation and correlation of health-query attributes such as length, clarity and specificity of either clinical or non
clinical queries. The knowledge gained from the study has an immediate
impact on the design of future health information seeking systems.

Keywords: Health Information Retrieval, Information Needs, Statistical Analysis.

1 Introduction

It is well known in information retrieval (IR) area that expressing queries that
accurately reflect the information needs is a difficult task either in general domains or specialized ones and even for expert users [14,17]. Thus, the identification of the users' intention hidden behind queries that they submit to a search
engine is a challenging issue. More specifically, according to the Pew Internet
and American Life Project, health-related queries are increasingly expressed by
a wide range of age groups with a variety of backgrounds [23]; consumer health
information through online environments support a variety of needs including
the promotion of health and wellness, use of health care services, information
about disease and conditions, and information about medical tests, procedures
and treatment. Unfortunately, it reveals from the literature that despite of the
diversity of the available health IR systems and the diversity of the used information sources, users still felt in retrieving relevant information that meet their
specific mental needs [2,21]. To answer this issue, several studies focused on the
analysis of health searchers' behaviour, including attitudes, strategies, tasks and
queries [11,16,18]. These studies involved large numbers of subjects within general web search settings, with uncontrolled experimental conditions, making it
difficult to generalize their findings to expert searches involved by physicians.

N. Peek, R. Marín Morales, and M. Peleg (Eds.): AIME 2013, LNAI 7885, pp. 48–57, 2013.

Moreover, most of these studies focused on search behaviour through search strategies and tactics. Unlike previous work, we address more specifically in this paper, domain expert health search through the analysis of query attributes namely length, specificity and clarity using appropriate proposed measures built according to different sources of evidence. For this aim, we undertake an in-depth statistical analysis of queries issued from IR evaluation compaigns namely Text REtrieval Conference (TREC)[1] and Conference and Labs of the Evaluation Forum (CLEF)[2] devoted for different medical tasks within controlled evaluation settings. Our experimental study includes a statistical pair-wise attribute correlation analysis and a multidimensional analysis across tasks.

The remainder of this paper is structured as follows. Section 2 presents related work on health information searching. Section 3 details the query attributes and section 4 describes the tasks and query collections analysed in the study. In section 5 we present and discuss the results analysis. Finally, section 6 summarizes the study findings, highlights design implications and concludes the paper.

2 Related Work

The increasing amount of health information available from various sources such as government agencies, non-profit and for-profit organizations, internet portals etc. presents opportunities and issues to improve health care information delivery for medical professionals [1], patients and general public [10]. One critical issue is the understanding of users' search strategies and tactics for bridging the gap between their intention and the delivered information. To tackle this problem, several studies investigated mainly the analysis of consumer health information behaviour in one side and their query formulations in the other side. Regarding consumer's health information behavior, several aspects have been investigated such as: (1) pattern of health information searching [16]: findings highlight in general that health IR obey to a trial-and-error process, or can be viewed as a serie of transitions between searching and browsing, (2) access results [16]: studies revealed that the majority of users access to top documents in the ranked outcome list of results, (3) goals, motivation and emotions particularly in social environments [13]: the authors emphasize that motivation is the main factor leading to the success or failure of health searches. More close to our work, the second category of research focused on query formulation issues by analysing query attributes such as length and topics. Several studies [11,14,20] highlighted that queries are short containing less than 3 terms with an average of 2 terms. For instance authors in [20] studied health related information searches on MedlinePlus and hospitals and revealed that queries lengths were in the range 1-3. The same general finding has been reported in [11] regarding queries submitted to Healthlink on the basis of 377000 queries issued from search logs. [14] reported quite analoguous results from health web searches studies. Through other observations at the topic level [8,19,22], where topics where

---

[1] http://trec.nist.gov/
[2] http://www.clef-initiative.eu/

identified using linguistic features or medical items, it seems that users may do not, in general, make use of terminologies and taxonomies; they use in contrast terms of their own-self leading to mispelling ones or abbreviations. However the above studies were conducted in the context of general web search involving participants with a variety of skills, backgrounds and tasks. Other studies looked at the differences in search strategies between domain experts and novices in the medical domain [3,4] or focused on expert information search behaviors [9,18]. In studies conducted in [3,4], the authors oberved significative differences in the way the users explore the search, beginning from key resources viewed as hubs of their domain for expert domain users rather than starting from general resources for novices. In [18], the author examined the search behavior of medical students at the beginning of their courses, the end of the courses and then six months later. The results suggest that search behaviour changes in accordance with domain expertise gain. In the work presented in this paper, we focus on the analysis of query formulations expressed by medical experts. The main underlying objective is not to explicitly compare expert health searches from novices, but to highlight the pecularities of expert search queries in attempt to customize the search which in turn, can impact medical education and clinical decisions. We address the following research questions: (1) How expert query attributes are correlated within a medical task and across different medical tasks? (2) Are clinical queries significantly different from non clinical queries?

3   Query Attributes

In our study, we consider a health-IR setting where an expert submits a query Q to a target collection of documents C. We propose and formalize in what follows various query attributes and justify their construction.

- **Query Length.** We retain two facets of query length: (1) length as the number of significant words, $LgW(Q)$, and (2) length as the number of terms referencing preferred entries of concepts issued from MESH[3] terminology, $LgC(Q)$. Our choice of MESH terminology is justified by its wide use in the medical domain. For this aim, queries are mapped to MESH terminology using our contextual concept extraction technique [6,7].
- **Query Specificity.** Specificity is usually considered as a criterion for identifying index words [12]. In our study, we are interested in two facets:
  1. *Posting specificity $PSpe(Q)$*: expresses the uniqueness of query words in the index collection; the basic assumption behind posting specificity is that less documents are involved by query words, more specific are the query topics. It is computed as follows:

$$PSpe(Q) = \frac{1}{LgW(Q)} \sum_{t_i \in words(Q)} -\log\left(\frac{n_i}{N}\right) \qquad (1)$$

---

[3] MEdical Subject Headings.

where $LgW(Q)$ is the query length in terms of words, $words(Q)$ is the set of query words, n_i is the number of documents containing the word t_i, N is the total number of documents in the collection C.

2. *Hierarchical specificity $HSpe(Q)$*: it is based on the query words deepness of meaning defined in MESH terminology. The basic underlying assumption is that a child word is more specific than its parent word in the terminology hierarchy. Hierarchical specificity is given by:

$$HSpe(Q) = \frac{1}{LgC(Q)} \sum_{c_i \in Concepts(Q)} \frac{level(c_i) - 1}{Maxlevel(MESH) - 1} \quad (2)$$

where $LgC(Q)$ is the query length in terms of concepts, $Concepts(Q)$ is the set of query concepts, $level(c_i)$ is the MESH level of concept c_i, $Maxlevel(MESH)$ is the maximum level of MESH hierarchy.

- **Query Clarity.** Broadly speaking, a clear query triggers a strong relevant meaning of the underlying topic whereas an ambiguous query triggers a variety of topics meanings that do not correlate each other. We propose to compute two facets of clarity:
  1. *Topic based clarity $TCla(Q)$*: The clarity score of a query is computed as the Kullback-Leiber divergence between the query language model and the collection language model, given by [15]:

$$TCla(Q) = \sum_{t \in V} P(t|Q) log_2 \frac{P(t|Q)}{P_{coll}(t)} \quad (3)$$

where V is the entire vocabulary of the collection, t is a word, $P_{coll(t)}$ is the relative frequency of word t and $P(t|Q)$ is estimated by: $P(t|Q) = \sum_{d \in R} P(w|D)P(D|Q)$ where d is a document, R is the set of all documents containing at least one query word.
  2. *Relevance based clarity $RCla(Q)$*: a query is assumed to be as much clear as it shares concepts with relevant documents assessed by experts. This assumption is the basis of IR models. Accordingly, $RCla(Q)$ is computed as:

$$RCla(Q) = \frac{1}{|R(Q)|} \sum_{d \in R(Q)} \frac{|Concepts(Q) \cap |Concepts(d)|}{LgC(Q)} \quad (4)$$

where $R(Q)$ is the set of relevant documents returned for query Q as assessed by experts, $|Concepts(d)|$ (resp. $|Concepts(Q)|$) is the number of document concepts (resp. query concepts).

- **Query Category.** We are interested in both clinical and non clinical queries. For this aim, we used the PICO model to classify queries [5]: P corresponds to patient description (sex, morbidity, race, age etc.), I defines an applied intervention, C corresponds to another intervention allowing comparison or control and O corresponds to experience results. According to this definition, we manually annotated all the test queries as clinical (C) if they contain at least 3 PICO elements, non clinical (NC) otherwise.

4   Data Sources

To perform this study, we used data issued from TREC and CLEF. We exploited queries (number is noticed $Nb.Q$), documents (number is noticed $Nb.D$) and physicians relevance assessments data with respect to various medical IR tasks described below:

- *TREC Medical records task ($Nb.Q = 35, Nb.D = 95.701$):* the retrieval task consists in identifying cohorts for comparative effectiveness research. Queries describe short disease/condition sets developed by physicians; documents represent medical visit reports.
- *TREC Genomics series task:* The TREC Genomics task was one of the largest and longest running challenge evaluations in biomedicine. This task models the setting where a genomics researcher entering a new area expresses a query to a search engine managing a biomedical scientific literature namely from Medline collection. TREC genomics queries evolved across years: gene names in 2003 ($Nb.Q = 50, Nb.D = 525.938$), information needs expressed using acronyms in 2004 ($Nb.Q = 50, Nb.D = 4.591.008$) and question-answering in the biomedical domain in 2006 ($Nb.Q = 28, Nb.D = 162.259$).
- *ImageCLEF case-based task ($Nb.Q = 10, Nb.D = 55.634$):* The goal of the task was to retrieve cases including images that a physician would judge as relevant for differential diagnosis. The queries were created from an existing medical case database including descriptions with patient demographics, limited symptoms, test results and image studies.

5   Results

5.1   Query Characteristics

To highlight the major differences between the collections (medical tasks), we first performed a descriptive analysis. Figure 1 shows the distributions of the six query attribute facets per collection and for all the queries presented by box-plots. Analysis of variance or non-parametric Kruskal-Wallis tests (adapted to small samples) were performed to compare attributes averages and to detect significative differences between the different collections (indicated by $p - value <$ 0.05). From figures 1.(a) and 1.(b), it is interesting to notice that similar trends are observed between the two facets of length. Moreover, the query length attribute is significantly different across the five query collections ($p - value <$ 0.0001), despite the fact that they all represent experts' information needs. The highest query length was observed for ImageCLEF queries with 24 terms and 5 concepts in average, versus lowest values for TRECGenomics2003 queries (4.6 terms and 1.4 concepts on average).

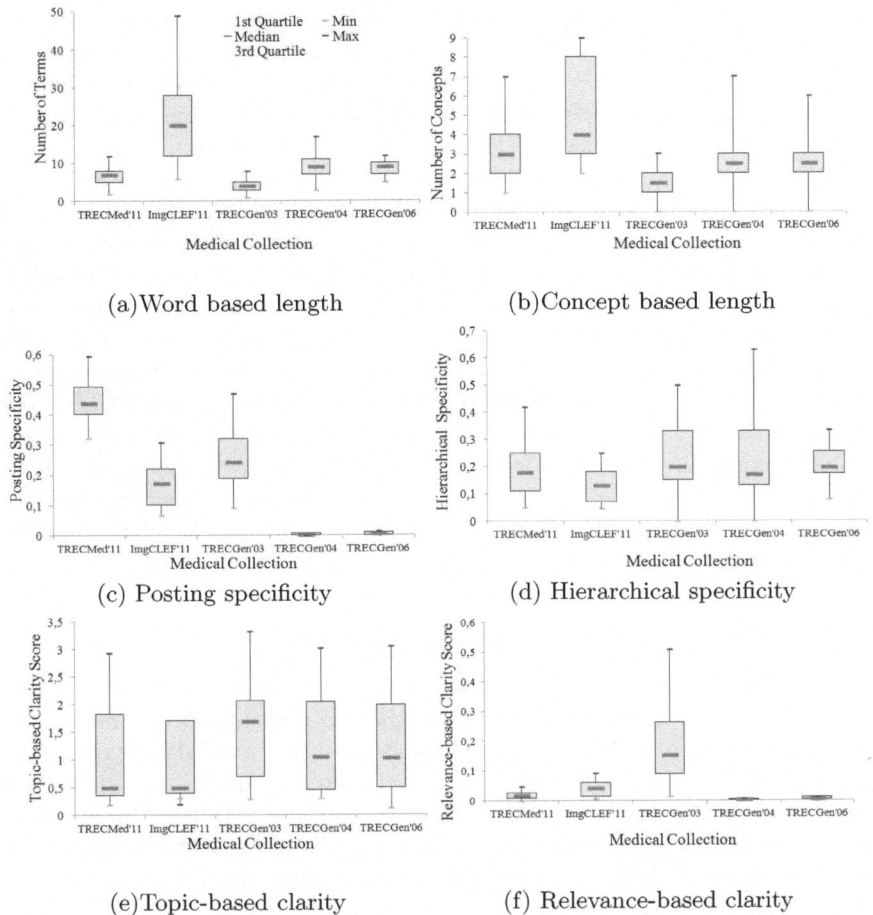

(a) Word based length

(b) Concept based length

(c) Posting specificity

(d) Hierarchical specificity

(e) Topic-based clarity

(f) Relevance-based clarity

Fig. 1. Query attribute facet distributions per collection

This can be explained by the main differences in the related tasks. Indeed, while in ImageCLEF, physicians express long technical descriptions of patient cases including images, biomedicine experts in TRECGenomics2003 express queries as gene names leading to relative short queries and consequently to a few number of concepts. Figures 1.(c) and 1.(d) represent respective distributions of query posting specificity scores and hierarchical specificity scores based on MESH terminology. As expected, given the definitions of these two facets, resulted scores are different. Significative differences of posting specificities were observed between the collections ($p-value < 0.0001$), whereas hierarchical specificities are not significantly different between the collections. As shown in Figure 1.(c), TRECGenomics 2004 and 2006 collections are characterized by relatively low values of posting specificity, compared with the three other collections. This can be also explained by the nature of the task: in TRECGenomics2004 collection, experts abuse of acronyms and abbreviations that are poorly distributed in Medline documents. In TRECGenomics2006, queries were expressed as specific entity-based questions about genes and proteins. Regarding hierarchical specificity, we observe that value ranges are wider for TRECGenomics2003 and TRECGenomics2004 (and potentially TRECMedical 2011) indicating that medical experts tend to make use of specialized terms through terminologies. Moreover, higher values of specificities indicate how much experts make use of their domain knowledge to point on their specific information needs. Analysing the clarity attribute from figures 1.(e) and 1.(f) conduct us to observe that the differences between the collections are more emphasized for the relevance based clarity score ($p-value < 0.0001$) than for the topical based one ($p-value > 0.05$), probably due to the larger variability of the latter score, as shown by the range of boxplots in figure 1.(e). However, some trends are similar: highest clarity scores are identified for TRECGenomics2003 queries, in opposition to ImageCLEF ones. This indicates that searching for genes and proteins favors the expression of unambiguous queries whereas medical case patient descriptions trigger various expert intents. We previously identified that queries on genes and proteins are short, so we can assume that even short expert queries can be clear depending on the task involved.

5.2   Correlation Analysis of Query Attributes

To study correlations between query attributes, we computed Spearman correlation coefficient (ρ) between the six quantitative query attribute facets. Only highly significative correlation pairs for each collection were displayed in Table 1. Given the differences highlighted above between the collections, we study the correlations between the query facets for each collection. In the four larger collections, we observe systematically a strong positive correlation between query length in number of words and query length in number of concepts ($p - value < 0.0001$). This was expected for two different reasons: the first one is related to the fact that a biomedical concept entry is generally, by definition, a set of words. The second reason, is as stated above, related to the search strategy of medical experts in searching for health information that favours the use of concepts relying on their domain knowledge. We can also notice that all significative correlations involve query length in number of words, reflecting the importance of this feature to characterize expert information needs. Other significative correlations are highlighted but not systematically on all the collections. In TRECMedical and TRECGenomics06 collections, a significative positive correlation is observed between the query length in number of words and posting specificity. This can be partly explained by the fact that, according to formula (1), longer is the query, higher is its posting specificity in general, the correlation is particularly higher for the two above tasks because of their comparable nature regardless of the form of the need: simple query or factual question related to a specific patient case. However, query length in terms and hierarchical query specificity facets are negatively correlated for TRECGenomics2003 ($p - value < 0.0001$). This is explained by the nature of the underlying task and the used terminology, namely MESH for concept recognition; it is probably not appropriate such as GENE

Table 1. Results of two-way significantly correlated facets

Collection	Facet1	Facet2	ρ	$p - value$
TREC Medical2011 ($N = 35$)	$LgW(Q)$	$LgC(Q)$	0.69	< 0.0001
	$LgW(Q)$	$PSpe(Q)$	0.39	< 0.02
TREC Genomics2003 ($N = 50$)	$LgW(Q)$	$LgC(Q)$	0.55	$< .0001$
	$LgW(Q)$	$HSpe(Q)$	−0.54	< 0.0001
TREC Genomics2004 ($N = 50$)	$LgW(Q)$	$LgC(Q)$	0.47	< 0.001
TREC Genomics2006 ($N = 28$)	$LgW(Q)$	$LgC(Q)$	0.67	< 0.0001
	$LgW(Q)$	$PSpe(Q)$	0.58	< 0.001

Ontology to point on specific terms. Finally, concerning ImageCLEF collection, no significative correlation is identified between query attributes.

5.3 Comparative Analysis of Clinical Vs. Non Clinical Queries

This part of our study aims to identify the attributes that can differentiate clinical queries from non clinical queries. According to TRECGenomics2004 and TRECGenomics2006 tasks, our manual annotation of clinical Vs. non clinical queries confirms that they do not include any clinical queries. Thus, given the low number of identified clinical queries this analysis will focus on all the 5 pooled collections (173 queries including 27 clinical ones). We modeled each attribute facet according to the query category and the collection by a two-way analysis of variance. No significative interaction between the collection and the clinical category was detected, indicating that the differences between clinical and non clinical queries, if they exist, are similar in the five collections, and justifying pooling collections for this analysis. Results displayed in Table 2 present mean (noted by m) and standard deviation (noted by $s.d.$) of each query attribute facet, for clinical and non clinical queries. In addition, a p-value (corresponding to the query category effect from the two-way analysis of variance) is given, allowing to assess differences between clinical and non clinical queries as significative ($p-value < 0.05$) or not. The results of the two-way analysis of variance revealed significative differences between clinical and non clinical queries. For length in words, the average number of words in clinical queries is estimated at 10 against 8 in non clinical queries ($p-value < 0.01$). As expected, there is also a significative difference in length in concepts ($p - value < 0.02$): clinical queries have on average three identified concepts against two for non clinical queries. The average score of relevance clarity is slightly higher for clinical queries ($p - value = 0.05$). For this attribute, the differences between clinical and non clinical queries are more highlighted per collection. Another comment relates to the posting specificity: the results of the analysis of variance with two attribute facets are in favor of no difference between specificity of clinical queries and those of non clinical queries ($p - value > 0.05$). But considering only query category factor in the model (without collection factor), we detect a highly significative effect of the clinical category on the posting specificity ($p - value < 0.0001$), more in accordance with average values of 0.32 for clinical queries and 0.15 for non clinical

Table 2. Clinical Vs. non clinical queries analysis

Facet	Clinical (n=27) m (s.d.)	Non clinical (n=146) m (s.d.)	p-value
LgW	10.0 (10.0)	8.0 (5.4)	< 0.01
LgC	3.2 (2.0)	2.3 (1.5)	< 0.02
PSpe	0.32 (0.13)	0.15 (0.18)	> 0.05
HSpe	0.19 (0.11)	0.24 (0.19)	> 0.05
TCla	1.27 (0.89)	1.31 (0.84)	> 0.05
RClar	0.07 (0.10)	0.065 (0.12)	0.05

queries. This can be explained by the fact that the TRECGenomics2004 and TRECGenomics2006 collections that have no clinical queries are characterized by very low values of specificity, as described above.

6   Findings Summary and Concluding Remarks

The analysis results issued from our study provide a picture of the pecularities of medical experts' queries with respect to different tasks. Our findings demonstrate, that unlike web health searchers [20], physicians' queries are relatively long and that length depends on the task at hand: medical case based search lead to longer queries than entity based search; moreover physicians make use of both their domain knowledge and semantic ressources for formulating queries, being specific particularly in medical case related information search. It has also been highlighted that clinical queries, compared to non clinical ones, are longer in both words and concepts, clearer according to the relevance facet, and more specific according to the posting facet. These findings suggest for the design of novel functionalities for future health IR systems including: query suggestion or query reformulation using appropriate levels of terminology to improve query clarity, search results personalization based on expertise level, query category, and task. Before designing such tools, we plan in future to undertake first, a large-scale user study that highlights the differences between expert search and novice search in the medical domain.

References

1. Andrews, J.E., Pearce, K.A., Ireson, C., Love, M.M.: Information-seeking behaviors of practitioners in a primary care practice-based research network (PBRN). Journal of the Medical Library Association, JMLA 93(2), 206–212 (2005)
2. Arora, N., Hesse, B., Rimer, B.K., Viswanath, K., Clayman, M., Croyle, R.: Frustrated and confused: the american and public rates its cancer-related information-seeking experiences. Journal of General Internal Medicine 23(3), 223–228 (2007)
3. Bhavnani, S.: Important cognitive components of domain-specific knowledge. In: Proceedings of Text Rerieval Conference TREC, TREC 2001, pp. 571–578 (2001)
4. Bhavnani, S.: Domain specific strategies for the effective retrieval of health care and shopping information. In: Proceedings of SIGCHI, pp. 610–611 (2002)

5. Boudin, F., Nie, J., Bartlett, J.C., Grad, R., Pluye, P., Dawes, M.: Combining classifiers for robust pico element detection. BMC Medical Informatics and Decision Making, 1–6 (2010)
6. Dinh, D., Tamine, L.: Biomedical concept extraction based on combining the content-based and word order similarities. In: Proceedings of the 2011 ACM Symposium on Applied Computing, SAC 2011, pp. 1159–1163. ACM, New York (2011)
7. Dinh, D., Tamine, L.: Combining Global and Local Semantic Contexts for Improving Biomedical Information Retrieval. In: Clough, P., Foley, C., Gurrin, C., Jones, G.J.F., Kraaij, W., Lee, H., Mudoch, V. (eds.) ECIR 2011. LNCS, vol. 6611, pp. 375–386. Springer, Heidelberg (2011)
8. Dogan, R., Muray, G., Névéol, A., Lu, Z.: Understanding pubmed user search behavior through log analysis. Database Journal, 1–19 (2009)
9. Ely, J.W., Osheroff, J.A., Ebell, M.H., Chambliss, M.L., Vinson, D.C., Stevermer, J.J., Pifer, E.A.: Obstacles to answering doctors' questions about patient care with evidence: qualitative study. BMJ 324(7339), 710 (2002)
10. Eysenbach, G.: Consumer health informatics. Biomedical Journal (3), 543–557 (2012)
11. Hong, Y., Cruz, N., Marnas, G., Early, E., Gillis, R.: A query analysis of consumer health information retrieval. In: Proceedings of Annual Symposium for Biomedical and Health Informatics, pp. 791–792 (2002)
12. Jones, S.: A statistical interpretation of term specificity and its application to retrieval. Journal of Documentation 28(1), 11–20 (1972)
13. Oh, S.: The characteristics and motivations of health answerers for sharing information, knowledge, and experiences in online environments. Journal of the American Society for Information Science and Technology 63(3), 543–557 (2012)
14. Spink, A., Jansen, B.: Web Search: Public Searching of the Web. Kluwer Academic Publishers (2004)
15. Steve, C.R., Croft, W.: Quantifying query ambiguity. In: Proceedings of the Second International Conference on Human Language Technology Research, HLT 2002, San Francisco, CA, USA, pp. 104–109 (2002)
16. Tomes, E., Latter, C.: How consumers search for health information. Health Informatics Journal 13(3), 223–235 (2007)
17. White, R., Moris, D.: How medical expertise influences seb search behaviour. In: Proceedings of the 31st International ACM SIGIR Conference on Research and Development in Information Retrieval, SIGIR 2008, pp. 791–792 (2008)
18. Wildemuth, B.: The effects of domain-knowledge on search tactic formulation, vol. 55, pp. 246–258 (2004)
19. Zeng, Q., Crowell, J., Plovnick, R., Kim, E., Ngo, L., Dibble, E.: Research paper: Assisting consumer health information retrieval with query recommendations. Journal of American Medical Informatics Associations 13(1), 80–90 (2006)
20. Zeng, Q., Kogan, S., Ash, N., Greenes, R., Boxwala, A.: Characteristics of consumer technology for health information retrieval. Methods of Information in Medicine 41, 289–298 (2002)
21. Zeng, Q., Kogan, S., Plovnick, R., Croweel, J., Lacroix, E., Greens, R.: Positive attitudes and failed queries: An exploration of the conundrums of health information retrieval. International Journal of Medical Informatics 73(1), 45–55 (2004)
22. Zhang, J., Wolfram, D., Wang, P., Hong, Y., Gillis, R.: Visualization of health-subject analysis based on query term co-occurrences. Journal of American Society in Information Science and Technology 59(12), 1933–1947 (2008)
23. Zickuhr, K.: Generations 2010. Technical report, Pew Internet & American Life Project (2006)

Comparison of Clustering Approaches through Their Application to Pharmacovigilance Terms

Marie Dupuch[1], Christopher Engström[2], Sergei Silvestrov[2],
Thierry Hamon[3], and Natalia Grabar[1]

[1] CNRS UMR 8163 STL, Université Lille 3, 59653 Villeneuve d'Ascq, France
[2] Division of Applied Mathematics, Mälardalen University, Västerås, Sweden
[3] LIM&BIO (EA3969), Université Paris 13, Sorbonne Paris Cité, France

Abstract. In different applications (*i.e.*, information retrieval, filtering or analysis), it is useful to detect similar terms and to provide the possibility to use them jointly. Clustering of terms is one of the methods which can be exploited for this. In our study, we propose to test three methods dedicated to the clustering of terms (hierarchical ascendant classification, *Radius* and maximum), to combine them with the semantic distance algorithms and to compare them through the results they provide when applied to terms from the pharmacovigilance area. The comparison indicates that the non disjoint clustering (*Radius* and maximum) outperform the disjoint clusters by 10 to up to 20 points in all the experiments.

1 Introduction

In different applications, such as information retrieval, filtering or analysis, it is useful to be able to detect similar terms. For instance, the terms *heart attack*, *myocardial infarction* and *heart disease* are semantically close: when they occur in a document or in a corpus, it may be useful indeed to provide the system with such knowledge, which may allow providing more complete results and also reducing the false negatives. Detection of semantically close words and terms is a very intensive research topics and several studies proposed various methods: paraphrasing [1–3]; term variation detection [4–6]; semantic similarity computing [7–12]; terminology structuring or alignment [13–16], etc. However, once the semantic relatedness between terms is computed, it shows often different degrees of relatedness. Hence, it may be important to distinguish between those terms which are more close and those which have broader and weaker semantic relatedness between them. Typically, the clustering methods are helpful and can be exploited for this. The objective of our work is to compare several clustering methods. The comparison is done with terms from the pharmacovigilance area (usually meaning adverse drug reactions), which have been previously processed with semantic distance and similarity algorithms.

2 Background

We distinguish three types of clustering methods, according to the types of the clusters they generate:

N. Peek, R. Marín Morales, and M. Peleg (Eds.): AIME 2013, LNAI 7885, pp. 58–67, 2013.
© Springer-Verlag Berlin Heidelberg 2013

- *Disjoint clusters*, in which a given object may belong to one cluster only. The disjoint clustering is done with algorithms such as *k-means* [17], *k-medoids* and *PAM* [18]. They are adapted to the processing of large data. These algorithms have two specificities: it is necessary to indicate the number of clusters to be generated and the generated clusters are disjoint;
- *Non disjoint clusters*, in which a given object may belong to more than one cluster. The non disjoint clustering is performed with so called fuzzy or soft algorithms. The fuzzy algorithms (*fuzzy c-means* [19], *fuzzy c-medoids* [20] or *axial k-means* [21]) state the degree up to which an object belongs to each concerned cluster. The difficulty with these algorithms is that they require to set up the thresholds, which may be a difficult step. The few existing soft clustering algorithms (*Radius* algorithm [22], PoBOC [23], OKM [24] or *Maximum* algorithm integrated within the *R project*) also allow an intersection between the generated clusters but without specifying the degree of relevance of each entity to a given cluster.
- *Hierarchical clusters* are considered as non disjoint when viewed through the dendrogram (smaller clusters are included into the larger clusters) or disjoint once the dendrogram is cut. Several hierarchical clustering algorithms have been proposed (AGNES [25, 26], BIRCH [27], CURE [28] and DIANA [26]). It is not necessary to set up the classes number, which eases the exploitation.

Our objective is to compare clustering algorithms within context related to the pharmacovigilance (detection and prevention of adverse drug reactions). The specificity of our data is that terms often show several semantic facets: because of their inherent semantics (*i.e.*, *Respiratory failure neonatal* is a malignancy, an abnormality of the respiratory system and a neonatal abnormality) and because of their medical manifestations (*i.e.*, *Respiratory failure neonatal* may appear as sign or symptom of several medical problems: *i.e.*, *Hypovolaemic shock conditions, Anaphylactic/anaphylactoid shock conditions, Hypoglycaemic and neurogenic shock conditions, Torsade de pointes*). For this reason, we put the priority on the non disjoint clustering methods, which allow one term to belong to more than one cluster, and compare them with the disjoint clustering.

3   Material

Pharmacovigilance Terms: ontoEIM Resource. The semantic resource ontoEIM [29] contains terms which describe the adverse drug reactions (*i.e.*, signs and symptoms, diagnostics, therapeutic indications, complementary investigations, medical and surgical procedures, medical and family history). The terms are provided by the MedDRA terminology [30]. The difference with MedDRA is that the ontoEIM terms have been restructured thanks to their projection on the terminology SNOMED CT [31], done through the exploitation of the UMLS [32], where an important number of terminologies are already merged and aligned, among which MedDRA and SNOMED CT. We exploit the preferred MedDRA terms *PT*. Their current rate of alignment with those from SNOMED CT is rather weak: 51.3% (7,629 terms). The restructuring of MedDRA terms makes

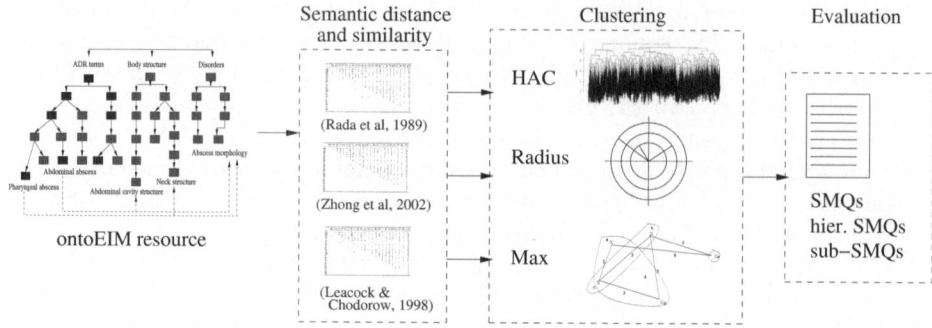

Fig. 1. General schema of the method

the structure more fine-grained: the SNOMED CT-like hierarchy within on-toEIM contains also terms added to fill in the intermediate levels absent among MedDRA terms. The maximal number of the hierarchical levels within ontoEIM reaches up to 14, while only five hierarchical levels are available in MedDRA.

Reference clusters: Standardized MedDRA Queries (SMQs). Currently, 84 Standardized MedDRA Queries (SMQs) are available, which have been created manually by international boards of experts. The SMQs gather MedDRA terms related to a given safety topic (or medical problem), such as *Cardiac arrhythmias, Malignancies* or *Hepatic disorders*. The SMQs are mostly plain lists of terms, but 20 SMQs have the particularity to provide a hierarchical structure. The number of the hierarchical levels they contain vary between 2 and 4. The hierarchically structured SMQs are composed of sub-SMQs (n=92). We exploit these different levels of the reference data: SMQs (n=84), hierarchical SMQs (n=20) and sub-SMQs (n=92).

4   Methods

Figure 1 presents the general schema of the method organized in three main steps: (1) semantic distance and similarity computing between MedDRA terms, (2) MedDRA terms clustering, (3) and evaluation of the obtained clusters against the reference data. For the implementation, we exploit Perl and R^1 languages.

4.1   Computing of the Semantic Distance and Similarity

Semantic distance and similarity algorithms state the semantic relatedness degree between two terms. For instance, *Respiratory failure neonatal* term is closer to term *Respiratory failure* than to *Cardiac failure*. The semantic distance and similarity algorithms may require the use of corpus and/or of terminologies. In our work, we use the terminological resource ontoEIM. Three measures are

---
[1] http://www.r-project.org

applied to the 7,629 *PT* MedDRA terms present in the ontoEIM resource in order to compute the distance and similarity values for each pair of terms *t1* and *t2*:

- the *Rada* algorithm [7] computes the semantic distance and relies on the detection and computing of the shortest path *sp*, which corresponds to the sum of the edges of this shortest path: $sp(t1, t2)$;
- the *LCH* Leacock and Chodorow algorithm [9] computes the semantic similarity and relies on the shortest path *sp* and on the maximal depth *MAX* found within the terminology (*MAX*=14 within ontoEIM): $-log[\frac{sp(t1,t2)}{2*MAX}]$;
- the *Zhong* approach [10] computes the semantic distance and relies on the absolute depth *depth* of terms and on their closest common parent *ccp*. The milestone value *m* is computed first for each term: $m(t) = \frac{1}{k^{depth(t)+1}}$, where *t* is a term, *depth* its absolute depth within a terminology and $k = 2$ (normalization coefficient). Then, the distance between two terms is computed: $2 * m(ccp(t1, t2)) - (m(t1) + m(t2))$, where *ccp* is the closest common parent and *m* milestone values obtained previously.

Further to the application of these three algorithms, we build three symmetrical matrices 7629*7629 (one for each algorithm). They contain the semantic distance and similarity values between the MedDRA PT terms from ontoEIM.

4.2 Clustering of Terms

Once the distances and similarities are computed, we use them for the creation of clusters of terms. We exploit and compare three methods for the clustering of the terms applied to matrices with the semantic distances and similarities:

- *HAC* hierarchical ascendant classification is performed through the *R Project* tools (*hclust* function). This method first chooses the best centers for clusters and then builds the hierarchy of terms by progressively merging smaller clusters to obtain the bigger ones and to build one unique dendrogram. The dendrogram is then segmented into *x* clusters. We test the following values: {100}, {200}, {300}, {400}, {500}, {1000}, {1500}, {2000} ... {7000}. After the segmentation, the obtained clusters are exclusive.
- *Radius* method, where every ADR term is considered as a possible center of a cluster and its closest terms are clustered together with it. We test several threshold values *x* with the three semantic measure approaches, *i.e.*, with *Rada*: $\forall x \in N, such\ as\ x \in [1; 5]$; with *Zhong*: $\forall x \in N, such\ as\ x \in [0.001; 0.002; \ldots ; 0.021]$. The obtained clusters are not exclusive;
- *Max* maximum method is similar to the *Radius* approach but is more permissive. Iteratively, it computes the cost of the clusters union, while the radius approach computes the cost of the inclusion of each term (it does not consider the notion of the cluster). The *Max* thresholds *x* tested: $\forall x \in N, such\ as\ x \in [2; 5]$. The following steps are repeated for each node:
  1. Assign a node a_1 to a cluster *c*;
  2. Create the list *l* containing all the remaining nodes;

3. For each node a_i from l, compute the cost of the union (c, a_i). The cost corresponds to $Maximum(distance)$ within a cluster, hence the name of the method. If there is more than one node with the same minimal distance value (step 6), then the comparison is done with the next greater value and so on;
4. Delete all nodes a_i, which belong to l and whose union cost with cluster c is above a given threshold;
5. If l is empty, terminate the algorithm;
6. The node from l which shows the lowest union cost is added to the cluster c and removed from the list l;
7. Restart from the step 3.

4.3   Generated Clusters Evaluation

Generated clusters evaluation is performed thanks to their comparison with all the SMQs, the hierarchical SMQs and the sub-SMQs. A cluster is associated to the SMQ with which it has the maximal F-measure. Setting of thresholds and of classes number is performed through a ten-fold cross-validation: the data are partitioned into ten subsets, one subset is used for the setting up the methods while the remaining nine subsets are used for the evaluation against the reference data. This process is done ten times with a different training subset each time. Values which show the best performance on training set are applied on the test set. Average performance is then computed with three classical measures (where *relevant* terms are those which are clustered together and which also belong to the corresponding SMQ): precision P (percentage of the relevant terms clustered divided by the total number of the clustered terms), recall R (percentage of the relevant terms clustered divided by the number of terms in the corresponding SMQ) and F-measure F (the harmonic mean of P and R). The final evaluation values are the mean values of those obtained at each cross-validation step. We perform also a detailed analysis of individual clusters and of failures.

5   Results and Discussion

Because the LCH and $Rada$ algorithms are similar (LCH adds the $log[2 * MAX]$ constant), values they provide are also close. Testing these two algorithms allowed to check out the performed computing correctness. In the following, we present and discuss results obtained with $Rada$ and $Zhong$ similarity distances.

In Table 1, the best settings defined, further to the cross-validation, for the two semantic algorithms and the clustering methods are presented. On the whole, we observe that settings, which lead to smaller clusters (lower $Rada$ and $Zhong$ thresholds and higher number of classes), prove to suit best the generation of sub-SMQs. On the contrary, the hierarchical SMQs require the largest clusters (high $Rada$ and $Zhong$ thresholds and lower number of classes). The threshold values required for the generation of the whole set of the SMQs (hierarchical and non hierarchical, but excluding separate sub-SMQs) are intermediate. Such

Table 1. Best clustering parameters (thresholds and number of classes) defined thanks to the cross-validation

		SMQs	Hier. SMQs	sub-SMQs
$Radius_{Rada}$	Threshold	4	4	2
$Radius_{Zhong}$	Threshold	0.006	0.019, 0.013	0.003, 0.004
HAC_{Rada}	Nb of classes	300, 400, 500, 2500	100, 200	3500
HAC_{Zhong}	Nb of classes	500	100	1500, 2500, 4000
Max_{Rada}	Threshold	4	5	4
Max_{Zhong}	Threshold	0.021	0.021	0.009

Table 2. Average performance on 0-100% scale (precision, recall, F-measure), against the three reference data sets, obtained with the best clustering parameters defined

	SMQs			Hier. SMQs			sub-SMQs		
	P(%)	R(%)	F	P(%)	R(%)	F	P(%)	R(%)	F
$Radius_{Rada}$	45	32	36	40	33	35	56	36	43
$Radius_{Zhong}$	34	24	27	26	36	30	36	27	30
HAC_{Rada}	44	11	17	26	12	16	60	20	29
HAC_{Zhong}	34	16	21	30	16	18	53	22	29
Max_{Rada}	49	30	37	56	26	36	46	38	39
Max_{Zhong}	38	24	29	36	26	30	59	23	33

an observation was expected. It is closely related to the size of the generated clusters and it follows the logics of the reference data: the sub-SMQs provide the smallest clusters, while the hierarchical SMQs the largest.

In Table 2, we indicate average evaluation values (precision, recall and F-measure) obtained with the three reference data sets (SMQs, hierarchical SMQs and sub-SMQs) and with the best parameters (Table 1). During cross-validation, we give advantage to F-measure. Compared to previous experiments without cross-validation, which gave advantage to precision [22], we obtain currently a best balance between precision and recall, and the whole performance is improved by 5 to 10%. Still, precision values remain higher than recall values. This is due to the fact that the generated clusters, whatever the methods and reference data, are smaller than the reference data. The generated clusters typically capture a given aspect of the reference SMQs: their recall is low, while precision may reach up to 60%. On the whole, the task related to the automatic creation of the SMQs remains difficult. With the currently exploited resources and methods we can capture but partially the terms relevant to a given medical condition.

With values indicated in Table 2, we can also propose a comparison between the three clustering methods tested in this work. Whatever the reference data, the non disjoint clusters outperform the disjoint HAC clusters by 10 to 20 points of F-measure. The only situation in which the HAC method is better is observed with precision obtained with the $Rada$ algorithm and sub-SMQs. Besides, this is the best precision we obtain with the presented experience: 60%. The next best precision is also obtained with the sub-SMQs but with Max method and

Table 3. Average, minimal and maximal values for precision, recall and F-measure obtained against the reference sub-SMQs with the best clustering parameters defined with the *Rada* algorithm

	Precision			Recall			F-measure		
	average	min	max	average	min	max	average	min	max
$Radius_{Rada}$	56	4	100	36	7	100	43	8	96
HAC_{Rada}	60	12	98	20	1	100	29	2	58
Max_{Rada}	46	7	100	38	8	100	39	14	74

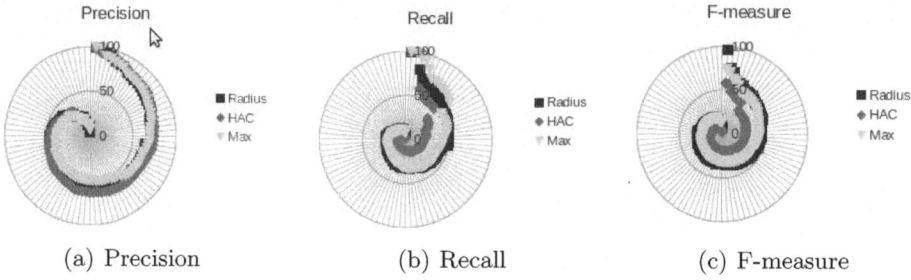

(a) Precision   (b) Recall   (c) F-measure

Fig. 2. Evaluation results against the 92 sub-SMQs (Precision, Recall and F-measure) and the three clustering methods applied to the *Rada* semantic distance matrix

Zhong algorithm: 59%. Our results seem to indicate that non disjoint clustering is more suitable for the aimed task. MedDRA terms may indeed be specific to more than one medical condition and belong to several clusters. Logically, this aspect is better captured when the non disjoint clusters are generated.

In Table 2, we presented the average values of the evaluation measures, while there is an important variability according to the clusters and the reference data. Hence, in Table 3, we present also, along with the average values, the minimal and maximal performance obtained with the reference sub-SMQs. We can see that the interval is very important and that there is indeed a very important variability across the sub-SMQs, as presented in Table 3, but the situation is similar with two other sets of the reference data. In relation to this observation, some of the SMQs are better reproduced than others. Among the best clusters, we have *Gastrointestinal obstruction, Liver-related coagulation and bleeding disturbances, Ischaemic cerebrovascular conditions*. Among the less competitive clusters, let's cite *Reproductive premalignant disorders* and *Pregnancy complications*.

In Figure 2, we present the evaluation values for individual sub-SMQs. In this circular lay-out, the results are not projected on the x and y axes. The 360 degrees correspond to the 92 reference sub-SMQs, while the radius 0-100 scale allows to position the evaluation measure values. For a given evaluation measure, the values are first sorted in a decreasing order and then projected. While reading the figures, it is necessary to notice that more a given line is closer to the outer border, the better the results for the corresponding method and measure. For

Table 4. Detailed performance for two randomly chosen clusters

	HAC_{Rada}			$Radius_{Rada}$			Max_{Rada}		
	P	R	F	P	R	F	P	R	F
Anaphylactic anaphylactoid shock conditions	100	8	14	60	23	33	43	23	30
Infectious biliary disorders		40	18	25	86	54	66	69	81	75

instance, we can see that precision values start with 100% performance, that more than 1/3 of the precision values are higher than 50%, and that less than 1/4 of the precision values are lesser than 50%. We can see also that the highest F-measure values do not start with 100%, but with lower values (see Table 3). Figure 2 provides several observations: (1) once again we can observe that there is an important variability between the SMQs; (2) very often, the precision is high while the recall is low (the generated clusters are smaller than the SMQs and show their different aspects); (3) the *HAC* clusters provide the lesser F-measure and recall performance (the red line, which correspond to this clustering is the closest to the center of the circles); (4) the *Radius* and *Max* clustering methods are comparable (the corresponding lines are often superimposed). We observe also that recall and F-measure are lower with *HAC* than with the other two clustering methods, which is due to the disjoint clusters generated by *HAC*.

We did a detailed analysis of two randomly chosen clusters (corresponding to two sub-SMQs), presented in Table 4: *Anaphylactic anaphylactoid shock conditions* and *Infectious biliary disorders*. *Anaphylactic anaphylactoid shock conditions* sub-SMQ contains 13 terms. The *HAC* method proposes only one relevant term (*Renal failure acute*). While *Radius* and *Max* method provide with respectively 5 and 7 relevant terms. Situation is very similar with the *Infectious biliary disorders* cluster: it contains 11 terms, among which 5 are also provided by *HAC*, 7 by *Radius* and 13 by *Max*. In both cases, the non disjoint clustering (*Radius* and *Max*) is more suitable for the aimed task than the disjoint clustering (*HAC*). Terms which are not collected with our methods are too distant in the exploited resource. Other methods and approaches should be used to capture them.

6   Conclusion and Perspectives

We presented an experiment on the comparison between three clustering methods (hierarchical ascendant classification, *Radius* and *Max*) applied to pharmacovigilance terms, which have been previously processed with the semantic distance and similarity algorithms. Our objective is to compare between disjoint and non disjoint clustering methods. The exploited reference data are composed of manually created sets of pharmacovigilance terms related to various medical conditions. The cross-validation allowed to define the best clustering parameters (thresholds and number of classes), which favor the global performance (F-measure) and which reach the best balance between precision and recall. As for the comparison between the clustering methods, the non disjoint clustering (*Radius* and *Max*) outperform the disjoint clusters by 10 to up to 20 points for nearly all the experiments and evaluation measures. Hence, the non disjoint clustering captures better the multi-facet characteristics of the pharmacovigilance terms. We assume these results are also relevant to other tasks and applications dealing with semantics and language data.

In the future, we plan to apply the proposed methods to other terminological resources, such as UMLS [32] or its subsets. In the current experience, only individual clusters have been considered, while we showed in past work that their merging is helpful as it allows increasing the recall almost without decreasing precision: merging of the clusters issued from the current study is a perspective. We also observed that there is a great variability across the clusters and the reference data. Currently, we apply the same setting to all the reference data, while we can distinguish several settings suitable for subsets of the medical conditions. We assume, this may capture better the inherent semantics of these subsets and to improve the overall results. Moreover, we plan to combine this method with other methods (exploitation of corpora and of Natural Language Processing methods...). Finally, we would like to test the proposed methods for the creation of novel SMQs describing not yet covered medical conditions.

Acknowledgement. The authors acknowledge the support of the French Agence Nationale de la Recherche (ANR) and the DGA, under the Tecsan grant ANR-11-TECS-012. The authors also would like to thank anonymous reviewers for their constructive remarks.

References

1. Barzilay, R., Elhadad, N.: Sentence alignment for monolingual comparable corpora. In: EMNLP, pp. 25–32 (2003)
2. Paşca, M.: Mining paraphrases from self-anchored web sentence fragments. In: Jorge, A.M., Torgo, L., Brazdil, P.B., Camacho, R., Gama, J. (eds.) PKDD 2005. LNCS (LNAI), vol. 3721, pp. 193–204. Springer, Heidelberg (2005)
3. Max, A., Bouamor, H., Vilnat, A.: Generalizing sub-sentential paraphrase acquisition across original signal type of text pairs. In: EMNLP, pp. 721–31 (2012)
4. Jacquemin, C.: A symbolic and surgical acquisition of terms through variation. In: Wermter, S., Riloff, E., Scheler, G. (eds.) IJCAI-WS 1995. LNCS, vol. 1040, pp. 425–438. Springer, Heidelberg (1996)
5. Daille, B., Habert, B., Jacquemin, C., Royauté, J.: Empirical observation of term variations and principles for their description. Terminology 3(2), 197–257 (1996)
6. Hahn, U., Honeck, M., Piotrowsky, M., Schulz, S.: Subword segmentation - leveling out morphological variations for medical document retrieval. In: Annual Symposium of the American Medical Informatics Association (AMIA), Washington (2001)
7. Rada, R., Mili, H., Bicknell, E., Blettner, M.: Development and application of a metric on semantic nets. IEEE Transactions on Systems, Man and Cybernetics 19(1), 17–30 (1989)
8. Wu, Z., Palmer, M.: Verb semantics and lexical selection. In: Proceedings of Associations for Computational Linguistics, pp. 133–138 (1994)
9. Leacock, C., Chodorow, M.: Combining local context and WordNet similarity for word sense identification. In: WordNet: An Electronic Lexical Database, pp. 305–332 (1998)

10. Zhong, J., Zhu, H., Li, J., Yu, Y.: Conceptual graph matching for semantic search. In: Priss, U., Corbett, D.R., Angelova, G. (eds.) ICCS 2002. LNCS (LNAI), vol. 2393, pp. 92–106. Springer, Heidelberg (2002)
11. Seco, N., Veale, T., Hayes, J.: An intrinsic information content metric for semantic similarity in wordnet. In: Proceedings of the 16th European Conference on Artificial Intelligence (ECAI 2004), pp. 1089–1090 (2004)
12. Nguyen, H., Al-Mubaid, H.: New ontology-based semantic similarity measure for the biomedical domain. IEEE Eng. Med. Biol. Proc., 623–628 (2006)
13. Maedche, A., Staab, S.: Mining ontologies from text. In: Dieng, R., Corby, O. (eds.) EKAW 2000. LNCS (LNAI), vol. 1937, pp. 189–202. Springer, Heidelberg (2000)
14. Bodenreider, O., Pakhomov, S.: Exploring adjectival modification in biomedical discourse across two genres. In: Workshop Natural Language Processing in Biomedical Applications of ACL, pp. 105–112 (2003)
15. Grabar, N., Zweigenbaum, P.: Lexically-based terminology structuring. Terminology 10, 23–54 (2004)
16. D'aquin, M., Euzenat, J., Le Duc, C., Lewen, H.: Sharing and reusing aligned ontologies with cupboard. In: K-CAP 2009, pp. 179–180 (2009)
17. MacQueen, J.: Some methods for classification and analysis of multivariate observations. In: Proceedings of 5th Berkeley Symposium on Mathematical Statistics and Probability, pp. 281–297 (1967)
18. Kaufman, L., Rousseeuw, P.: Clustering by means of medoids. In: Statistical Data Analysis based on the L1 Norm, pp. 405–416 (1987)
19. Bezdek, J.: Pattern Recognition with Fuzzy Objective Function Algoritms. Plenum Press, New York (1981)
20. Krishnapuram, R., Joshi, A., Nasraoui, O., Yi, L.: Low complexity fuzzy relational clustering algorithms for web mining. IEEE Trans. Fuzzy System, 595–607 (2001)
21. Lelu, A.: Modles neuronaux pour lanalyse de donnes documentaires et textuelles. Phd thesis, Universite de Paris VI, Paris, France (1993)
22. Dupuch, M., Bousquet, C., Grabar, N.: Automatic creation and refinement of the clusters of pharmacovigilance terms. In: ACM IHI, pp. 181–190 (2012)
23. Cleuziou, G., Martin, L., Vrain, C.: PoBOC: An overlapping clustering algorithm. application to rule-based classification and textual data. In: ECAI, pp. 440–444 (2004)
24. Cleuziou, G.: OKM: Une extension des k-moyennes pour la recherche de classes recouvrantes. In: EGC, pp. 691–702 (2007)
25. Johnson, S.: Hierarchical clustering schemes. Psychometrika 32, 241–254 (1967)
26. Kaufman, L., Rousseeuw, P.: Finding Groups in Data: An Introduction to Cluster Analysis. Wiley, New York (1990)
27. Zhang, T., Ramakrishnan, R., Livny, M.: Birch: An efficient data clustering method for very large databases. In: ACM SIGMOD, pp. 103–114 (1996)
28. Guha, S., Rastogi, R., Shim, K.: Cure: An efficient clustering algorithm for large databases. In: ACM SIGMOD, pp. 73–84 (1998)
29. Alecu, I., Bousquet, C., Jaulent, M.: A case report: Using snomed ct for grouping adverse drug reactions terms. BMC Med. Inform. Decis. Mak. 8(1), 4 (2008)
30. Brown, E.G., Wood, L., Wood, S.: The medical dictionary for regulatory activities (MedDRA). Drug Saf. 20(2), 109–117 (1999)
31. Stearns, M.Q., Price, C., Spackman, K.A., Wang, A.Y.: SNOMED clinical terms: Overview of the development process and project status. In: AMIA, pp. 662–666 (2001)
32. NLM: UMLS Knowledge Sources Manual. National Library of Medicine, Bethesda, Maryland (2008), http://www.nlm.nih.gov/research/umls/

Trusting Intensive Care Unit (ICU) Medical Data: A Semantic Web Approach

Laura Moss[1,2,3], David Corsar[1], Ian Piper[3], and John Kinsella[2]

[1] Department of Computing Science, University of Aberdeen, Aberdeen, AB24 3FX
[2] School of Medicine, University of Glasgow, Glasgow, G12 8QQ
[3] Department of Clinical Physics, University of Glasgow, Glasgow, G12 8QQ

Abstract. The Intensive Care Unit (ICU) domain generates large volumes of patient data which can be used in medical research. However, inaccuracies often exist in this data and due to the data's size and domain complexity, automated approaches are required to associate a level of quality and trust with the data. We describe a computational framework to perform such assessments based on semantic web technologies. Linked data enables integration with other datasets, which can be used along with details of the data's provenance and medical domain knowledge from appropriate ontologies. We have successfully applied the framework to two types of ICUs: general medical and traumatic brain injury.

Keywords: Data Quality, Semantic Web, Ontologies, Critical Care.

1 Introduction

Increasing use of patient monitoring equipment in medicine is generating large repositories of patient data, which are recorded manually and/or automatically. Trusting this data is important: along with being used for medical decision making, the data is often stored for offline analysis. However, error rates of between 2.3% and 26.9% are common [5]. Various methods have been proposed to improve the quality of medical data (e.g.[6]), which may help avoid certain errors (e.g. physiologically impossible values). However, detailed domain knowledge and human judgement is often required to identify other, more subtle errors, e.g. a recorded heart rate of 120 may be identified as an error by a simple threshold based rule, but if the patient was suffering from sepsis at the same time, then the value may actually be a symptom of that disorder.

Recently, interlinked datasets have been made openly available on the Web of Linked Data. These datasets are described by ontologies, published according to a set of principles, and linked through the use of technologies such as URIs, HTTP, and RDF. This enables provision of contextual information about any piece of data, along with enabling machines to access, browse, and reason with it[1]. Most existing approaches to assessing the quality of linked data focus on the application of simple rules or policies; e.g. the WIQA framework, which

---

[1] http://www.w3.org/DesignIssues/LinkedData.html

N. Peek, R. Marín Morales, and M. Peleg (Eds.): AIME 2013, LNAI 7885, pp. 68–72, 2013.
© Springer-Verlag Berlin Heidelberg 2013

adopts the *"fitness for use"* perspective to data quality, applies a set of policies to filter RDF data that does not meet requirements [1]. In contrast, the SWIQA framework adopts the *"free of defects"* perspective, using a series of rules to perform common data quality checks on RDF datasets including: completeness (e.g. provision of mandatory values), syntactic and semantic accuracy, timeliness, and uniqueness [3]. However, we argue these assessments do not consider the complexities of real world datasets and need to be extended to include context dependent assessments.

In this paper, Section 2 describes our novel approach and framework that applies Semantic Web technologies to assess the quality of medical datasets, by considering the data, its provenance, and relevant clinical knowledge; Section 3 describes the application of our framework to two different medical domains; and Section 4 concludes by discussing our findings and future work plans.

2   Approach

Our approach consists of three stages: converting the medical data into RDF; optionally annotating the data with provenance information; and finally, assessing the data (Figure 1). Ideally, all of the datasets we describe below would be reused from the Web of Linked Data or open data repositories. However, some of the required information is not available; in these cases we have created our own datasets, which we intend to contribute to the Linked Open Data cloud.

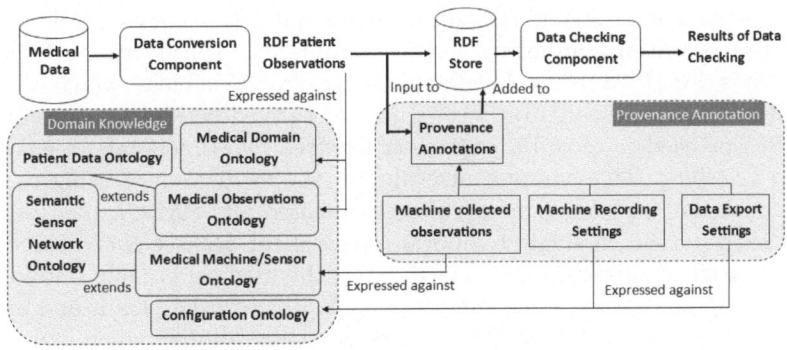

Fig. 1. Overview of the approach to medical data assessment

Data Conversion. In this stage an RDF version of the medical data, expressed against the Patient Data and Medical Observations ontologies is created. For the two case studies described in this paper, we have developed a program that generates a series of SPARQL update statements to produce the desired RDF dataset; RDB2RDF was considered but was not appropriate for how a case study dataset was represented (as a spreadsheet). The Patient Data (pd) ontology [2] provides classes for representing Patients, Sessions, and Timepoints. Each Timepoint is associated with a set of Readings which refer to the Parameter being observed and its value. The Medical Observations ontology defines a series of axioms that integrate our patient ontology with the W3C Semantic Sensor Network (ssn) Incubator Group's sensor ontology [4] and allows the pd:Readings to be linked to the machines/sensors that produced them. We define pd:Reading as a subclass of ssn:ObservationValue (which represents the value produced by some sensing process); pd:Parameter (representing things that were recorded) as a subclass of ssn:Property; and pd:Patient as a ssn:FeatureOfInterest. To represent a pd:Timepoint as a set of observations, we use the Observation Collection pattern [4], defining pd:Timepoint as a subclass of mo:ObservationCollection, which has an associated set of ssn:Observations.

Provenance Annotation. This optional, semi-automatic stage involves annotating the patient observations with provenance, considered as *"a description of the entities and processes involved in producing ... that resource"* [4]. Providing provenance information increases the available types of assessments compared to solely using the observations. In this framework, we capture details of the sensors that were responsible for producing the pd:Readings. Our Medical Machine/Sensor ontology (mms), extends the SSN ontology with classes and individuals representing the machines used in our medical evaluation. We have defined mms:Machine as a subclass of ssn:Platform, and various subclasses of ssn:Sensor for the different types of sensors on the machine. Each sensor is then described in terms of the ssn:Sensing process that is implements, the ssn:Property it observes, and its ssn:MeasurementCapability. The machine recording settings annotate the observations with knowledge about how the sensors were configured to record the data; this knowledge is provided by the Configuration ontology (c). For example, the specification of the sampling rate is described using the c:MachineConfiguration class, which references a set of c:RecordingConfigurations, which, in turn, describe the mms:Machine or ssn:Sensor used to record a parameter between two timepoints in a session.

Data Checking. This component evaluates the medical data using the available information and assessment rules represented as SPARQL queries (Table 1). For each patient, a single temporary assessment dataset is created consisting of the patient observations RDF dataset, the medical domain ontology, the SSN ontology, and provenance annotations. A program then loads and executes each assessment query, storing the results in a separate file which is used later to generate a summary of the analysis. If a value is identified as an error it is annotated with 'Possible Error' (PoE) or a 'Probable Error' (PrE); where PrE is more likely to be an error than PoE. Definitions of acceptable values, sensor accuracies, and medical conditions & treatments are provided by ontologies, enabling reuse of existing knowledge and as the rules are expressed at the ontological level, their reuse across multiple domains without modification; whereas other approaches e.g. complex event processing and rule engines do not easily allow for this. RDF also provides a common representational formalism, allowing data to be provided in a proprietary format, e.g. database or spreadsheet.

Table 1. Example assessments

Name	Details of Rule	Conclusion
Missing Data 3	If, for every sequential pair of readings, the time period between them does not equal the sampling rate	PrE
Acceptable Range 1	If the recorded value is less than the min. acceptable value	PrE
Acceptable Range 2	If the recorded value is greater than the max. acceptable value	PrE
Acceptable Range 3	If an accuracy value (defining a +/- value or %) is associated with the sensor AND the recorded value minus accuracy value is below the min. acceptable value	PoE
Acceptable Range 4	If an accuracy value (defining a +/- value or %) is associated with the sensor AND the recorded value plus the accuracy value is above the min. acceptable value	No longer an error
Acceptable Range 5	If an accuracy value (defining a +/- value or %) is associated with the sensor AND the recorded value plus the accuracy value is above the max. acceptable value	PoE
Medical Disorders Rule 1	If the recorded value is outwith its acceptable range AND is associated with a symptom of a disorder, AND at the same time other symptoms associated with the disorder	Reclassify from PrE to PoE
Treatments Rule 1	If the recorded value is outwith its acceptable range AND is associated with an effect of a treatment AND that treatment was administered previous to that value	Reclassify from PrE to PoE

3 Evaluation

We have applied our framework to data taken from two types of ICUs: general medical and traumatic brain injury (TBI)[2]. In both cases, time series physiological data was collected from patient monitoring equipment, but the machines used, parameters recorded, and frequency of data collection differs. We were able to reuse the same clinical domain ontology for both evaluations. For the Medical Disorders rule, we created specific queries for hypotension and hypertension; and for the Treatments rule, queries for effects of noradrenaline and adrenaline.

For the TBI domain, we used data consisting of 37 patients, 595,439 distinct timepoints, 4,467,949 observations for 14 parameters, and the resulting RDF consists of 52,093,104 triples. Glasgow Royal Infirmary's (GRI) general medical ICU dataset consisted of 209 patients, 68,142 distinct timepoints, 687,393 observations for 14 parameters, and the resulting RDF consists of 41,819,163 triples. In both domains, data is collected every minute, exported every minute in the TBI domain, and exported hourly in the GRI domain; the machine recording and export configuration tools were set accordingly.

Missing Data Rule 3 found 27,002 ($\geq$0.6%) and 64,307 ($\geq$9.4%) sequences of missing data points for the TBI and GRI datasets respectively. In the TBI dataset, 376,389 (9.4%) values were found to be less than the min. acceptable for a parameter, and 1,386,262 (31%) were found to be higher than the max.; when

---

[2] Further evaluation results are available at: http://www.abdn.ac.uk/~csc316

sensor accuracies were considered 18,839 additional errors were found and 19,604 of the original errors removed. In the GRI dataset, 129,716 (18.9%) values were found to be less than the min. acceptable for a parameter, and 189,601 (27.6%) were found to be higher than the max.; when sensor accuracies were considered 272,357 additional errors were found and 159,219 of the original errors removed. In the GRI dataset, a number of readings identified by Acceptable Range Rules 1 & 2 may have been affected by hypertension (91%), hypotension (85.6%), noradrenaline (24.2%) and adrenaline (6.7%)[3]. A number of TBI values may also be affected by hypertension (92.1%) and hypotension (80.5%).

4 Discussion and Future Work

We have shown that our approach can be successfully applied to assess medical data and illustrates the benefit of additional contextual information provided by linking data. Using a simple approach, a large number of acceptable range errors are identified; however, when the context of the data is considered, many are re-classified or new errors are identified. In the future we plan to investigate: further context dependent rules; detection of interventions that have been carried out on a patient but not recorded; and using High Performance Computing to improve performance times, e.g. it took 2 hours 8 mins to apply the Medical Disorders rules which clearly would not be practical if used regularly in a clinical setting.

Acknowledgements. The staff and patients of the ICU Unit, GRI. This work was an extension of the routine audit process in GRI's ICU; requirements for further Ethical Committee Approval have been waved. The authors would like to acknowledge the work of the BrainIT group investigators and participating centres to the BrainIT dataset.

References

1. Bizer, C., Cyganiak, R.: Quality-driven information filtering using the WIQA policy framework. Journal of Web Semantics 7(1), 1–10 (2009)
2. Corsar, D., Moss, L., Sleeman, D., Sim, M.: Supporting the Development of Medical Ontologies. In: Frontiers in Artificial Intelligence and Applications: Formal Ontologies Meet Industry, pp. 114–125 (2009)
3. Furber, C., Hepp, M.: SWIQA - A Semantic Web Information Quality Assessment Framework. In: Proc. of ECIS (2011)
4. Gil, Y., Cheney, J., Groth, P., Hartig, O., Miles, S., Moreau, L., Pinheiro da Silva, P. (eds.): Provenance xg final report. W3C Incubator Group Report (December 2010)
5. Goldberg, S.I., Niemierko, A., Turchin, A.: Analysis of data errors in clinical research databases. In: AMIA Annu. Symp. Proc., vol. 6, pp. 242–246 (2008)
6. Hogan, W.R., Wagner, M.M.: Accuracy of Data in Computer-based Patient Records. J. Am. Med. Inform. Assoc. 4(5), 342–355 (1997)

---

[3] The rule was not applied to the TBI dataset as it contains sparsely collected treatment information.

Learning Formal Definitions for SNOMED CT from Text

Yue Ma* and Felix Distel

Institute of Theoretical Computer Science, Technische Universität Dresden,
Dresden, Germany
{mayue,felix}@tcs.inf.tu-dresden.de

Abstract. SNOMED CT is a widely used medical ontology which is formally expressed in a fragment of the Description Logic $\mathcal{EL}++$. The underlying logics allow for expressive querying, yet make it costly to maintain and extend the ontology. In this paper we present an approach for the extraction of SNOMED CT definitions from natural language text. We test and evaluate the approach using two types of texts.

1 Introduction

SNOMED CT [6] is a medical ontology and now a widely accepted international standard. It describes concepts such as anatomical structures, disorders, organisms among others. It has been adopted in many countries worldwide as a standard for electronic health records and is also used in clinical decision support systems. Users can access SNOMED CT through browsers such as NIH Browser (cf. Table 1).

Unlike simpler medical vocabularies SNOMED CT has a formal logic-based foundation, based on Description Logics (DL), more precisely the lightweight DL $\mathcal{EL}++$ [1], a fragment of the standard OWL2EL[1]. While this is hidden to most users, it is a key advantage of SNOMED CT compared to other systems. The formal semantics results in a computer processable knowledge base that can be extended, debugged and queried through reasoning services.

While setting SNOMED CT apart from medical vocabularies such as MeSH the formal semantics also comes at a cost. Adding new concepts to a formal ontology is a tedious, costly and error-prone process, that needs to be performed manually by specially trained knowledge engineers [5]. Thus, researchers have developed services providing assistance in ontology design and maintenance, some of which can extract formal DL-based definitions from text [3,7,8,2].

DL vocabulary consists of concept names such as Baritosis, Lung_structure, etc. and relationships, typically called roles, such as Causative_agent, Finding_Site. Roles link concepts to one another. Using concept constructors, new concepts can be defined using existing ones. $\mathcal{EL}++$ provides the constructors conjunction ($\sqcap$) and existential restrictions ($\exists$) among others. Table 2 shows how the relationships from Table 1 can be expressed in the DL syntax.

---

* We acknowledge financial support by the DFG Research Unit FOR 1513, project B1.
[1] http://www.w3.org/TR/owl2-profiles

N. Peek, R. Marín Morales, and M. Peleg (Eds.): AIME 2013, LNAI 7885, pp. 73–77, 2013.

Table 1. The concept Baritosis as displayed by NIH Snomed CT Browser

Concept: [50076003] Baritosis

Relationships from *this* concept (9)

Baritosis | Causative agent | Barium dust (Defining)

Baritosis | Associated morphology | Deposition of foreign material
Baritosis | Finding site | Lung structure (Defining)

Baritosis | Associated morphology | Inflammation
Baritosis | Finding site | Lung structure (Defining)

Baritosis | Is a | Pneumoconiosis due to inorganic dust

Baritosis | Clinical course | Courses (Qualifier)
Baritosis | Episodicity | Episodicities (Qualifier)
Baritosis | Severity | Severities (Qualifier)

Table 2. The concept description of Baritosis in $\mathcal{EL}$-syntax

Baritosis $\equiv$
$\exists$Causative_agent.Barium_dust
$\sqcap$ $\exists$Associated_morphology.
    Deposition_of_foreign_material
$\sqcap$ $\exists$Finding_site.Lung_structure
$\sqcap$ $\exists$Associated_morphology.Inflammation
$\sqcap$ $\exists$Finding_site.Lung_structure
$\sqcap$ Pneumoconiosis_due_to_inorganic_dust
$\sqcap$ $\exists$Clinical_course.Courses
$\sqcap$ $\exists$Episodicity.Episodicities
$\sqcap$ $\exists$Severity.Severities

Existing approaches for ontology generation mostly focus on learning superclass or subclass relations [8] and therefore fail to make use of existential restrictions allowed by $\mathcal{EL}{+}{+}$. To overcome this, we propose an approach, named *Snomed-supervised relation extraction*, for automatically extracting relationships for concepts (or existential restrictions in DL lingo) from natural language texts. A key advantage of our approach is that no manually labeled training data is required by profiting from the large amount of existing formal knowledge in Snomed CT. It uses a multiclass classifier to classify sentences according to the relationships they describe (if any). To test the approach we use text data from Wikipedia, as well as textual definitions found by the tool Dog4Dag [8].

Task Description

Our approach is based on the observation that in Snomed CT the set of roles remains relatively stable while the set of concepts constantly increases. To facilitate adding new concept descriptions, we create a system that for a given input sentence annotated with two Snomed CT concepts is able to decide if the sentence describes a relationship between the two concepts and which relationship. Since systems for learning subclass and superclass relations already exist, this will eventually enable us to obtain formal definitions for new concepts as in Table 2.

For example, for the target concept Baritosis we expect the Causative_agent relation to Barium_dust and the Finding_site relation to Lung_structure to be recognizable from the following two sentences: (1) "Baritosis is a benign type of pneumoconiosis, which is caused by long-term exposure to barium dust." (2) "Baritosis is due to inorganic dust lies in the lungs."

2   Related Work

Formal ontology generation is an important but non-trivial task [3]. It is particularly challenging for specific domains, such as Snomed CT. [7] describes some first approaches which apply syntactic transformation rules to generate OWL DL concept definitions for generic domains. When directly applying their approaches to SNOMED CT concept definition generation, we may encounter unresolved reference roles such as ∃Of. Moreover, different formal expressions (e.g. ∃Caused_by, ∃Due_to, ...) will be generated from variant expressions (e.g. "caused by", "due to", ...), even though they all express the same relation ∃Causative_agent in SNOMED CT. By contrast, our approach naturally avoids unresolved reference roles and the lexical variant problems by the prefixed set of SNOMED CT roles.

In addition, [7] does not specifically consider $\mathcal{EL}++$ constructors, while [2] is similar to the present work where $\mathcal{EL}++$ is the target language. However, [2] is based on the inductive logic programming technique and requires a large amount of facts about individual entities (called ABox in DL lingo) instead of merely conceptual descriptions of concepts as in the case of SNOMED CT.

Relation extraction is often used to construct ABoxes from ontologies [3]. We extend this idea to generate formal definitions of SNOMED CT concepts. Among the approaches for relation extraction, ours is similar to *distance supervision* [4] in that no manually labelled data is required. However, [4] is not proposed for formal concept definition purposes and works at the entity level. Moreover, we use features independently instead of feature conjunctions as in [4] because of the limited data available for the medicine domain. And we show that medicine domain specific features (SNOMED CT types) are important for the system.

3 Architecture

Textual information from the medical domain is widely available from publicly accessible resources, such as the web or textbooks. The methodology used in our system makes use of both textual data and existing SNOMED CT definitions. In the following we describe the three steps used in our method.

Automatic Data Preparation. During data preparation SNOMED CT roles and SNOMED CT concept labels are aligned to textual sentences. We achieve this automatically as follows.

Relationship extraction: Through DL reasoning we generate the set of all relationships $A|R|B$ that logically follow from SNOMED CT: $\mathcal{RB} = \{A|R|B :$ SNOMED $\models A \sqsubseteq \exists R.B\}$. Reasoning provides a way to use implicit information encoded in SNOMED CT. For example, for Finding_site 630,547 relation pairs are obtained through reasoning compared to only 43,079 explicitly given ones.

Annotation: Using the tool *Metamap* developed at the U.S. National Library of Medicine we annotate the textual sentences with SNOMED CT concepts to identify all concepts occurring in a sentence.

Relationship Alignment: Annotated sentences are aligned with a relationship if they contain two concepts that are in a relationship in SNOMED CT. This is illustrated in Table 3, where "Baritosis" and "barium dust" in the sentence are annotated with concepts Baritosis_(disorder) and Barium_Dust_(substance), respectively, by Metamap. The inferred role base $\mathcal{RB}$ contains the relationship Baritosis_(disorder) | Causative_agent | Barium_dust_(substance). The sentence is thus aligned with Causative_agent, with the latter called an aligned role.

Table 3. Text Alignment and Features

Annotated Sentence	"*Baritosis*/Baritosis_(disorder) is pneumoconiosis caused by *barium dust*/Barium_Dust_(substance)."		
SNOMED CT relationship	Baritosis_(disorder) | Causative_agent | Barium_Dust_(substance)		
Features	left type	between-words	right type
	disorder	"is pneumoconiosis caused by"	*substance*

Training Phase. Once the relationship alignment is done, features will be extracted from the corresponding sentences. The assumption here is that such sentences likely represent role relationships of the aligned role. Since several sentences can be aligned to the same role, weights for different features extracted from different sentences will be learned by a multi-class classifier. For the features, besides the standard lexical features (between-words of annotated phrases [4]), we use eleven semantic types, including *organism*, *finding*, and *disorder*, which are provided by SNOMED CT for each concept. A flag denotes if the two concepts occur in the same order in the sentence as in SNOMED CT.

Test Phase. Test data consists of textual sentences that are candidates for describing a relation. Such sentences are first annotated with SNOMED CT concepts by Metamap, and then features are extracted. Based on these a multi-class classifier can predict role relationships between the target concept and other concepts appearing in the sentences. Note that the roles considered in the current system are disjoint, i.e. no pair of concepts can be related via two different roles. However, for one target concept different roles can be predicted for the same successor concept, which conflicts the above fact. For aggregation we select the role which maximizes the predicted weight according to the classifier.

4   Evaluation and Conclusion

The two corpora chosen for experiments are named WIKI and D4D. WIKI is obtained by querying Wikipedia with one-word SNOMED CT concept names, resulting in around 53,943 distinct sentences with 972,038 words. D4D contains textual definitions extracted by querying DOG4DAG[2] [8] over concepts that occur in the relationships of three well populated roles (i.e., Causative_agent, Associated_morphology, Finding_site) examined in this paper, obtaining 7,092 sentences with 112,886 words. MIX is a combination of WIKI and D4D.

The SNOMED CT relationship set is divided for testing and training: only relationships not concerning a target concept can be considered for training. Negative examples are generated for the classifier to recognize sentences which do not describe any relationship. We test the approach on two test datasets: TW and TD.

---

[2] DOG4DAG is a system that can retrieve and rank textual definitions from the web. However, it has query number restrictions.

Table 4. Evaluation over training datasets WIKI, D4D, and MIX and test datasets TW, and TD with and without the type features

	TW			TD		
	WIKI	D4D	MIX	WIKI	D4D	MIX
Without Type	0.00	0.40	0.20	0.27	0.45	0.59
With Type	0.40	**0.80**	0.60	0.50	**0.64**	0.59

TW contains sentences from Wikipedia about the concepts to be defined and TD is TW combined with sentences from DOG4DAG for the same concepts. The Stanford maximum entropy classifier[3] is used for the implementation and micro average F-measure is the evaluation metric. Different feature settings (with/without type information) are explored. Table 4 compares the results based on different training and test data. We can have the following conclusions:

- The semantic type information described in Section 3 significantly improved the results for all the experiments except for the MIX training data with the TD test data. This suggests that type is an important feature to be used in our system for predicating formal definitions of concepts.
- D4D training data outperformed WIKI and MIX on both of the test data. This shows that precomputed textual definitions by DOG4DAG are helpful for generating formal definitions of concepts of SNOMED CT.

In the future, we will improve the system by using logic reasoning to avoid unreasonable predicted relationships. Text quality appears to be crucial with D4D outperforming WIKI. So we will consider high quality MeSH textual definitions.

References

1. Baader, F., Brandt, S., Lutz, C.: Pushing the $\mathcal{EL}$ envelope. In: Proceedings of IJCAI 2005. Morgan Kaufmann (2005)
2. Chitsaz, M., Wang, K., Blumenstein, M., Qi, G.: Concept Learning for $\mathcal{EL}^{++}$ by Refinement and Reinforcement. In: Anthony, P., Ishizuka, M., Lukose, D. (eds.) PRICAI 2012. LNCS, vol. 7458, pp. 15–26. Springer, Heidelberg (2012)
3. Cimiano, P.: Ontology learning and population from text - algorithms, evaluation and applications. Springer (2006)
4. Mintz, M., Bills, S., Snow, R., Jurafsky, D.: Distant supervision for relation extraction without labeled data. In: Proceedings of ACL/AFNLP 2009, pp. 1003–1011 (2009)
5. Paslaru Bontas Simperl, E., Tempich, C., Sure, Y.: ONTOCOM: A cost estimation model for ontology engineering. In: Cruz, I., Decker, S., Allemang, D., Preist, C., Schwabe, D., Mika, P., Uschold, M., Aroyo, L.M. (eds.) ISWC 2006. LNCS, vol. 4273, pp. 625–639. Springer, Heidelberg (2006)
6. SNOMED Clinical Terms. College of American Pathologists, Northfield (2006)
7. Völker, J.: Learning expressive ontologies. PhD thesis, Universität Karlsruhe (2009)
8. Wächter, T., Fabian, G., Schroeder, M.: Dog4dag: Semi-automated ontology generation in OBO-Edit and Protégé. In: Proceedings of SWAT4LS 2011, pp. 119–120 (2011)

---

[3] http://nlp.stanford.edu/software/classifier.shtml

Towards Automatic Patient Eligibility Assessment: From Free-Text Criteria to Queries

Krystyna Milian and Annette ten Teije

VU University Amsterdam, the Netherlands

Abstract. The presented work contributes to bridging the representation of clinical trials and patient data. Our ultimate goal is to support the trial recruitment, by automating the process of formalizing eligibility criteria of clinical trials, starting from free text of criteria and leading to a computable representation. This paper discusses the final step in the pipeline i.e. generating queries from the structured representation consisting of detected patterns and semantic entities. The queries allow to evaluate patient eligibility for a given trial. To enable easy incorporation of semantic reasoning using medical ontologies, we built the queries in SPARQL and use the OWL representation of one the standards for patient data storage - openEHR archetypes and NCI ontology. The available public repository of archetypes and the expressivity of SPARQL allow to create template queries for the majority of patterns.

Keywords: query generation, semantic reasoning, clinical trials, medical ontologies, patient data representation.

1 Introduction

Clinical trials evaluate new approaches to diagnosis, treatments or prevention, and are essential for the progress of medicine. The recruitment is based on eligibility criteria, related to the current health situation of a patient (age, diagnosis, medications used, etc.) and history of treatment. Since criteria are expressed in natural language, the recruitment is time and effort consuming. Many clinical trials are not finalized due to insufficient participation. Our research aims to support the recruitment, by providing a generic method that interprets free text of criteria leading to computable representation. The pipeline of processing steps is depicted in Figure 1. The first step of structuring the criteria is described in section 2, it consists of detection of contextual patterns and semantic entities and was previously reported in [1]. Section 3 describes the main contribution, the process of transforming the structured representation into queries determining patient eligibility. Since this step requires the linkage with patient data, to enhance the reusability we conform to one of medical data standards, the openEHR archetypes[1]. We describe the mapping of structured representation to archetypes, used for constructing the query templates (the dashed line in Figure 1), and their instantiation. Section 4 discusses and concludes presented work.

---

[1] http://www.openehr.org/home.html

N. Peek, R. Marín Morales, and M. Peleg (Eds.): AIME 2013, LNAI 7885, pp. 78–83, 2013.

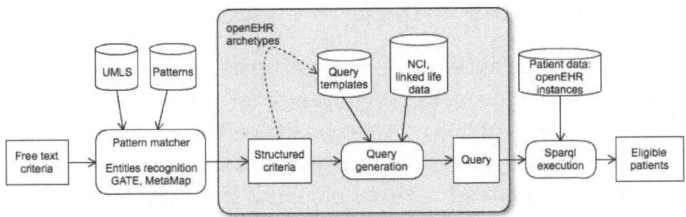

Fig. 1. Transforming criteria to queries. The rectangle indicates the focus of this paper.

2   Structuring Eligibility Criteria

The method for structuring eligibility criteria consists of several steps, initially described in [1,2]. We start with the preprocessing i.a. delimiting the sentences using GATE [3]. Next, we detect the patterns providing the context, finally, we detect semantic entities (ontology concepts, thresholds etc.). For instance, in "No prior chemotherapy except for tamoxifen", first we detect the pattern "No prior () except for ()", and then the concepts "chemotherapy" and "tamoxifen".
Detecting Patterns. The set of patterns was defined after analyzing trials published at ClinicalTrials.gov. It contains 165 items reflecting the typically occurring constraints related to patient characteristics e.g. "Age over ()", disease characteristics e.g. "T () stage" and therapies e.g. "No prior () for ()". The majority of patterns is generic, a few are specific for oncology (e.g. cancer staging), or breast cancer. The algorithm of pattern detection uses regular expressions.
Detecting Semantic Entities. The detection of semantic entities (e.g. diseases, treatments, value or temporal constraints) is performed using GATE, providing relevant semantic taggers i.a. Number, Measurement and MetaMap [4], an UMLS annotator. This step enables generating a normalized representation (concepts are replaced by UMLS codes, measurements by normalized values and units).

3   From Structured Criteria to Queries

The proposed representation of criteria covers coding using medical ontologies, and is independent on a patient data model. The final step in the pipeline (Figure 1) requires the linkage to patient data. To enhance the reusability, we use a clinical data standard and medical ontologies, serving as a bridge between semantics of criteria and patient data. We chose openEHR archetypes over CDA[2], as they provide higher granularity of data specification and due to the availability of their OWL representation [5,6] enhancing semantic reasoning. openEHR is adopted by research projects, healthcare and non-profit organizations[3].

---

[2] http://hl7book.net/index.php?title=CDA
[3] http://www.openehr.org/who_is_using_openehr/

3.1 Mapping Structured Criteria to openEHR Archetypes

Mappings for Simple Patterns. Some patterns of eligibility criteria indicate a value of some implicit parameter (e.g "pregnant") or a parameter - value pair (e.g. "Required diagnosis of ()"). A majority of these (28 patterns) could be directly mapped to archetypes and their parameters, some examples are below. Constructing query templates for these patterns is straightforward.

Pattern	openEHR archetype	parameters
Age over (); Age under ()	openEHR-DEMOGRAPHIC-ITEM_TREE. person_details.v1	Birth date
Estrogen status Her2-neu status	openEHR-EHR-CLUSTER. microscopy_breast_carcinoma.v1	Hormone Receptor assays
T () stage N() stage	openEHR-EHR-CLUSTER. tnm_staging_7th-breast.v1	Primary tumour Regional lymph nodes
() diagnosis by () Diagnosis within ()	openEHR-EHR-EVALUATION. problem-diagnosis.v1	Diagnosis, Diagnostic criteria, Date recognized

Semantic Type Dependent Mappings for Complex Patterns. In case of complex patterns, providing the context, one pattern can correspond to multiple templates, choosing one depends on the semantic type of instantiating data. For instance a query related to a pattern "History of ()" instantiated with "radiotherapy" should address data represented with an archetype related to procedure, with "diabetes" - archetype related to diagnosis. We identified 8 archetypes that could be used to represent concepts having 12 semantic types, e.g:

Semantic Type	openEHR Archetype
Disease or Syndrome Neoplastic process	openEHR-EHR-EVALUATION.problem-diagnosis.v1 OR openEHR-EHR-EVALUATION.exclusion-problem_diagnosis.v1
Organic chemical Pharmacologic substance	openEHR-EHR-ACTION.medication.v1 AND openEHR-EHR-ITEM_TREE.medication.v1
Laboratory Procedure Laboratory or Test Result	openEHR-EHR-OBSERVATION.lab_test.v1 OR openEHR-EHR-EVALUATION.excluded-intervention.v1

Concept Dependent Mappings. Finally, because of the broad range of available archetypes, some diseases or findings might be modeled with specialized archetypes. We analyzed 50 most frequent concepts of selected semantic types, detected in our previous study of over 2000 breast cancer trials [7], and found 4 additional relevant archetypes, e.g. openEHR-EHR-OBSERVATION.lab_test-full_blood_count.v1 for 'Platelet count', which is one of the attributes.

In total we identified 21 relevant archetypes, that model data items from eligibility criteria to various level of detail. Among them only 2 are strictly related to breast cancer, others are applicable for representing eligibility criteria of clinical trials related to other diseases. However, we could not map all the patterns and concepts, either because of missing expressivity or inability to find. This regards i.a. criteria requiring specific type of confirmation and findings e.g. "cytologically confirmed () by ()", "recovery from ()" or a gene mutation.

3.2 Query Templates

Data Model. Selected archetypes were transformed using the adapted ADL (Archetype Definition Language) to OWL tool [5], described in [6]. Next, they were merged into one ontology using Protege. Our approach assumes that patient data are also transformed into OWL, stored as instances of classes related to corresponding archetypes and annotated with ontology codes.

Generating Queries. The query generation involves several steps. First, the UMLS concepts detected in criteria are related to codes in patient file, in our case it is NCI Thesaurus[4], but could be as well other ontology. To get NCI codes, the program queries Linked life data[5] using Jena[6]. Next, the algorithm chooses a template corresponding to the extracted pattern. It is either straightforward, or depends on the semantic type of detected concepts (section 3.1). Semantic type is extracted from MetaMap annotation, so this step is also automatic. An example below presents a template query, related to the pattern "At least (threshold) since (procedureCode)". It uses the NCI hierarchy to reason about the subtypes of procedures, and recalculates units enabling temporal comparison.

```
SELECT distinct ?patient
WHERE {
    ?patient a archetypes:at0000_1_Patient ;
    c:links> ?procedure .
    ?procedure a p:at0000_Procedure_undertaken ;
    archetypes:time_value_ ?procedureTime ;
    c:items ?procedureName .
    ?procedureName a p:at0002_Procedure .
    c:value_element> ?procedureCode .
    ?subclass rdfs:subClassOf nci:procedureCode .
    BIND (86400*(day(now()) + 30*month(now()) + 360*year(now()))) AS ?now).
    BIND (xsd:dateTime(?procedureTime) AS ?t)
    BIND (86400*(day(?t) + 30*month(?t) + 360*year(?t)) AS ?procTimeInS).
    FILTER ((?procedureCode = nci:procedureCode || ?code = ?subclass)
            && ?now - ?procTimeInS> threshold)
}
```

The expressiveness of SPARQL and archetypes allows to construct the template queries for the majority of patterns.

4 Discussion, Conclusions and Future Work

Discussion. Currently we use the simplistic approach and processes only the criteria that are mapped exclusively to one of patterns, and with entities that get the maximal MetaMap mapping score. Our previous work [2] reports that it leads to rather low recall (approx. 18 %). Presented approach requires the manual definition of query templates. Although it is effort consuming task, it leads to the generic solution, which might be reused for various clinical trials. Reuse of templates in other institutes applying openEHR might require some editions, as the standard leaves some freedom for adaptation and extension.

Related Work. The support for trial recruitment is active research area. Recently published [8,9] describe the structuring of criteria, and represent them as semantic dependency trees. The latter focuses on the temporal constraints. The authors of [10] address the transformation of free text criteria to queries. Our approach has lower recall, but is automatic and bounded to openEHR standard. Additionally, we use NCI ontology hierarchy allowing to reason also about

---

[4] http://nciterms.nci.nih.gov/ncitbrowser/index.jsp
[5] http://linkedlifedata.com/
[6] http://jena.apache.org

subtypes of diseases and procedures. Semantic techniques have been applied in several studies e.g. [11,12]. Both transform patient data into ABox of a medical ontology (SNOMED CT and NCI Thesaurus respectively), and eligibility criteria are manually transformed into queries. With respect to using openEHR, authors of [6] present a case study, where they adopt and extend ADL to OWL translator [5], and describe the calculation of medical quality indicators.

Conclusions. This paper describes the approach of transforming eligibility criteria written in natural language to computable representation. We investigated the applicability of openEHR archetypes to cover frequently occurring data items mentioned in eligibility criteria. Our findings indicate that the expressivity of archetypes is sufficient to model data items of eligibility criteria to big extent. The expressivity of SPARQL 1.1. allowed to construct template queries reflecting various complex temporal or semantic constraints. Choosing OWL representation of patient data, and SPARQL for template queries, allowed for straightforward incorporation of semantic reasoning using medical ontologies. The study was performed with the focus on breast cancer, but the approach could be directly reused for eligibility criteria of trials studying other diseases.

Future Work. Next steps will cover the evaluation of the approach with patient data. To deal with missing items we plan to incorporate domain knowledge, e.g. by exploiting the ontologies, that provide many semantic relations (currently we use only the hierarchy) and apply probabilistic reasoning. Moreover, we will need to complete the set of templates. We might also extend the algorithm of pattern detection by using semantic parsers to process combined patterns.

References

1. Milian, K., Bucur, A., ten Teije, A.: Formalization of clinical trial eligibility criteria: Evaluation of a pattern-based approach. In: BIBM (2012)
2. Milian, K., Bucur, A., van Harmelen, F.: Building a Library of Eligibility Criteria to Support Design of Clinical Trials. In: ten Teije, A., Völker, J., Handschuh, S., Stuckenschmidt, H., d'Acquin, M., Nikolov, A., Aussenac-Gilles, N., Hernandez, N. (eds.) EKAW 2012. LNCS, vol. 7603, pp. 327–336. Springer, Heidelberg (2012)
3. Cunningham, H., Maynard, D., Bontcheva, K., Tablan, V., Aswani, N., Roberts, I., Gorrell, G., Funk, A., Roberts, A., Damljanovic, D., Heitz, T., Greenwood, M.A., Saggion, H., Petrak, J., Li, Y., Peters, W.: Text Processing with GATE (2011)
4. Aronson, A.R.: MetaMap: Mapping Text to the UMLS Metathesaurus. In: AMIA, pp. 17–21 (2001)
5. Lezcano, L., Sicilia, M.-A., Rodríguez-Solano, C.: Integrating reasoning and clinical archetypes using OWL ontologies and SWRL rules. JBI 44(2), 343–353 (2011)
6. Dentler, K., ten Teije, A., Cornet, R., de Keizer, N.: Semantic Integration of Patient Data and Quality Indicators Based on *open*EHR Archetypes. In: Lenz, R., Miksch, S., Peleg, M., Reichert, M., Riaño, D., ten Teije, A. (eds.) ProHealth 2012/KR4HC 2012. LNCS, vol. 7738, pp. 85–97. Springer, Heidelberg (2013)
7. Milian, K., Bucur, A., van Harmelen, F., ten Teije, A.: Identifying most relevant concepts to describe clinical trial eligibility criteria. Health Inf. (2013)

8. Weng, C., Wu, X., Luo, Z., Boland, M.R., Theodoratos, D., Johnson, S.B.: EliXR: An Approach to Eligibility Criteria Extraction and Representation. JAMIA

9. Boland, M., Tu, S., Carini, S., Sim, I., Weng, C.: EliXR-TIME: A Temporal Knowledge Representation for Clinical Research Eligibility Criteria. In: AMIA (2012)

10. Tu, S.W., Peleg, M., Carini, S., Bobak, M., Ross, J., Rubin, D., Sim, I.: A practical method for transforming free-text eligibility criteria into computable criteria. JBI 44(2), 239–250 (2011)

11. Besana, P., Cuggia, M., Zekri, O., Bourde, A., Burgun, A.: Using semantic web technologies for clinical trial recruitment. In: Patel-Schneider, P.F., Pan, Y., Hitzler, P., Mika, P., Zhang, L., Pan, J.Z., Horrocks, I., Glimm, B., et al. (eds.) ISWC 2010, Part II. LNCS, vol. 6497, pp. 34–49. Springer, Heidelberg (2010)

12. Patel, C., Cimino, J., Dolby, J., Fokoue, A., Kalyanpur, A., Kershenbaum, A., Ma, L., Schonberg, E., Srinivas, K.: Matching patient records to clinical trials using ontologies. In: Aberer, K., et al. (eds.) ISWC/ASWC 2007. LNCS, vol. 4825, pp. 816–829. Springer, Heidelberg (2007)

Biomedical Knowledge Extraction Using Fuzzy Differential Profiles and Semantic Ranking

Sidahmed Benabderrahmane

INRIA Research Center, Campus Scientifique, France
sidahmed.benabderrahmane@gmail.com

Abstract. Recently, technologies such as DNA microarrays allow to generate big scale of transcriptomic data used to the aim of exploring background of genes. The analysis and the interpretation of such data requires important databases and efficient mining methods, in order to extract specific biological functions belonging to a group of genes of an expression profile. To this aim, we propose here a new approach for mining transcriptomic data combining domain knowledge and classification methods. Firstly, we propose the definition of Fuzzy Differential Gene Expression Profiles (FG-DEP) based on fuzzy classification and a differential definition between the considered biological situations. Secondly, we will use our previously defined efficient semantic similarity measure (called IntelliGO), that is applied on Gene Ontology (GO) annotation terms, for computing semantic and functional similarities between genes of resulting FG-DEP and well known genetic markers involved in the development of cancers. After that, the similarity matrices will be used to introduce a novel Functional Spectral Representation (FSR) calculated through a semantic ranking of genes regarding their similarities with the tumoral markers. The FSR representation should help expert to interpret by a new way transcriptomic data and infer new genes having similar biological functions regarding well known diseases.

Availability: The semantic similarity measure and the ranking method are available at http://plateforme-mbi.loria.fr/intelligo/ranking.php.

1 Introduction

Nowadays, the pharmaceutical industries require large volume of biological data and need a sophisticated computational methods to manage and extract relevant knowledge. Recently, DNA microarrays were used for measuring the expression levels of thousands of genes under various biological conditions. Hence, gene expression data analysis proceeds in two steps: Firstly, expression profiles are produced by grouping genes displaying similar expression levels under biological situations [1]. Secondly, a functional analysis, based on functional annotations, is applied on genes sharing the same expression profile, in order to identify their relevant biological functions [2]. In fact, the main goal of this functional analysis is to identify and characterize genes that can serve as diagnostic signatures or prognostic markers for different stages of a disease. One of the interesting source

N. Peek, R. Marín Morales, and M. Peleg (Eds.): AIME 2013, LNAI 7885, pp. 84–93, 2013.
© Springer-Verlag Berlin Heidelberg 2013

of functional annotations in the biological domain is the Gene Ontology (GO) [3]. The interpretation of transcriptomic data requires efficient mining methods for extracting specific biological functions belonging to genes of an expression profile. In this context, we introduce here, by an innovative way, a cascade of methods for mining such data combining domain knowledge and classification methods. Firstly, we propose the definition of Fuzzy Differential Gene Expression Profiles (FD-GEP) based on fuzzy classification and a differential definition of the expression between the considered biological situations. This classification approach affects genes through fuzzy sets when there are differential physiological relations between the studied biological situations. Secondly, we will use our previously defined efficient semantic similarity measure (called IntelliGO), that is applied on Gene Ontology (GO) annotation terms, for computing semantic and functional similarities between genes of resulting FD-GEP and set of well known genetic markers involved in the development of cancers. After that, the similarity matrices will be used to introduce a novel Functional Spectral Representation (FSR) calculated through a semantic ranking of genes regarding their similarities with the tumoral markers. This new paradigm for visualizing expression data displays as a bar code, genes of a given FD-GEP w.r.t. disease markers. Genes that are at the top of the sorted list are functionally similar to these markers and can hence be explored by biologists to verify experimental hypothesis.

This paper is organized as follows. The next section, outlines the presentation of the used dataset and introduce the new proposed method for profiles extraction. The next subsections present the new gene functional analysis based IntelliGO similarity and semantic Ranking. Finally, we discuss in the last section the relevance of the obtained results of the proposed methods.

2   Material and Methods

2.1   DNA Microarrays Dataset

In this work, we will use a list (L) of 222 differentially expressed genes of colorectal cancers. An Affymetrix HGU133+[1] microarray was used for experiments. In this dataset, we dispose of three biological situations in the gene expression matrix (M) that correspond to three biological samples: (i) healthy tissue (normal); (ii): tumor tissue (cancer); (iii) cell line. We name these situations: $S1$, $S2$, $S3$ respectively. Each situation represents the average of multiple replicates and multiple specimens in each type of tissue during experiences [4]. An example of the expression data in the matrix M is illustrated in Table 1. The expression value for a given gene g from a set of genes G in a situation S_i is given by ν_{si}. The selected 222 genes represent a significant fold change observed between $S2$ and $S1$. Thus biologists are interested by genes for which the expression varies between these two situations, i.e., found deregulated in cancer tissues.

---

[1] www.affymetrix.com/products_services/arrays/specific/hgu133plus.affx

Table 1. Example of the expression matrix M of the 222 genes relative to colorectal cancer, used in this study. This matrix is used for extracting gene expression profiles.

Gene	Healthy : S_1	Cancer: S_2	Cell line: S_3
KIAA1199	33,6	827,87	735,75
FOXQ1	65,36	1240,21	2631,71
PSAT1	89,03	1019,0	3025,66
CLDN1	12,15	119,9	78,5
SLC6A6	56,6	551,1	568,6
....	...	...	...
Gene g	ν_{s1}	ν_{s2}	ν_{s3}
....	...	...	...
PSAT1	113,1	407,1	1258,0

2.2 Definition of the Fuzzy Differential Genes Expression Profiles: FD-GEP

In the state-of-the-art methods for extracting expression profiles [1], there is no prior exploitable knowledge between the nature of biological situations. However, the interpretation of groups of genes in an expression profile is usually guided by hypothesizes related to the objectives of the study. This is the case in particular when relations exist between the biological situations. Such kind of relations could be temporal when expression levels are measured at different time stamp, or kinetic when a kind of a tissue is considered but in different physiological states (e.g. stages of tumor). In this last case, the differences existing between pairs of situations may interest biologists, and it would be interesting to regroup together genes with the same variations between two situations regardless of the level of expression they have each in one situation. This observation conducts us to introduce here the notion of a priori definition of *Differential Genes Expression Profiles* (D-GEP). It is the first contribution of this paper. Constructed from pairs of situations chosen by the user, these profiles can be considered as combinations, for each pair of situations, of the *Differential Expression Sets* (DES), to regroup genes having similar variations (over-expression, or even under-expression) between two situations. The membership of a gene to a given profile begins by studying its membership to a particular DES for each pair of situations. Here we use a fuzzy modeling of the expression level variations between two situations to consider noise in the data and provide an opportunity for a gene to belong to more than one profile. With our data set, and having three situations, we have 3 possible pairs of situations (S_3, S_1) (S_2, S_1) and (S_3, S_2), respectively. For n situations, we can have $n(n-1)/2$ pairs of situations. Identifying a D-GEP for a gene g leads us to affect this gene, for each pair of situation (S_i, S_j), either in the set of genes over-expressed in S_i with respect to S_j (which we denote $\text{Over}_{i,j}$), or in the set of genes under-expressed in S_i compared to S_j (which we denote $\text{Under}_{i,j}$), or rather in set of genes with similar expression in S_i w.r.t. S_j (which we denote $\text{Iso}_{i,j}$). By extension, the sets $\text{Over}_{i,j}$, $\text{Under}_{i,j}$, $\text{Iso}_{i,j}$ are called *Differential Expression Sets* (DES), and allow to represent the differential expression of genes between two situations of interest S_i and S_j. Consequently, the formal definition of a D-GEP is a K-uplet of DES, where K is the number of pairs of situations. For example, in our case, the profile $(\text{Over}_{3,1}$, $\text{Over}_{2,1}, \text{Under}_{3,2})$, is a D-GEP in which genes are: over expressed in Cell Line

(S_3) w.r.t. Normal tissue (S_1), over expressed in cancer (S_2) w.r.t. Normal tissue (S_1), and under expressed in the Cell Line (S_3) w.r.t. Cancer (S_2). As we said before, the affectation of genes in the different DES is performed with fuzzy logic. Firstly, we need to define a value of variation of expression noted $\xi_{i,j}$ to represent the difference of the expression of a gene g in two situations (S_i, S_j): $\xi_{i,j}(g) = \frac{\nu_{s_i} - \nu_{s_j}}{\min_{k=1..n} \nu_{sk}}$ for all i, j in k situations. The proposed fuzzy model conducts to define a threshold value σ for the expression variation value $\xi_{i,j}(g)$, and for each pair of situations (S_i, S_j). Three membership functions of three fuzzy sets allow to define the affectation of genes to DES depending on the value of $\xi_{i,j}(g)$. These membership functions are defined as:

$$Over_{i,j} : G \longrightarrow [0,1] \quad Over_{i,j}(g) = \begin{cases} 1 & if & \xi_{i,j}(g) \geq \sigma \\ \frac{1}{\sigma} \times \xi_{i,j}(g) & if & 0 < \xi_{i,j}(g) < \sigma \\ 0 & otherwise \end{cases}$$

$$Under_{i,j} : G \longrightarrow [0,1] \quad Under_{i,j}(g) = \begin{cases} 1 & if & \xi_{i,j}(g) \leq -\sigma \\ \frac{-1}{\sigma} \times \xi_{i,j}(g) & if & -\sigma < \xi_{i,j}(g) < 0 \\ 0 & otherwise \end{cases}$$

$$Iso_{i,j} : G \longrightarrow [0,1] \quad Iso_{i,j}(g) = \begin{cases} 0 & if \ \xi_{i,j}(g) < -\sigma \ or \ \xi_{i,j}(g) > \sigma \\ \frac{1}{\sigma} \times \xi_{i,j}(g) + 1 & if \ -\sigma < \xi_{i,j}(g) < 0 \\ \frac{-1}{\sigma} \times \xi_{i,j}(g) + 1 & if \ 0 < \xi_{i,j}(g) < \sigma \end{cases}$$

The defuzzification process allows the final classification of a gene g to one or more DES in accordance to a given threshold value μ. This is done with the following constraint: if the value taken by function $Over_{i,j}(g)$, $Under_{i,j}(g)$ or $Iso_{i,j}(g)$ is $\geq \mu$, thus the gene is classified in the corresponding DES. The figure (1) represents the three membership functions $Over_{i,j}$, $Under_{i,j}$, $Iso_{i,j}$. For example, for the gene g, we have $Over_{i,j}(g) = 0.25$, $Under_{i,j}(g) = 0$, $Iso_{i,j}(g) = 0.75$. We observe that for $\mu = 0.5$, this gene is classified in the DES $Iso_{i,j}$ only, otherwise for $\mu = 0.25$ it will be affected both in $Iso_{i,j}$ with membership probability of 0.75 and $Over_{i,j}$ with a complementary membership value of 0.25. We can remark that with this modelization, the bi-classification criteria of a gene in two DES is possible for $\mu \leq 0.5$. Hence, a D-GEP is a combination of DES, and the fuzzy modelization introduced here allows to genes to be affected to more than one D-GEP. By consequence a Fuzzy differential genes expression profile (FD-GEP) is a D-GEP where the affectation of genes in DES is performed with fuzzy logic. Note that, with 3 situations, and with 3 DES, we can obtain 27 possible FD-GEP. As we can observe, there are two parameters that can be taken into account during the classification algorithm, namely: σ and μ. The different values affected to these variables depend on the used datasets. We performed an exploratory analysis by testing different values for $\mu=\{0.1, 0.2, 0.3, 0.4, 0.5\}$ and $\sigma=\{0.1, 0.2, 0.3, 0.4, 0.5, 0.6, 0.7, 0.8, 0.9, 1\}$. Each pair of values of the two parameters were tested for extracting the possible FD-GEP profiles. Results for the different combination are not shown

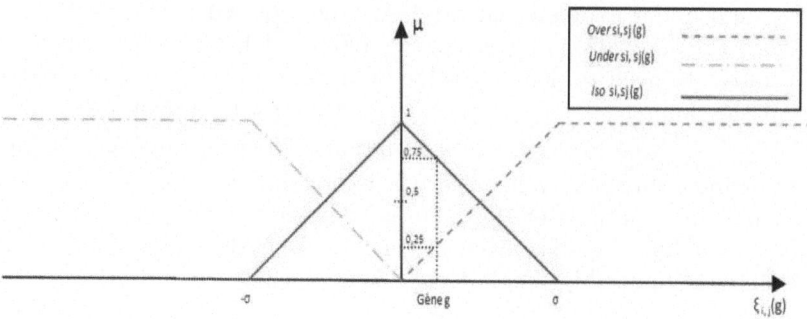

Fig. 1. Representation of the membership functions defining the affectation of a gene to the differential expression sets $Over_{i,j}$, $Under_{i,j}$, $Iso_{i,j}$ used for defining the FD-GEP profiles.

here. Although, we used some prior knowledge to eliminate certain values that generate outliers FD-GEP profiles. For example, for $\sigma \geq 0.6$ we observed that some genes were classified in the DES $Iso_{2,1}$ (same expression in cancer and normal tissues), even if in our dataset the genes are differentially expressed between the two situations (S2) and (S1). We decided after multiple testing, to keep the combination $(\mu,\sigma)=(0.3, 0.4)$ which expects a reasonable number of genes in the obtained profiles. With this pair of values, and from the list of 222 colorectal cancer genes, we extracted the FD-GEP expression profiles presented in Table 2. The number of genes in each profile is displayed in the diagonal of the matrix, while overlaps (due to fuzzy classification) are observed between some profiles in terms of number of shared genes are displayed in the rest of cells of the matrix.

Table 2. Distribution of genes in the obtained expression profiles. Note that if a cell is empty then the two corresponding FD-GEP profiles do not share any gene. The diagonal represents the number of genes in each FD-GEP.

Name of the FD-GEP	Definition of the FD-GEP	Profile 1	Profile 2	Profile 3	Profile 4	Profile 11	Profile 13	Profile 14	Profile 15	Profile 20	Profile 21
Profile 1	$Over_{2,1},Over_{3,1},Over_{3,2}$	51		2							
Profile 2	$Over_{2,1},Over_{3,1},Under_{3,2}$		108	17						24	1
Profile 3	$Over_{2,1},Over_{3,1},Iso_{3,2}$			30						1	1
Profile 4	$Over_{2,1},Under_{3,1},Over_{3,2}$				1						
Profile 11	$Under_{2,1},Over_{3,1},Under_{3,2}$					1					
Profile 13	$Under_{2,1},Under_{3,1},Over_{3,2}$						9	1			
Profile 14	$Under_{2,1},Under_{3,1},Under_{3,2}$							7	1		
Profile 15	$Under_{2,1},Under_{3,1},Iso_{3,2}$								5		
Profile 20	$Iso_{2,1},Over_{3,1},Under_{3,2}$									56	
Profile 21	$Iso_{2,1},Over_{3,1},Iso_{3,2}$										1

2.3   Gene Expression Functional Analysis

Calculating Semantic and Functional Similarity between Genes: A lot of functional analysis methods have been proposed using either statistical enrichment [5] or gene functional clustering [6]. In this last case, a semantic similarity is used for grouping genes regarding Gene Ontology (GO) functions [3]. We admit that the performance of the used similarity will have an impact on the clustering results. Recently, we proposed an hybrid functional analysis method combining both fuzzy clustering and statistical enrichment analysis [7,8,9], using our *IntelliGO* measure [10]. Our second contribution in this paper (after having defined FD-GEP), is to propose a complementary visualization method that should help biologists to investigate interesting genes during the transcriptomic data study. The principle of the technique is detailed below.

In the rest of the experiments, we will use the same list of 222 colorectal cancer genes, for computing the IntelliGO similarity matrices. As a first step, and in order to have a global overview of the distribution of the biological annotations of the used list of genes, we produced a Heatmap with a two way hierarchical clustering. The results are shown in figure (2). Despite the change in color intensity in different regions of the heatmap, several clusters can be distinguished in its diagonal. Homogeneous cluster in the upper left of the heatmap and with very little cross similarity with other genes in the data set has been studied from the point of view of its gene content. The strong functional similarity between these genes can be explained by recurrent Biological Process annotations on transport processes. Transport processes are important in the physiology of the digestive system and cluster genes are already known to be deregulated in colorectal cancer. This is the case of gene AQP8 aquaporin 8 whose expression is no longer detectable in colorectal tumors [11]. In fact AQP8 gene is found in the FD-GEP Profile_14 corresponding to genes under-expressed in tumor vs the normal situation. Another gene (ATP11A) is also present in the functional cluster analyzed here, with an annotation transport of phospholipids, and was recently described as a new predictive marker of metachronous metastasis of colorectal cancer [12]. Associated in our study to FD-GEP Profile_1, it actually appears as over-expressed in tumor position relative to the healthy situation. These two genes can be considered as positive controls, confirming the validity of classification results.

Functional Spectral Representation: A Genes Functional Ranking Approach: As reported above, to enhance the analysis of the transcriptomic data, we propose a new functional spectral representation of genes. The main idea of the proposition is summarized in the Figure (3). Firstly, we proceed by ranking with descending order (from most to less similar) an input list of genes regarding their IntelliGO functional semantic similarity with given well known biological markers. After the ranking step, we identify for a given FD-GEP profile, the position of its genes in the ranked list. The position of each gene of this profile is marked with a red line. Blue line indicates the 0.5 functional similarity threshold. The main objective here is to verify if the genes belonging to the profile

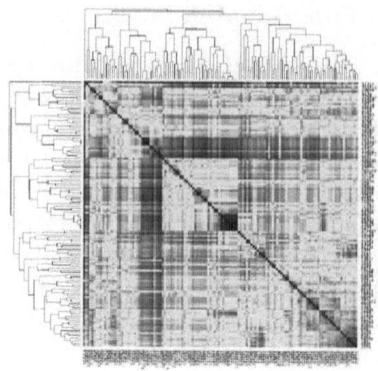

Fig. 2. Generated Heatmap with 222 colorectal cancer

(marked with red lines) are top ranked in the list or not, i.e., the number of red lines over the blue line is important or not. If it is the first case, these genes are judged to be functionally similar to the well-known biological markers and therefore they could be suggested to biologists for further analysis.

In preliminary experiences, we have selected 6 genes involved in target WNT signaling pathway[2] known as transcriptionally repressed in colorectal cancer [13]. Genes of this pathway are known as contributors in mutations in degenerative diseases and cancers. Namely we have chosen: AXIN2 (The Axin-related protein), CD44 (Cell-surface glycoprotein), MET (MNNG HOS Transforming gene), MYC (v-myc myelocytomatosis viral oncogene homolog), SOX9 (SRY (sex determining region Y)-box 9) and ASCL2.

Results for FD-GEP profile1 are presented in Figure (4). We can observe that with AXIN2, MET, MYC, SOX9 markers, the blue line (50% of similarity) is positioned in low levels of the ranked list. It means that genes of this profile are very functionally similars to these markers, in particular with MET and MYC ($\geq$60% of genes of the profile) as it is shown in figure 5. We recall that these two biomedical markers are confirmed to be catalyst in the colorectal cancer, and we know that the studied data set is relative to this kind of cancer [14]. Thus, these results confirm the pertinence of the proposed approach. For deepening the analysis, we processed the same analysis for FD-GEP 2, 3, 14, 20 since genes in these profiles are dysregulated in the cancer situation vs normal (either Over or Under in S_2 vs S_1). We calculated for each profile its FSR and also the average percentage of its genes having functional similarity w.r.t. the used cancer biomedical markers over than 0.50. Results are shown in figure 5. We can observe that all FD-GEPs except Profile 14 have similar functional background regarding the used markers, and it appears very clearly that genes of the used data set share biological processes that are very similar to MET and MYC cancer genes (more than 40 %). Hence, we can suggest to biologists the top positioned genes in the produced ranked lists of the FSRs of each profile, in order to verify their

---

[2] http://www.genome.jp/kegg/pathway/hsa/hsa04310.html

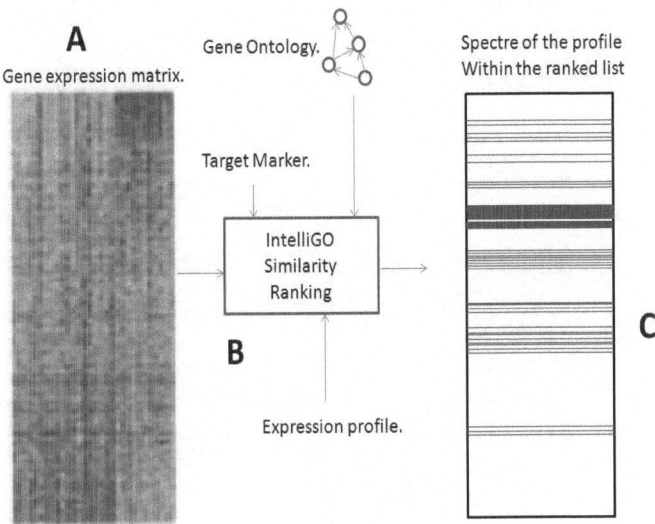

Fig. 3. A Functional Spectral Representation (FSR) overview illustrating the method. A: An expression data matrix is used as input. B: The IntelliGO functional similarity is calculated within all genes of the input list and a given bio-marker. C: The ranked list is displayed by highlighting with red lines genes of a studied expression profiles. A blue line is used to identify the 0.5 functional similarity threshold.

sequence similarity with the used markers. It could be then possible to extend the WNT signaling pathway with those genes, and verify other hypothesis of their involvement in the colorectal cancers.

3   Conclusion and Perspectives

In this paper, we proposed data mining methods combining classification and visualization for analyzing transcriptomic data by an innovative way. In a first step, we propose a new definition of the Fuzzy Differential Genes Expression Profiles FD-GEP, for classifying genes through fuzzy sets when there are differential physiological relations between biological situations. After the step of profiles extraction, a gene functional analysis is essential to give sense to the affected genes in the profiles. We propose a new functional analysis approach, with a new paradigm for visualizing expression data through a process of semantic ranking regarding interesting disease markers. Indeed, the proposed FSR displays as a bar code, genes of a given FD-GEP w.r.t. disease markers. Genes that are at the top of the sorted list are functionally similar to these markers and can hence be explored by biologists to verify experimental hypothesis.

Further, we would consider the idea of performing the same study on genes belonging to other disease processes. Indeed, the OMIM database (Online

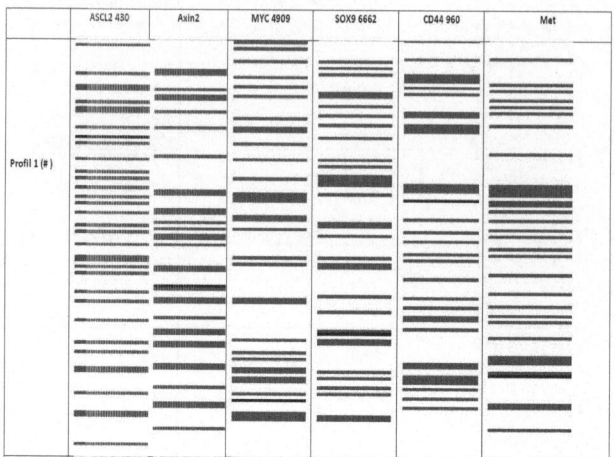

Fig. 4. Functional Spectral Representation (FRS) using genes of FD-GEP Profile 1

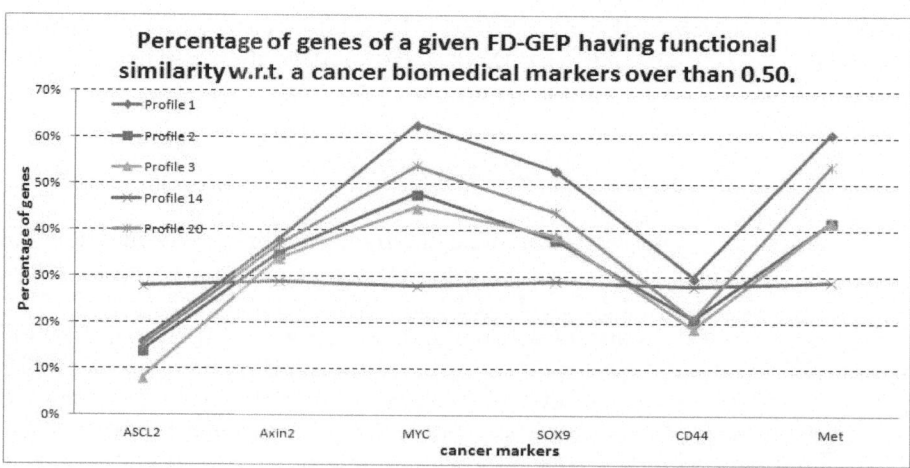

Fig. 5. Average percentage of genes of an FD-GEP having functional similarity w.r.t. a cancer biomedical markers over than 0.50. Values are varying from a marker to another for the considered FD-GEPs. We can observe that majority of the FD-GEP have similar biological behavior regarding their functional similarities with biological functions of the markers.

Mendelian Inheritance in Man)[3] provides markers for different types of diseases that are listed in this database. One can test these markers with different lists of gene expression data.

References

1. Eisen, M.B., Spellman, P.T., Brown, P.O., Botstein, D.: Cluster analysis and display of genome-wide expression patterns. Proceedings of the National Academy of Sciences of the United States of America 95(25), 14863–14868 (1998)
2. Khatri, P., Draghici, S.: Ontological analysis of gene expression data: current tools, limitations, and open problems. Bioinformatics 21(18), 3587–3595 (2005)
3. Daniel, B., et al.: The GOA database in 2009–an integrated Gene Ontology Annotation resource. Nucl. Acids Res. 37(suppl. 1), D396–D403 (2009)
4. Benabderrahmane, S., Devignes, M.-D., Smaïl-Tabbone, M., Napoli, A., Poch, O., Nguyen, N.-H., Raffelsberger, W.: Analyse de données transcriptomiques: Modélisation floue de profils dexpression différentielle et analyse fonctionnelle. In: INFORSID, pp. 413–428 (2009)
5. Martin, D., Brun, C., Remy, E., Mouren, P., Thieffry, D., Jacq, B.: GOToolBox: functional analysis of gene datasets based on Gene Ontology. Genome Biology 5(12) (2004)
6. Dennis, G., Sherman, B., Hosack, D., Yang, J., Gao, W., Lane, H., Lempicki, R.: David: Database for annotation, visualization, and integrated discovery. Genome Biology 4(9), R60 (2003), A previous version of this manuscript was made available before peer review at http://genomebiology.com/2003/4/5/P3
7. Benabderrahmane, S.: Ontology-based gene set enrichment analysis using an efficient semantic similarity measure and functional clustering. In: Proceedings of the 4th International conference on Web and Information Technologies (ICWIT 2012), Sidi Bel Abbes, Algeria, April 29-30, pp. 151–159 (2012)
8. Benabderrahmane, S., et al.: Functional classification of genes using semantic distance and fuzzy clustering approach: evaluation with reference sets and overlap analysis. I. J. Computational Biology and Drug Design 5(3/4), 245–260 (2012)
9. Sidahmed, B., et al.: Ontology-based functional classification of genes: Evaluation with reference sets and overlap analysis. In: 2011 IEEE International Conference on Bioinformatics and Biomedicine Workshops (BIBMW), pp. 201–208 (November 2011)
10. Sidahmed, B., et al.: Intelligo: a new vector-based semantic similarity measure including annotation origin. BMC Bioinformatics 11(1), 588 (2010)
11. Helene, F., et al.: Differential expression of aquaporin 8 in human colonic epithelial cells and colorectal tumors. BMC Physiology 1(1), 1 (2001)
12. Miyoshi, N., et al.: Atp11a is a novel predictive marker for metachronous metastasis of colorectal cancer. Oncology Reports 23(2), 505–510 (2010)
13. Jiang, X., et al.: Dact3 is an epigenetic regulator of wnt b catenin signaling in colorectal cancer and is a therapeutic target of histone modifications. Cancer Cell 13(6), 529–541 (2008)
14. Hiroya, T., et al.: c met expression level in primary colon cancer a predictor of tumor invasion and lymph node metastases. Clin. Cancer Res. 9(4), 1480–1488 (2003)

---

[3] http://www.omim.org/

Knowledge-Based Identification of Multicomponent Therapies

Francesca Vitali[1], Francesca Mulas[1], Pietro Marini[2], and Riccardo Bellazzi[1]

[1] Dipartimento di Ingegneria Industriale e dell'Informazione,
University of Pavia, Italy
[2] Demetra Pharmaceutical, Piacenza, Italy
francesca.vitali03@ateneopv.it, francesca.mulas@unipv.it,
scientifico@demetrapharmaceutical.it, riccardo.bellazzi@unipv.it

Abstract. In recent years, several approaches have been proposed to improve the capacity of pharmaceutical research to support personalized care. An approach that takes advantages of the large amount of biological knowledge continuously collected in different repositories could improve the drug discovery process. In this context, networks are increasingly used as universal platforms to integrate the knowledge available on a complex disease. The objective of this work is to provide a knowledge-based strategy to support polypharmacology, a new promising approach for drug discovery. Given a specific disease, the proposed method is able to identify the possible targets by analysing the topological features of the related network. The network-based analysis defines a score aimed at ranking the targets and selecting their best combinations. The results obtained on Type 2 Diabetes Mellitus highlight the ability of the method to retrieve novel target candidates related to the considered disease.

Keywords: polypharmacology, network-based bioinformatics, drug discovery, target ranking.

1 Introduction

With the growing understanding of complex diseases, the focus of drug discovery has shifted from the traditional "one target, one drug" model, designed to act on a single molecular target, to a new "multi-targets, multi-drugs" model, aimed at systemically modulating multiple targets to better treat diseases. In this context, polypharmacology has emerged as a new paradigm able to effectively implement personalized care. Network-based approaches represent elective strategies to deal with multicomponent therapeutics in complex diseases, as they "naturally" offer new therapeutic views and recommendations for drug repositioning [2].

Complex -omics interactions of the underlying disease can be conveniently represented as networks (graphs) with nodes (vertices) and links (edges) which denote molecules and interaction between them, respectively. The analysis of such networks provides insights into the disease of interest and allows identifying novel targets and drug candidates. Two key challenges facing the development

N. Peek, R. Marín Morales, and M. Peleg (Eds.): AIME 2013, LNAI 7885, pp. 94–98, 2013.

of network pharmacology are i) identifying the nodes in a biological network whose perturbation results in a desired therapeutic outcome and ii) discovering agents with the desired polypharmacology profile to perturb those nodes. A number of recent studies analysing multi-target drug discovery with a network-based approaches are reviewed in [2]. Among them Li et al. [3] utilize a biological network-based multi-target computational estimation scheme to screen anticoagulant activity of specific molecules based on affinity predictions from their multi-target docking scores and on a network efficiency analysis. The authors built a network by using the Reactome repository and designed a method for selecting targets that can be applied only to the proteins whose virtual screening is known.

In a related paper, Li, Zhang and colleagues prioritize synergistic drug combinations on the basis of a scoring function [4]. Their "target network" is built with the idea of mapping the relationships among pharmacological agents and their targets into a biological *gene* network specific for a disease. Using a similar approach, we built a *protein* network based on reliable physical interaction between proteins.

A detailed description of the proposed approach and the results obtained for the selected disease follow. Given the social impact and scientific interest and the high number of open access data, we chose to test our methods on type 2 Diabetes Mellitus (T2DM) a noteworthy example of multi-factorial and complex disease.

2   Methods

We developed a heuristic network-based method for the identification of the core disease causative pathways and the combinations of targets where it is desirable to act with a multicomponent therapy.

The method starts with the network design representing the disease as follows. Reactome [1] and STRING [2] were previously utilized to build a network whose nodes are proteins and two proteins are connected by a weighted edge if there is evidence of their association. The weights are equal to the association confidence (we considered *confidence score* > 0.7, corresponding to high confidence for the interaction predicted by STRING). Gene Expression Omnibus [3] and Stanford Microarry Database[4] were subsequently used to select the up- or down- regulated proteins by analysing human microarray data. Considering that such proteins correspond to the nodes of the network where the drug should act, we called them *disease proteins* (DP).

Afterwards, the network targeting was performed to select the candidates nodes for a multi-target therapy. We called these proteins $source_T$, because they are the sources of a potential synergistic pharmacological effect.

---

[1] http://www.reactome.org

[2] http://string-db.org/

[3] http://www.ncbi.nlm.nih.gov/sites/entrez?db=geo

[4] http://smd.stanford.edu/

2.1 Target Features

Instead of selecting all the network nodes as $source_T$ targets in order to restrict the space of the variables to the most interesting nodes, we introduced the following constraints.

First, we discarded the hub nodes, i.e. highly connected nodes. Given the high number of hub neighbours, acting on these nodes might provoke a large number of side effects. The hub identification in the network was performed by applying a method proposed by [5].

As a second constraint, we considered a variant of the bridging centrality (C_r) which can discriminate the nodes with more information flowing through them and located between highly connected regions. In our approach, $C_r(i)$ for the node i is the product of its Random Walk Betweenness Centrality (RWBC) and the bridging coefficient (BC), which measures global and local properties of i, respectively [1]. RWBC quantifies the influence of a node on the spread of information through the network, while BC assesses the node local bridging properties and penalizes nodes with high degree (hubs).

The last constraint for the $source_T$ nodes is the druggability, i.e. the ability of a protein to be targeted by a drug. To classify a protein as druggable, it had to be included in STITCH [5] and to be located in the extracellular space or in the cell membrane.

The nodes in the network with the three previously described features were identified as possible targets ($source_T$). It should be noted that a $source_T$ could be a generic protein in the network as well as a disease protein (DP).

2.2 Scoring System

The selection of the significant target combinations was performed by defining a score function *Topological Score of Drug Synergy* (TSDS) that automatically extracts protein combinations eligible for a synergistic therapy on the basis of the topological network properties. The TSDS was calculated in 3 steps.

Node reachability. A function $T_{to}DP$ assigns a score to every $source_T$ target on the basis of the topological reachability of a known DP. The $T_{to}DP$ was calculated as follows:

$$T_{to}DP(t,d) = \frac{\sum_{sh=1}^{N_{sh}} \prod_{i,j} w_{i,j}}{N_{sh}} \qquad \forall (i,j) \in sh \qquad (1)$$

where N_{sh} is the total number of shortest paths between the target t and the *Disease Node d*, *(i,j)* is a pair of nodes that belongs to the shortest path sh and $w_{i,j}$ is the edge weight between the two nodes. The function multiplies the edge weights of a shortest path ($\prod_{i,j} w_{i,j}$). Indeed a $source_T$ node t showing high weights in its own shortest paths will obtain a higher score. In this way, the best nodes are the ones with the highest confidences in their predicted relationships.

---

[5] http://stitch.embl.de/

Global Effect. The Eq.2 assigns a score to each target in relation to their global effect on all the DPs in order to construct a ranked list of targets.

$$T_{toall}DP(t) = \sum_{d=1}^{N_d} \frac{T_{to}DP(t,d)}{N_d} \tag{2}$$

where N_d is the total number of DPs and $T_{to}DP(t,d)$ is calculated as in Eq.1.

Synergistic Effect. The TSDS function, by applying the concept of polypharma-cology, assigns a score to each $source_t$ combination. This simulates simultaneous actions of multiple-agents which potentially could act on these combinations. For computational and therapeutic compliance reasons, the multi-target approach has been restricted to triplets of targets. The proposed TSDS score is given as:

$$TSDS(A,B,C) = \prod_{t \in (A,B,C)} T_{toall}DP(t) \tag{3}$$

where (A,B,C) is a triplet of targets $source_T$ and $T_{toall}DP(t)$ is obtained using the equation 2. The score is calculated for all the possible combinations of 3 $source_t$.

To validate the robustness of our constraints, the identification of the best target combinations was assessed as follow. We compute the TSDS for 50000 combinations of 3 proteins randomly selected from the complete set of nodes. With this procedure a TSDS null distribution was made and its evaluation allowed to select the significant combinations (p-value< 0.01).

3   Result and Discussion

The network built for the T2DM, following the method described in section 2, was made of 587 nodes (proteins) and 3683 edges (associations). The weights distribution of the network's edges is shown in Fig.1a.

The over- or down- expressed nodes in the network were identified from 19 and 6 data sets available in SMD and GEO. With this procedure, 87 *disease proteins* DP were selected (61 down-expressed and 26 up-expressed). The disease network is shown in Fig.1b. The nodes $source_T$ showing the features introduced by the method (see section 2.1) result 47 in total. They are the common proteins among 14 hub proteins (discarded), 314 druggable nodes and 147 bridging proteins.

The $TSDS_{norm}$ for each possible combination of 3 $source_T$ was calculated using equation 3. The null distribution construction computed allowed to select 88 significant $source_T$ triplets with a p-value< 0.01.

Among the targets identified, none with the exception of the insulin receptor is a standard target for T2DM therapy, but each of them has a strong relation with the T2DM resulting from indirect experimental observations. This absence is due to the fact that we built and analysed the network identifying the genes and consequently the proteins whose differential expression is an effect of the disease. In this way, instead of considering only the reduced insulin production and supply, which represent only one of the factors, we took into account the whole disease framework allowing the identification of novel targets.

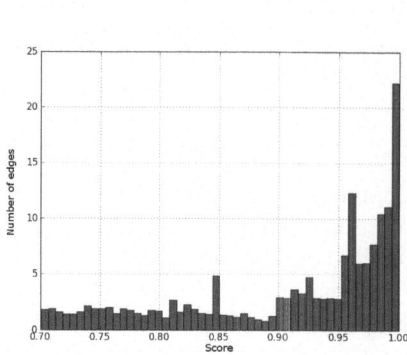

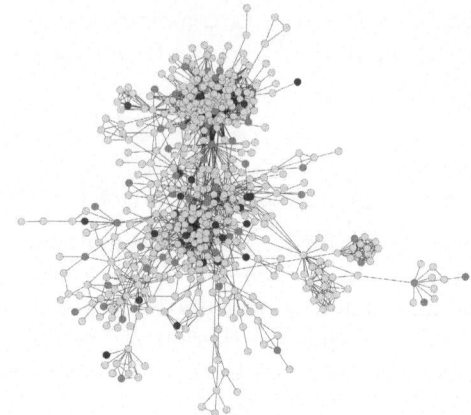

(a) Histogram of the network weights   (b) T2DM network. Up- and down- regulated nodes are respectively shown in red and green.

Fig. 1. T2DM network

4   Conclusion

The method developed in this work implemented a computational platform that integrates pathways, protein-protein interactions, transcriptional analysis to result in a comprehensive network for new multi-target discovery. Higher integration across different system biology platforms could provide mutual-support and validate data as well as speed up multi-target drug discovery. The findings obtained on Type 2 Diabetes Mellitus network demonstrate that the method could elucidate the interactions of the complex disease under study and the potential drug intervention on the target identified.

References

1. Hwang, W., Cho, R.M.: Bridging centrality: Identifying bridging nodes in scale-free networks. Technical Report, Department of Computer Science and Engineering, University at Buffalo (2006)
2. Leung, E.L., Cao, Z.W., Jiang, Z.H., Zhou, H., Liu, L.: Network-based drug discovery by integrating systems biology and computational technologies. Briefings in Bioinformatics (2012)
3. Li, Q., Li, X., Li, C., Chen, L., Song, J., Tang, Y., Xu, X.: A network-based multi-target computational estimation scheme for anticoagulant activities of compounds. PLoS ONE 6(3), e14774 (2011)
4. Li, S., Zhang, B., Zhang, N.: Network target for screening synergistic drug combinations with application to traditional chinese medicine. BMC Systems Biology 5(suppl. 1), S10 (2011)
5. Vallabhajosyula, R.R., Chakravarti, D., Lutfeali, S., Ray, A., Raval, A.: Identifying hubs in protein interaction networks. PLoS ONE 4(4), e5344 (2009)

Enhancing Random Forests Performance
in Microarray Data Classification

Nicoletta Dessì, Gabriele Milia, and Barbara Pes

Università degli Studi di Cagliari, Dipartimento di Matematica e Informatica,
Via Ospedale 72, 09124 Cagliari, Italy
{dessi,milia.ga,pes}@unica.it

Abstract. Random forests are receiving increasing attention for classification of microarray datasets. We evaluate the effects of a feature selection process on the performance of a random forest classifier as well as on the choice of two critical parameters, i.e. the forest size and the number of features chosen at each split in growing trees. Results of our experiments suggest that parameters lower than popular default values can lead to effective and more parsimonious classification models. Growing few trees on small subsets of selected features, while randomly choosing a single variable at each split, results in classification performance that compares well with state-of-art studies.

Keywords: Microarray data classification, Random Forests, Feature selection.

1   Introduction

As observed in [1], the random forest performance tends to decline when the number of features is huge and the proportion of truly informative features is small, such as with gene expression data. Thus, applying random forests in microarray data analysis presents an interesting research goal due to the additional issue of reducing the contribution of trees whose nodes are populated by non-informative features.

Pre-filtering features is a popular procedure that has proved to be useful to face the curse of dimensionality of gene expression data. When applied before growing a random forest, this process has to face an additional issue: asserting values for the two critical parameters of the random forest, i.e. the number of variables randomly chosen at each split, namely *mtry*, and the number of the trees in the forest, namely *ntree*.

This paper evaluates the effects of a filtering process on the predictive performance of a random forest classifier as well as on the choice of its critical parameters. Using two popular microarray datasets, we carried out classification experiments by growing random forests both on the whole set of features and on different subsets of pre-filtered features: different parameter settings were explored in order to investigate the optimal trade-off between the number of trees and the number of variables randomly chosen at each split. Our results suggest that growing few trees on small subsets of pre-filtered features, with only one variable randomly chosen at each split, presents results which compare very well with state-of-art studies in literature.

N. Peek, R. Marín Morales, and M. Peleg (Eds.): AIME 2013, LNAI 7885, pp. 99–103, 2013.

2   Experiments and Results

We experimented with two public microarray datasets: *Leukemia* [2] and *Colon* [3]. The overall analysis was performed using the Weka data mining environment [4]. For performance estimation, we used a standard cross-validation procedure (LOOCV), as in the majority of the papers, though it has been observed that a cross-validation setting can produce overoptimistic results on small sample size domains [5]. The performance was evaluated using the AUC (area under the ROC curve) metric in order to synthesize the information of sensitivity and specificity.

The experiments were divided into two classes:

1. *Tuning on the whole dataset.* We grew different random forests within the following parameters values: (i) *ntree* = 10, 20, 30, 50, 100, 200, 300, 500, 1000, 1500; (ii) *mtry* = 1, 2, 3, 5, 10, 20, 30, 40, 50, 80. Both the choices (i) and (ii) aim to finely explore parameters values smaller than the common default values.
2. *Tuning on filtered subsets.* First, we ranked the features of the original dataset using two popular ranking methods, i.e. *Information Gain* (IG) and *Chi Squared* (χ^2). Based on their outputs, we selected different subsets of highly-ranked features denoted in the following as TOP10 (i.e. the first 10 top-ranked features), TOP20 (i.e. the first 20 top-ranked features) and so on. Then, we used these subsets for growing random forests within the following parameter configurations: (i) *ntree* = 10, 20, 30, 50, 100, 200, 300; (ii) *mtry* = 1, 2, 3, 5, 10, 20, 30.

Results about Tuning on the Whole Dataset. Fig.1 and Fig. 2 show, for different values of *mtry*, the effects of changes in the parameter *ntree* on the AUC. As asserted by [6], the behavior of AUC is asymptotic: as the number of trees increases, the AUC value converges to a limit. Interestingly, in both *Leukemia* and *Colon*, we observed this asymptotic trend for *ntree* > 100, while previous studies [7][8] on microarray datasets made use of *ntree* values in the order of thousands. Globally, results in Fig. 1 and Fig. 2 suggest that, even on high-dimensional domains, the choice *ntree* = 100 can be quite adequate, with further increases having negligible effects and smaller values leading to more unstable AUC performance.

As regards the influence of *mtry* parameter on random forest behavior, Fig. 1 and Fig. 2 show that, for small values (≤ 50) of *ntree*, the choice of high values of *mtry* (*mtry* >= 30 for *Leukemia* and *mtry* >= 5 for *Colon*) results in higher values of AUC. This seems to suggest that, when we choose to grow a forest with a small number of trees, we need to set higher values for *mtry* in order to increase the probability of randomly selecting informative variables. On the other hand, if the forest is sufficiently large (*ntree* >= 100), the influence of *mtry* parameter decreases. In particular, no improvement in AUC performance can be observed when setting values of *mtry* > 20 and *mtry* > 10 for *Leukemia* and *Colon* respectively. Hence, as previously observed for the *ntree* parameter, the common default setting of *mtry* = sqrt(M) [7][8], where M is the dataset dimensionality, seems to be unnecessary large, with smaller values ensuring a good predictive performance at a lower computational cost.

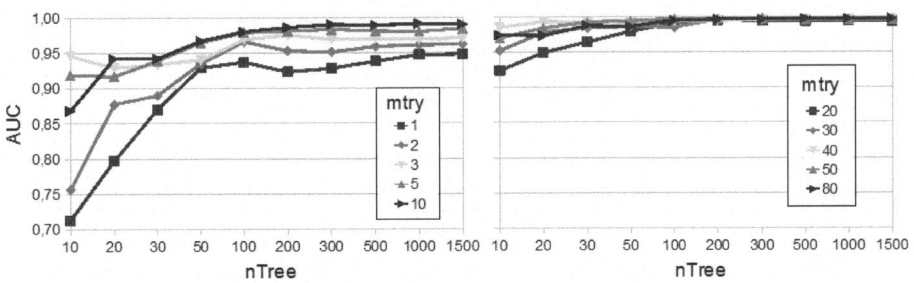

Fig. 1. Tuning on *Leukemia* dataset: AUC versus *ntree* for *mtry* = 1, 2, 3, 5, 10 (left) and *mtry* = 20, 30, 40, 50, 80 (right)

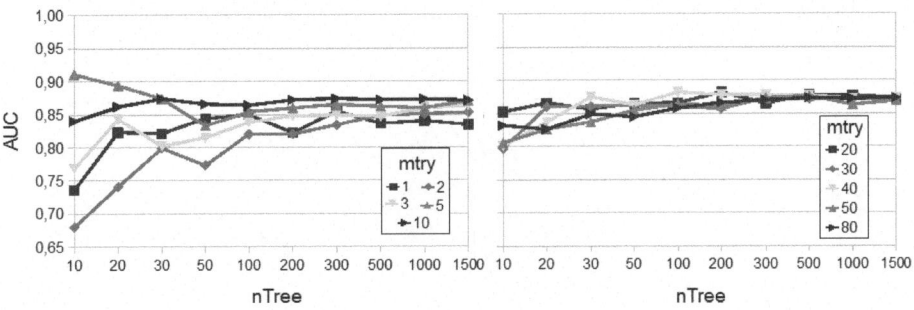

Fig. 2. Tuning on *Colon* dataset: AUC versus *ntree* for *mtry* = 1, 2, 3, 5, 10 (left) and *mtry* = 20, 30, 40, 50, 80 (right)

Results about Tuning on Filtered Subsets. As said before, we applied two ranking methods (IG and χ^2) and, for each ranking method, we performed tuning experiments on pre-filtered subsets of increasing size (TOP10, TOP20, etc). Table 1 summarizes the "optimal" values of both parameters *ntree* and *mtry*, i.e. the lowest values leading, on a given subset, to the best AUC result. As we can see, in most cases, the value *mtry* = 1 is sufficient to maximize the predictive performance of random forests. The optimal number of trees is also quite low, especially for *Leukemia*, where the AUC is maximized with at most 30 random trees. More trees (a few hundred at most) can be needed for *Colon* which is recognized to be a more noisy dataset. Results in Table 1 globally confirm what previously observed on the overall datasets: parameter values lower than common default values can lead to effective and more parsimonious classification models. Although surprising, the goodness of the choice *mtry* = 1 is also supported (for datasets of low-moderate dimensionality, as the pre-filtered datasets here considered) by some considerations reported in [6].

Additionally, the pre-filtering process significantly improves the predictive performance. As regards *Leukemia*, our experiments gave excellent AUC results in all the subsets from TOP10 to TOP500. Only for larger subsets (TOP1000), the AUC decreases if the number of random trees is not sufficiently large, as we can see in Fig. 3.a, where the AUC behavior is shown for some subsets filtered by IG (an analogous trend has been registered for χ^2) within the "optimal" setting *mtry* = 1.

Table 1. Optimal values of *mtry* and *ntree* for pre-filtered subsets of increasing size, as obtained by IG and χ^2 ranking methods, for both *Leukemia* and *Colon* datasets

Pre-filtered subset	Leukemia				Colon			
	IG		χ^2		IG		χ^2	
	mtry	*ntree*	*mtry*	*ntree*	*mtry*	*ntree*	*mtry*	*ntree*
TOP10	1	30	1	20	1	30	10	20
TOP20	1	10	1	10	1	10	1	200
TOP30	1	10	1	10	1	20	1	10
TOP50	1	10	1	20	10	10	1	10
TOP100	1	20	1	20	1	100	1	200
TOP300	1	30	1	20	1	100	1	300
TOP500	1	10	1	20	1	200	3	50

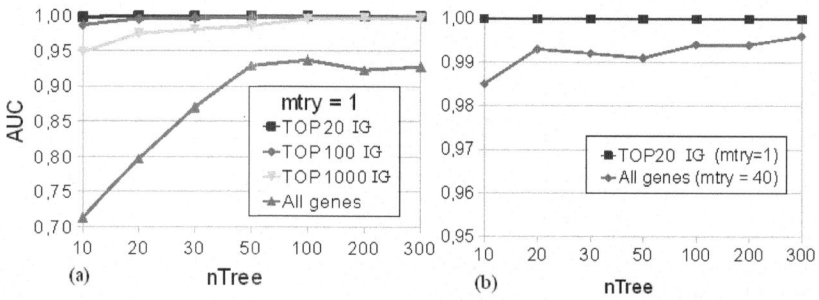

Fig. 3. Leukemia dataset: (a) AUC versus *ntree* for some pre-filtered subsets and for the whole dataset (*mtry* = 1 for all the curves); (b) AUC versus *ntree* for the subset TOP20 (*mtry* = 1) and for the whole dataset (*mtry* = 40)

Again, we notice the asymptotic behavior of AUC. The effectiveness of pre-filtering is considerable as the random forests grown on the reduced subsets greatly outperform the random forests built on the original dataset. However, the setting *mtry* = 1, optimal for the filtered subsets, is not so optimal for the whole dataset, where the best AUC performance is registered for *mtry* ≥ 30, as shown in Fig.1. Hence, a further demonstration of the effectiveness of the pre-filtering process is given in Fig. 3.b where the performance on the TOP20 subset (*mtry* = 1) is compared with the performance on the whole dataset, based on *mtry* = 40 (this value corresponds to the "best" AUC curve in Fig.1). The advantages deriving from pre-filtering are confirmed by the analysis on *Colon* dataset (here omitted for the sake of space).

Finally, Table 2 shows the effectiveness of our approach when compared to the most cited studies that applied random forests to microarray data [7] [8]. In particular, [8] reports an error rate of 0,051 for the *Leukemia* dataset (in a slightly different version) using the random forest method with *mtry* = sqrt(M) and *ntree* = 5000 and without a preliminary gene selection. Within the same settings, the error rate reported for *Colon* is 0.127. By integrating a variable selection approach, the best error rates given in [8] for *Leukemia* and *Colon* are 0,075 and 0,159 respectively. In [7], the AUC performance for *Colon* is 0.867 on the full dataset and 0,917 with gene selection; here, the best-performing configuration is selected among the following values of parameters: *ntree* = 500, 1000, 2000 and *mtry* = 0,5·sqrt(M), 1·sqrt(M), 2·sqrt(M).

Table 2. Our best results on Leukemia and Colon, both in terms of AUC and accuracy

Dataset	On the full set of genes		Using a filtered subset	
	AUC	*Accuracy*	*AUC*	*Accuracy*
Leukemia	0,997	0,986	1,00	1,00
Colon	0,911	0,855	0,939	0,903

3   Conclusions

The experimental analysis performed on two public microarray datasets reveals that a pre-filtering process positively impacts both on random forest performance and on its optimal parameterization, leading to very effective and more parsimonious classification models. Our future research will address a further potentiality of the random forest method: it can be used not only for classification but also for feature selection, due to its capacity of deriving a variable importance index.

Acknowledgments. This research was supported by RAS, Regione Autonoma della Sardegna (Legge regionale 7 agosto 2007, n. 7), in the project *"DENIS: Dataspaces Enhancing the Next Internet in Sardinia"*.

References

1. Amaratunga, D., Cabrera, J., Lee, Y.S.: Enriched random forest. Bioinformatics 24, 2010–2014 (2008)
2. Golub, T.R., et al.: Molecular Classification of Cancer: Class Discovery and Class Prediction by Gene Expression Monitoring. Science 286, 531–537 (1999)
3. Alon, U., et al.: Broad patterns of gene expression revealed by clustering analysis of tumor and normal colon tissues probed by oligonucleotide arrays. In: PNAS, vol. 96, pp. 6745–6750 (1999)
4. http://www.cs.waikato.ac.nz/ml/weka/
5. Braga-Neto, U., Dougherty, E.: Is cross-validation valid for small-sample microarray classification? Bioinformatics 20, 374–380 (2004)
6. Breiman, L.: Random forests. Machine Learning 45, 5–32 (2001)
7. Statnikov, A., Wang, L., Aliferis, C.F.: A comprehensive comparison of random forests and support vector machines for microarray-based cancer classification. BMC Bioinformatics 9, 319 (2008)
8. Dìaz-Uriarte, R., Alvarez de Andrés, S.: Gene selection and classification of microarray data using random forest. BMC Bioinformatics 7, 3 (2006)

Copy–Number Alterations
for Tumor Progression Inference

Claudia Cava[1,*], Italo Zoppis[2,*], Manuela Gariboldi[3,4], Isabella Castiglioni[1],
Giancarlo Mauri[2], and Marco Antoniotti[2]

[1] IBFM-CNR, 20090 Segrate (MI), Italy
claudia.cava@unimib.it, castiglioni.isabella@hsr.it
[2] Department of Informatics, Systems and Communications,
University of Milano–Bicocca, Milano, Italy
{zoppis,antoniotti,mauri}@disco.unimib.it
[3] Department of Experimental Oncology,
Fondazione IRCCS Istituto Nazionale dei Tumori, Milano, Italy
[4] Ifom, Fondazione Istituto FIRC Oncologia Molecolare, Milano, Italy
manuela.gariboldi@ifom.eu

Abstract. Copy–number alterations (CNAs) represent an important
component of genetic variations and play a significant role in many human diseases. Such alterations are related to certain types of cancers,
including those of the pancreas, colon, and breast, among others. CNAs
have been used as biomarkers for cancer prognosis in multiple studies,
but few works report on the relation of CNAs with the disease progression. In this paper, we provide cases where the inference on the disease
progression improves when exploiting CNA information. To this aim, a
specific dissimilarity-based representation of patients is given. The employed framework outperforms a typical approach where patients are
represented through a set of available attribute values. Three datasets
were employed to validate the results of our analysis.

Keywords: CNAs, tumor progression, dissimilarity representation.

1 Introduction

The development and progression of many solid cancers is a multi-step process, generally leading to the accumulation of chromosomal instability occurring
over the lifetime of a tumor. An important component of these instabilities
are *Copy–Number Alterations* (CNAs), i.e. regions of aberrantly increased or
decreased DNA sequences. CNAs leads to malignant transformation and progression in certain types of cancers, including those of the pancreas, colon, and
breast, among others [8]. The need for better understanding of tumor genesis
and its relationship with CNAs has led many studies to attack the problem
from different prospectives (e.g. [1]). Almost of the studies concerning CNAs
investigate the use of aberrations as biomarkers for cancer prognosis, but few

---

* C. Cava and I. Zoppis contributed equally to this work.

N. Peek, R. Marín Morales, and M. Peleg (Eds.): AIME 2013, LNAI 7885, pp. 104–109, 2013.
© Springer-Verlag Berlin Heidelberg 2013

works report on the relationship of CNAs with disease progression. In this paper we provide cases where a state-of-the-art inference method, i.e. Support Vector Machine (SVM), improves performance when using CNA-based information to forecast the tumor progression, as reflected by either the clinical *stage* classification system (CRC data) or the *histological grade* (breast data). To the best of our knowledge, we note that many studies in this context still do not consider that most real domains are best described by *structured* data where instances of multiple types are related to each other in complex ways. Following this evidence, we are interested in providing cases where a SVM-based *standard approach* (SA)[1] to predict the disease progression improves performance when explicitly exploiting CNA relationships among patients. This way, we give to the inference method a source of information that has been proved useful for both classification and clustering in many application fields [9]. Moreover, when the relationships are addressed through dissimilarities [7], the resulting patient representation is intuitively effective and is supported by the fact that classification methods can be suitably applied in the resulting "dissimilarity space". Briefly, the framework we apply quantifies relationships by defining *dissimilarities* (i.e., distances) over "advanced-stage" (patient) groups and specific "representative" base groups, e.g. patients with the lowest stage (which we will refer to as "prototype" group) [2]. Given the above concern, this paper is laid out as follows. First, in Sec. 2.1 we reports the dissimilarity-based formulation. Then, we describe three real datasets (Sec. 2.2). The first was provided, from a case-control study, by our authors at the "Fondazione IRCCS Istituto Nazionale dei Tumori" (INT), Milano, Italy. The two other datasets was downloaded from GEO to investigate further the validity of our results. In Sec. 3 we report the numerical experiments. We conclude this work in Sec. 4 by discussing some issues for future analysis.

2 Materials and Methods

2.1 Dissimilarity-Based Representation

Single nucleotide polymorphisms (SNP) is a widely used technology to detect chromosomal CNAs. SNPs are DNA sequence variations occurring when a single nucleotide (or other shared sequences) in the genome differs between either members of a biological species or paired chromosomes in an individual. To formulate the framework mentioned above, let us call CNA_c a set of m CNAs of different lengths over the chromosome c, i.e. $CNA_c = \{s_1, s_2, \ldots, s_m\}$. We assume that, for each patient x, our data consists of a CNAs' collection $\{CNA_1, CNA_2, \ldots, CNA_{22}\}$ observed over the whole set of his/her chromosomes[3]. In this paper, we summarize this information giving a *standard approach* (SA) of each case/control patient x by counting the number of such alterations over

---

[1] Where subjects are assumed to be independent and identically distributed.

[2] A detailed description, providing mathematical foundation and designed procedures based around *dissimilarities* may be found in [7].

[3] To avoid gender-related issues, we do not consider the gender-linked chromosomes.

his chromosomes. This way we represent any given patient x_1 by the vector $(x_{1,1}, x_{1,2}, \ldots, x_{1,22})$ whose jth component provides the number of alterations observed over the chromosome j, i.e. $x_{1,j} = |\text{CNA}_j|$. Our final interest is to give a *dissimilarity representation* (RA), which can express, through a function $D(x, y)$, CNA-based dissimilarity values for the pair of patients x and y. By extending $D(x, y)$ for all pairs (of patients), we can formulate a dissimilarity matrix whose rows can be assessed also by representing any patient $x \in \mathcal{X}$ through the mapping $(\mathcal{X}, \mathcal{P}) \to \mathcal{R}^n$ defined as $\varphi(x, \mathcal{P}) = [D(x, y_1), D(x, y_2), \ldots, D(x, y_n)]$ where, $\mathcal{X}$ and $\mathcal{P}$ respectively denote a set of *case/control patients* and a set of n *prototype patients*. Here the difference between $\mathcal{X}$ and $\mathcal{P}$ reflects the need to discriminate case/control patients in $\mathcal{X}$ as compared to a common set of n prototype patients in $\mathcal{P}^4$. A critical aspect of this representation concerns the definition of a well-discriminating dissimilarity function D for non-trivial learning problems. In this paper we empirically evaluate the following two ordinary metrics. (i) *Euclidean distance* and (ii) *Manhattan distance*.

2.2   Datasets and Inference Procedure

The framework described in the previous sections was applied on the following three (GEO) datasets. (i) GEO16125 [5]: 10 stage-II patients (*Duke* stage classification system), 10 stage-III patients and 23 stage-IV patients. (II) GSE11417: 3 patients with stage 1 (*Duke* system), 46 patients with stage 2, 37 patients with stage 3 and 8 patients with stage 4. (III) GSE16619: 9 patients with histological grade I, 38 with grade II and 66 with grade III [6]. To evaluate the performances of RA as compared with SA, we designed a *Rapid Miner* (RM) *workflow* (WF) [6]. RM is a software environment for rapid prototyping of machine learning and knowledge discovery processes. It is currently used for classification, clustering, and also data integration tasks (e.g., [10]). Basically, we implement standard Support Vector Machine (SVM) as "black box" inference processes to score each input *datatype* according to the inference performance of the algorithm [3]. The main issues of this WF are characterized by the following (sub)processes. (I) **Parameter Optimization**. We employed this (sub)process to optimize the inference *accuracy* and to find the best parameter combination for the SVM learning process. (II) **Cross Validation** encapsulates a *k-fold cross validation process*. First a classifier is built describing a predetermined set of data classes. Then a trained SVM is used for testing new classification examples.

---

[4] The choice of a correct prototype set can be critical in this approach. Here we use the group with the lowest stage (CRC) or the lowest grade (breast). As our data does not provide a sufficient number of stage-I patients, we use the stage-II patients as the *prototype set* for CRC.

[5] Provided by our authors at the INT and deposited on GEO.

[6] GSE11417 and GSE16619 have been previously used in [5] and [4]. In these works new CNAs linked to patient prognosis and new amplified loci in primary breast tumor are relieved.

3   Results

The main issue of our investigation was to provide cases where the inference on the disease progression improves performance when exploiting CNA information. All numerical experiments were evaluated through sensitivity (*sens*), specificity (*spec*), positive predictive value (*PPV*), negative predictive values (*NPV*), accuracy (*acc*) and balanced accuracy (*blacc*) [2][7]. In order to give an overall judgment, for each dataset we compared RA (d_1 and d_2) and SA (d_0) by averaging the performances over the three considered tasks (see *Average Performances*). For a better visualization, we highlighted those RA values which are lower than their corresponding SA performance indexes, thus reporting lower RA performances. First we notice that dataset GSE16619 is the one where RA has a better behavior, outperforming SA for all the considered indexes. On the contrary, GSE11417 reports for *stage II vs III* the worst RA behavior. In this case, d_2 is not able to increase the performance of d_0, while d_1 is quite comparable with d_0 reporting, at most, an increase of specificity not higher than 2.17%. Differently, the other two tasks are complexively better for RA. Also, we notice that in GSE16125, d_1 and d_2 (even with a lower sensibility) are able, for the *stage II vs IV* task, to balance better the accuracy of d_0 which, in turn, is sensibility biased (sensibility 100% vs specificity 30%). The remaining indexes are (out of 4 values) favorable for RA. Finally we notice that the average performances are clearly better for RA which improves (out of 1 time) all the considered performances. From the above observations, we can say that RA, with the provided distances, have an overall better (average) behavior when compared with the considered typical approach on the employed datasets.

	GSE16125 stage II vs III			stage II vs IV			stage III vs IV			GSE11417 stage II vs III			stage II vs IV			stage III vs IV		
	d0	d1	d2	d0	d1	d2	d0	d1	d2	d0	d1	d2	d0	d1	d2	d0	d1	d2
sens	80	*70*	80	100	*95.65*	*95.65*	82.61	95.65	95.65	72,97	*70,27*	72,97	37,50	37,50	37,50	37,50	62,50	37,50
spec	80	90	90	30	70	60	70	80	80	71,74	73,91	*67,39*	95,65	100	100	100	*97,30*	100
PPV	80	87.5	88.89	76.67	88	84.62	86.36	91.67	91.67	67,50		*64,29*	60	100	100	100	*83,33*	100
NPV	80	*75*	81.82	100	*87.5*	*85.71*	63.64	88.89	88.89	76,74	*75,56*	*75,61*	89,80	90,20	90,20	88.1	92,31	88,10
acc	80	80.95	85.71	78.79	87.88	84.85	78.79	90.91	90.91	72,22	72,35	*69,97*	87,04	90,74	90,74	88.89	91,11	88,89
blacc	80	80	85	65	82.83	77.83	76.31	87.83	87.83	72,36	*72,09*	*70,18*	66,58	68,75	68,75	68.75	79,90	68,75

	GSE16619 grade II vs III			grade I vs II			grade I vs III			AV PERF. GSE16125			GSE11417			GSE16619		
	d0	d1	d2	d0	d1	d2	d0	d1	d2	d0	d1	d2	d0	d1	d2	d0	d1	d2
sens	84.85	87,88	84.85	97.37	100	100	11.11	44.44	33.33	87.54	87.1	90.43	49.32	56.76	49.32	94.07	95.95	94.95
spec	55.26	68.42	65.79	55.56	66.67	55.56	100	100	100	60	80	76.77	89.13	90.4	89.13	40.64	59.84	51.56
PPV	76.71	82.86	81.16	90.24	92.68	90.48	89.19	92.96	91.67	81.01	89.06	88.39	75.83	83.92	88.1	85.38	89.5	87.77
NPV	67.74	76.47	71.43	83.33	100	100	100	100	100	81.01	83.8	85.47	84.88	86.02	*84.64*	83.69	92.16	90.48
acc	74.03	80.76	77.93	89.44	93.61	91.53	89.33	93.33	92	79.19	86.58	87.16	82.72	84.73	83.2	84.27	89.23	87.15
blacc	70.06	78.15	75.32	76.47	83.84	77.78	55.56	72.22	66.67	73.77	83.55	83.55	69.23	73.58	69.23	67.36	77.9	73.26

Fig. 1. Performances. d_0: SA; d_1: Euclidean distance; d_2: Manhattan distance

---

[7] The following values are used in RM. *kernel.γ*: from 0 to 5, step 35; *kernel.C*: from 0 to 5, step 35; *kernel.type* ∈ {ANOVA, DOT, RADIAL}. See http://rapid-i.com

4   Conclusion

Previous studies integrating gene expression and CNA data have shown that changes in gene expression level between normal and tumor tissue can be associated with, and presumably caused by, changes in copy number of contiguous genes along chromosome segments. In this paper, we demonstrated that even a prediction analysis, concerning the disease progression as characterized by the considered *progression's marker* (stage or grade) improves performance when using CNA-based information and RA representation of patients. Our approach allowed SVMs to outperform SA of representation where patients are expressed by their set of available attribute values. The choice of a correct prototype set can be critical in this context. We did not study the best possible prototype set, instead we used the group with the lowest available progression's marker. An interesting extension to this work could be provided by integrating different CNA-based information, e.g. concerning chromosome specific regions or the *probe* number used for each aberrant region.

References

1. Bomme, L., Bardi, G., Pandis, N., Fenger, C., Kronborg, O., Heim, S.: Clonal karyotypic abnormalities in colorectal adenomas: clues to the early genetic events in the adenoma-carcinoma sequence. Genes Chrom. Cancer 10(3), 190–196 (1994)
2. Davis, J., Goadrich, M.: The relationship between precision-recall and roc curves. In: Proc. of the 23rd Int. Conf. on Machine Learning, ICML 2006, pp. 233–240 (2006)
3. Guyon, I., Gunn, S., Nikravesh, M., Zadeh, L.: Feature Extraction: Foundations and Applications. Springer (2006)
4. Kadota, M., Sato, M., Duncan, B., Ooshima, A., Yang, H.H., Diaz-Meyer, N., Gere, S., Kageyama, S.I., Fukuoka, J., Nagata, T., Tsukada, K., Dunn, B.K., Wakefield, L.M., Lee, M.P.: Identification of novel gene amplifications in breast cancer and coexistence of gene amplification with an activating mutation of pik3ca. Cancer Res. 69(18), 7357–7365 (2009)
5. Kurashina, K., Yamashita, Y., Ueno, T., Koinuma, K., Ohashi, J., Horie, H., Miyakura, Y., Hamada, T., Haruta, H., Hatanaka, H., Soda, M., Choi, Y.L., Takada, S., Yasuda, Y., Nagai, H., Mano, H.: Chromosome copy number analysis in screening for prognosis-related genomic regions in colorectal carcinoma. Cancer Sci. 99(9), 1835–1840 (2008)
6. Mierswa, I., Wurst, M., Klinkenberg, R., Scholz, M., Euler, T.: Yale: Rapid prototyping for complex data mining tasks. In: KDD 2006, pp. 935–940 (2006)
7. Pekalska, E., Duin, R.P.W.: The Dissimilarity Representation for Pattern Recognition: Foundations and Applications. In: Machine Perception and Artificial Intelligence. World Scientific Publishing Company (2005)
8. Reid, J.F., Gariboldi, M., Sokolova, V., Capobianco, P., Lampis, A., Perrone, F., Signoroni, S., Costa, A., Leo, E., Pilotti, S., Pierotti, M.A.: Integrative approach for prioritizing cancer genes in sporadic colon cancer. Genes Chrom. Cancer 48(11), 953–962 (2009)

9. Zoppis, I., Borsani, M., Gianazza, E., Chinello, C., Rocco, F., Albo, G., Deelder, A.M., van der Burgt, Y.E.M., Magni, F., Antoniotti, M., Mauri, G.: Analysis of correlation structures in renal cell carcinoma patient data. In: BIOINF, pp. 251–256. SciTe Press (2012)

10. Zoppis, I., Gianazza, E., Borsani, M., Chinello, C., Mainini, V., Galbusera, C., Ferrarese, C., Galimberti, G., Sorbi, S., Borroni, B., Magni, F., Antoniotti, M., Mauri, G.: Mutual information optimization for mass spectra data alignment. IEEE/ACM Trans. Comp. Biol. Bioinf. 9(3), 934–939 (2012)

Constraining Protein Docking with Coevolution Data for Medical Research

Ludwig Krippahl, Fábio Madeira, and Pedro Barahona

CENTRIA, FCT-UNL
{ludi,pb}@fct.unl.pt

Abstract. Protein interaction is essential to all biological systems, from the assembly of multimeric complexes to processes such as transport, catalysis and gene regulation. Unfortunately, the prediction of protein-protein interactions is a difficult problem, often with modest success rates, in part because docking algorithms must filter a very large number of possibilities and then attempt to identify a correct model among many incorrect candidates. This paper presents a scoring function to estimate contacts in coevolving proteins, shows how the predicted contacts can constrain the filtering stage and significantly reduce the number of incorrect candidates, and illustrates the application of this method to the docking of two complexes of medical relevance, one involving a chromosome condensation regulator homologous to a protein responsible for retinitis pigmentosa and the other a cyclin-dependent kinase, a likely target for cancer therapy.

Keywords: Protein docking, coevolution, constraints.

1 Introduction

Although approximately twenty thousand non-redundant structures are deposited in the Protein Data Bank (PDB), less than 1% are experimentally determined non-obligatory protein complexes [1]. Given the importance of protein interaction for medical research and drug design (e.g. [2,3]), the prediction of these structures is an important computational problem. Protein docking methods consist of two main stages [4]: a search stage that filters a set of billions of models for the interaction of the two proteins and a scoring stage to select, and possibly refine, the most promising candidates from a sub-set of thousands retained during the first stage. Thus, one way of improving the process is to reduce the number of models that need to be retained in the first stage without losing the correct models, which can be done in BiGGER (Bimolecular complex Generation with Global Evaluation and Ranking) [5,6] by propagating contact constraints derived from estimates of coevolution in Multiple Sequence Alignments (MSA). This is the motivation for the work reported in this paper.

N. Peek, R. Marín Morales, and M. Peleg (Eds.): AIME 2013, LNAI 7885, pp. 110–114, 2013.
© Springer-Verlag Berlin Heidelberg 2013

2   Method

From the protein-protein docking benchmark version 4.0 [1], we selected the 14 binary complexes that were not antibody-antigen interactions, had at least 90% of the residues in the structure file and for which homologous sequences were found in at least 100 different organisms. For these 14 complexes (28 proteins) we collected related sequences using PSI-BLAST [7] and calculated the MSA using ClustalW [8]. The sequences were then matched by source organism to screen the MSA for coevolution across the interaction partners using 13 published measures (see Results, below) using Pycoevol [9]. The ranking of the highest scoring correct contact in each case was compared to the ranking obtained with our Estimated Coevolution Score (ECS). ECS evaluates each pair of residues, one residue from each partner, by the weighted average of three factors. The first, with relative weight one, is sequence conservation measured as the fraction of sequences containing the same amino acid residue at that position. The second factor, with relative weight of two, is the average contact propensity for the pair of residues (one from each partner) in those positions measured across all sequences. The third factor, with weight three, is the average contact propensity for the patches of surface residues formed by the immediate neighbors at the surface of the protein. These relative weights model the increasing importance from conservation to single amino acid interaction to the interaction of the neighboring surface patch. For scoring contact propensities we used the contact propensity matrix in [10], but ignoring Cys-Cys contacts, generally involved in covalent bonds. We illustrate the application of this method to medically relevant protein interactions with a complex of human cyclin-dependent kinase 2 (CDK2) and a cell-cycle regulatory protein (CKSHS1), a likely target for anti-cancer drugs, and a complex of chromosome condensation regulator (RCC1) with a GTP-binding nuclear protein involved in retinitis pigmentosa (RAN). All docking simulations were run on an AMD Phenom II processor, at 3.1GHz. The times reported are CPU processing times for the search stage, including constraint propagation.

3   Results

Table 1 compares the mean, median and maximum positions of the highest scoring correct contact for ECS and the other scores found in the literature. The two closest to ECS, contact preferences volume normalized (CPVN) [17] and residue-residue volume derived matrix (VOL) [19] have similar medians but significantly higher average and maximum values. Since the objective is to restrict the docking search space without losing correct models, the best measure is the ECS, which allows us to use the smallest set of predicted contacts that still contain at least one correct contact. Table 2 compares the ranking of the top scoring correct contact in our method (ECS) and the two closest measures (CPVN and VOL) for the 14 test cases. While ECS scores a correct contact in the top 100 in all cases, the upper bound for the other estimates is significantly higher, which would require the retention of a much larger set of candidates.

Table 1. Summary of the coevolution score results, showing the mean, median and maximum ranking of the top scoring correct contact, for each method, over the 14 tested complexes. In order, our ECS; Mutual Information (MI) [11]; normalized MI (NMI) [12]; Row and Column Weighed MI (RCW) [13]; Pearson's correlation (PC) [14]; Spearman's rank correlation (SRC) [15]; McLachlan Based Substitution Correlation (BASC) [16];contact preferences volume normalized (CPVN) [17]; contact PDB-derived likelihood matrix (CLM) [18]; and a residue-residue volume derived matrix (VOL) [19]; Observed Minus Expected Squared (OMES) [20];Quartets (QTETS) [21]; Statistical Coupling Analysis (SCA) [22]; Explicit Likelihood of Subset Covariation (ELSC) [23].

	ESC	MI	NMI	RCW	PC	SRC	BASC	CPVN	CLM	VOL	OMES	QTETS	SCA	ELSC
Mean	35	1194	870	935	611	765	524	68	573	116	990	1217	409	828
Median	22	730	298	273	252	443	224	26	411	17	208	712	159	745
Max	91	5801	4596	5721	3504	4291	3490	380	2352	883	3886	6306	1499	2416

The rankings of the top scoring correctly predicted interface residues are shown only for ECS because these are derived from the pairwise contact scores.

The unconstrained docking of RCC1 and RAN (1i2m in Table 2) took 107 minutes. From the 5000 models retained at the search stage only 5 had a backbone rmsd below 3Å when compared to the 1i2m structure, the highest ranking of which was ranked by BiGGER in position 375 in the shape complementarity score used to screen candidates during the search stage. In contrast, imposing the residue contact identified in position 17 on our contact prediction score (Val96-Met77) to restrict the search space, there were 3 models with a rmsd below 3Å in just 10 models retained, the highest ranking one in second place, with a search time of 5 minutes. This means that even screening the 100 highest ranking contacts, keeping 10 models for each, would reduce the candidate set by 80%, from 5000 to 1000, while retaining at least one correct model. Though computation time would increase fivefold, to approximately 8 hours, this is a less important aspect than the improvement in the results, especially since these are all independent docking runs and trivial to compute in parallel.

In the case of the human cyclin-dependent kinase 2 complex with CKSHS1 (structure 1buh in Table 2), the first correctly predicted contact is only ranked in 78th place. While the unconstrained docking took 66 minutes and resulted in 5 models with less than 3Å RMSD within the set of 5000 models retained (the top ranking one in position 658), restricting the search to the correct contact (Phe213-Tyr12) predicted in rank 78 resulted in 2 models below 3Å RMS within a set of 10 in 7 minutes of CPU time. A screening of the top 100 predicted pairwise contacts would still reduce by 80% the number of models to retain, though it would require approximately 12 hours of CPU time. An alternative constraint is to require at least one contact between the sets of the top scoring predicted interface residues. This allowed a 90% reduction in the total number of models to consider (500 instead of 5000) while still retaining 4 models below the 3Å rmsd threshold and also cut computation time to 38 minutes from 66 for the unconstrained docking.

Table 2. For each complex in the test set, this table shows the PDB identifier; the ranking of the top correctly predicted interface residues for monomers A and B with the ECS (ECS-A and ECS-B); the ranking of the top correctly predicted pairwise contact with ECS; and the ranking and of the top correctly predicted pairwise contact for our ECS and the two best scores from the literature [17,19]

PDB	ECS-A	ECS-B	ECS	CPVN	VOL	PDB	ECS-A	ECS-B	ECS	CPVN	VOL
2cfh	2	2	38	13	177	2pcc	17	2	84	128	273
3cph	1	1	1	1	3	2z0e	2	1	9	29	2
1i2m	1	1	17	100	34	1ewy	1	1	3	17	11
1buh	4	3	78	27	4	2o8v	12	4	39	3	1
1jk9	1	1	1	8	23	1f6m	7	1	27	60	6
1gpw	1	1	17	1	5	1gla	20	2	91	380	883
1e6e	3	1	12	24	164	2ido	8	3	67	157	35

4   Conclusions

This paper addresses an important problem in protein docking, which is how to minimize the set of candidate models from which the correct complex structures must be obtained without risking the loss of those correct structures. To this end, we present a method that uses readily available sequence information to estimate contacts between surface residues from the traces that coevolution left in the sequences of homologous proteins in different organisms. One contribution of this paper is the score itself, which outperforms, for this particular purpose, all 13 scores we tested from the literature. The other contribution is the application of these predicted contacts as constraints to prune the docking search. For this, we present two different approaches. The first is to screen specific contacts individually, each constraining the search to a small set of possibilities, and then aggregating the models obtained from all searches. The second is to predict interface residues from coevolution data and then constrain the docking search by requiring contacts between any residues in the predicted sets. In both cases we show a significant reduction in false positives in the candidate models retained during the search stage of docking.

Aknowledgments. This work was supported by portuguese national funds from Fundação para a Ciência e Tecnologia under project PTDC/EIA-CCO/115999/2009.

References

1. Hwang, H., Vreven, T., Janin, J., Weng, Z.: Protein-protein docking benchmark version 4.0. Proteins 78(15) (November 2010)
2. Arkin, M.R., Wells, J.A.: Small-molecule inhibitors of protein-protein interactions: progressing towards the dream. Nat. Rev. Drug Discov. 3(4) (April 2004)

3. Archakov, A.I., Govorun, V.M., Dubanov, A.V., Ivanov, Y.D., Veselovsky, A.V., Lewi, P., Janssen, P.: Protein-protein interactions as a target for drugs in proteomics. Proteomics 3(4) (April 2003)
4. Janin, J.: Protein-protein docking tested in blind predictions: the capri experiment. Mol. Biosyst. 6(12) (December 2010)
5. Palma, P.N., Krippahl, L., Wampler, J.E., Moura, J.J.: Bigger: a new (soft) docking algorithm for predicting protein interactions. Proteins 39(4) (June 2000)
6. Krippahl, L., Barahona, P.: Applying constraint programming to rigid body protein docking. In: van Beek, P. (ed.) CP 2005. LNCS, vol. 3709, pp. 373–387. Springer, Heidelberg (2005)
7. Altschul, S.F., Madden, T.L., Schäffer, A.A., Zhang, J., Zhang, Z., Miller, W., Lipman, D.J.: Gapped blast and psi-blast: a new generation of protein database search programs. Nucleic Acids Res. 25(17) (September 1997)
8. Chenna, R., Sugawara, H., Koike, T., Lopez, R., Gibson, T.J., Higgins, D.G., Thompson, J.D.: Multiple sequence alignment with the clustal series of programs. Nucleic Acids Res. 31(13) (July 2003)
9. Madeira, F., Krippahl, L.: Pycoevol - a python workflow to study protein-protein coevolution. In: Schier, J., Correia, C.M.B.A., Fred, A.L.N., Gamboa, H. (eds.) Bioinformatics, pp. 143–149. SciTePress (2012)
10. Jha, A.N., Vishveshwara, S., Banavar, J.R.: Amino acid interaction preferences in proteins. Protein Sci. 19(3) (March 2010)
11. Martin, L.C., Gloor, G.B., Dunn, S.D., Wahl, L.M.: Using information theory to search for co-evolving residues in proteins. Bioinformatics 21(22) (November 2005)
12. Gloor, G.B., Martin, L.C., Wahl, L.M., Dunn, S.D.: Mutual information in protein multiple sequence alignments reveals two classes of coevolving positions. Biochemistry 44(19) (May 2005)
13. Gouveia-Oliveira, R., Pedersen, A.G.: Finding coevolving amino acid residues using row and column weighting of mutual information and multi-dimensional amino acid representation. Algorithms Mol. Biol. 2 (2007)
14. Göbel, U., Sander, C., Schneider, R., Valencia, A.: Correlated mutations and residue contacts in proteins. Proteins 18(4) (April 1994)
15. Pazos, F., Helmer-Citterich, M., Ausiello, G., Valencia, A.: Correlated mutations contain information about protein-protein interaction. J. Mol. Biol. 271(4) (August 1997)
16. Fodor, A.A., Aldrich, R.W.: Influence of conservation on calculations of amino acid covariance in multiple sequence alignments. Proteins 56(2) (August 2004)
17. Glaser, F., Steinberg, D.M., Vakser, I.A., Ben-Tal, N.: Residue frequencies and pairing preferences at protein-protein interfaces. Proteins 43(2) (May 2001)
18. Singer, M.S., Vriend, G., Bywater, R.P.: Prediction of protein residue contacts with a pdb-derived likelihood matrix. Protein Eng. 15(9) (September 2002)
19. Esque, J., Oguey, C., de Brevern, A.G.: A novel evaluation of residue and protein volumes by means of laguerre tessellation. J. Chem. Inf. Model. 50(5) (May 2010)
20. Kass, I., Horovitz, A.: Mapping pathways of allosteric communication in groel by analysis of correlated mutations. Proteins 48(4) (September 2002)
21. Galitsky, B.: Revealing the set of mutually correlated positions for the protein families of immunoglobulin fold. In Silico Biol. 3(3) (2003)
22. Lockless, S.W., Ranganathan, R.: Evolutionarily conserved pathways of energetic connectivity in protein families. Science 286(5438) (October 1999)
23. Dekker, J.P., Fodor, A., Aldrich, R.W., Yellen, G.: A perturbation-based method for calculating explicit likelihood of evolutionary co-variance in multiple sequence alignments. Bioinformatics 20(10) (July 2004)

Single- and Multi-label Prediction of Burden on Families of Schizophrenia Patients

Pablo Bermejo[1,*], Marta Lucas[2], José A. Rodríguez-Montes[3],
Pedro J. Tárraga[4], Javier Lucas[5], José A. Gámez[1], and José M. Puerta[1]

[1] University of Castilla-La Mancha, Albacete, Spain
Pablo.Bermejo@uclm.es
[2] Almansa General Hospital, Almansa, Spain
[3] La Paz University Hospital, Madrid, Spain
[4] Primary Care Management Office, Albacete, Spain
[5] Primary Care Consultation, Elche de la Sierra, Spain

Abstract. Whereas there exist questionnaires used to measure the level of anxiety or depression in caregivers of schizophrenia patients, sometimes these symptoms take too long to be detected and the treatment needed is more difficult than it would have been if the burden had been detected at an earlier stage. In this paper we propose the use of automatic classification techniques to predict the output of such questionnaires (Hamilton and ECFOS-II), making it possible to anticipate an appropriate treatment or advice for the family caregivers from Primary Care consultations. In particular, we apply standard (one class variable) and multi-dimensional classification approaches to predict caregiver anxiety, depression and answers to questionnaires. Our study has been carried out with a dataset containing data from 180 schizophrenia patients and their caregivers, and the results are very promising, obtaining accuracies of approximately 96%.

Keywords: burden prediction, multi-label, Primary Care consultation.

1   Introduction

After the Psychiatric Reform was implemented in Spain at the beginning of the last century, the deinstitutionalization of patients with severe mental illness and their consequent return to their homes, led to an increase in the burden experienced by their caregivers; and this is an area of particular interest. Family caregivers of patients with schizophrenia experience high levels of burden. The treatment and care of schizophrenic patients is predominantly at community level; patients who are symptomatic have many psychiatric hospitalizations but the continuity of care and supervision rests with families.

The prevalence of schizophrenia is between 1 and 1.9% of the population. It is a disorder with a complex and highly variable clinical expression that is caused by a combination of genetic and environmental factors. Schizophrenia usually

---

* Corresponding author.

N. Peek, R. Marín Morales, and M. Peleg (Eds.): AIME 2013, LNAI 7885, pp. 115–124, 2013.
© Springer-Verlag Berlin Heidelberg 2013

starts between one's late teens and mid-30s, the onset in men being a few years earlier than in women [1].

An estimated 50 to 80% of schizophrenic patients live with, or have regular contact with, a family caregiver. Because of the emotional, social and financial impacts that schizophrenia has on a family, members of the family should support each other. The family burden experienced by caregivers of people with schizophrenia is one of the most significant consequences of this disorder. The greatest impact occurs in physical, psychological, economic, family, social, and occupational aspects; this may lead to limitations in daily life, with high levels of dependency, suffering, disagreement, family disruption and restricted social activity [7,4]. It is easy for a family caregiver to burn out.

To evaluate the impact of schizophrenia on primary caregivers we use scales with several limitations: they are not specific to the actual caregivers, they are not adapted to their mother tongue, they do not include subjective aspects and they need a long time to complete. It would be useful to be able to predict the levels of anxiety and depression before the caregivers start to take responsibility for the patients. We could thus choose the appropriate treatment and, consequently, early treatment intervention would shorten the length of the episode.

In the literature we can find two different studies related with the prediction of burden on schizophrenia caregivers [3,5]. These cases a regression model is built from 70 and 101 caregivers, respectively. The model in [3] achieves an R^2 statisticns of 0.4, while the one used in [5] raises this figure to 0.77. In both cases, all the data is used to learn the model and no validation scores are provided.

In this article we present a predictive study on a database of 180 patients diagnosed with schizophrenia and their caregivers in the province of Albacete (Spain) during 2006-2011. Unlike the two studies mentioned above, we based our study on supervised classification instead of regression. In our study we can distinguish two different parts: (1) prediction of depression and anxiety levels in caregivers, which is tackled by means of standard classification; and (2) prediction of caregivers' answers to the ECFOS-II questionnaire. This second task needs to simultaneously deal with several class (target) variables, so we approach the problem as a multi-dimensional classification one [11] which aims to predict not the value of a class variable, but to simultaneously predict several variables or labels given another set of input values.

From our experiments, validated by using leave-one-out cross-validation, reach an important conclusion: it is possible to predict the level of depression and anxiety in caregivers by using the usual and easy-to-acquire variables obtained during clinical interviews.

The rest of the paper is organized as follows. The next section describes the input and output data over which we carried out the study. Then Sections 3 and 4 describe the two classification tasks dealt with in our work. Finally, in Section 5 we present our conclusions.

2   Data

As mentioned above, our goal is to predict the output of two different questionnaires (Hamilton and ECFOS-II), without the patients and/or caregivers having to fill them in. To acheive this we count on a set of input variables that have been selected by the doctors as relevant, and which are also *easy* to obtain: patient or caregiver history data, test-based data, and data obtained by direct interview of doctor-caregiver/patient. Below we describe both the input data and the two target questionnaires (output data).

2.1   Input Data

During the years 2008-2011, a database of 180 cases was compiled at the *Hospital Universitario of Albacete, (Spain)*, where each case corresponds to a set of variables describing both the schizophrenia patients and the main caregiver registered. The variables are shown in Table 1. The 30 collected variables are evenly divided, 15 are related with the patient and 15 with the main associated caregiver.

Regarding patients, the variables are mainly related with schizophrenia, including:

- EEAG (Evaluation Scale for Global Activity) [2]: a numeric scale (0 through 100) used by mental health clinicians and physicians to subjectively rate the ability of adults to function in daily life. It considers psychological, social, and occupational functioning on a hypothetical continuum of mental health-illness. The scale is divided into 10 ranges of functioning.
- PANSS (Positive and Negative Syndrome Scale) [8]: a medical scale used for measuring symptom severity in patients with schizophrenia. The PANSS is obtained via a relatively brief interview, requiring 45 to 50 minutes to administer. All sixteen items in the PANSS range from one to seven, resulting in a minimum total score of sixteen; this implies that the PANSS is an interval scale.

Regarding caregivers, most outcomes are qualitative and easy to obtain, as we can observe in Table 1. From here on we will refer to these variables as $\mathbf{X} = \{P_1, \ldots, P_{15}, CG_1, \ldots, CG_{15}\}$, which will be used as predictive attributes in our classification tasks.

2.2   Output Data - Evaluation Questionnaires

As output data we will work with two different questionnaires: the Hamilton Rating Scale for Depression and Anxiety, and the Subjective and Objective Family Burden Interview (ECFOS II). Although our goal is to avoid the need of filling in these questionnaires for our training data we do of course need that information. Thus, for the 180 cases of patients with schizophrenia mentioned above, their caregivers were interviewed in order to fill in both questionnaires. Special care was taken in this process. A brief description of the two questionnaires is given below:

Table 1. Descriptive variables of caregiver (c-) and patient (p-)

Name	Type	Description
c-AGE	Numeric	Caregiver's age
c-TSH	Numeric	Caregiver's TSH levels
c-T4	Numeric	Caregiver's T4 levels
c-RELATIONSHIP_DEGREE	Spouse, Parent, Child, Brother-Sister, Other	Patient-Caregiver relationship
c-ORIGIN	Rural, Urban	Caregiver's social origins
c-LIVETOGETHER	Yes, No	Patient and Caregiver live together
c-GENDER	Male, Female	Caregiver's gender
c-EMPLOYMENT_STATUS	Full, Partial, Unemp	Caregiver's employment status
c-STUDIES_DEGREE	Illiterate, Read_Write, Basic, Medium, High	Caregiver's studies degree
c-HYPOTHYROIDISM	Yes, No	Patient's and Caregiver's hypothyroidism
c-RELATIONSHIP_FREQ	1h/week, $< 0.5h/day, 0.5 - 1h/day, 1 - 2h/day, 2 - 3h/day, 3 - 4h/day, > 4h/day$	Frequency of relationship between patients and Caregiver's
c-CAREGIVER_QUALITY	Excel,good,normal,not bad,bad,very bad	Quality of patient's relationship
c-PATIENT_QUALITY	Excel,good,normal,not bad,bad,very bad	Quality of caregiving relationship
c-THYROID_TREATMENT	Yes, No	Caregiver's hypothyroidism treatment
c-PSICOFARM_TREATMENT	Yes, No	Caregiver's psychopharmacology treatment
p-GENDER	Male,Female	Patient gender
p-ORIGIN	Rural, Urban	Patient's social origin
p-EMERGENCY_last_6months	Yes, No	Psych. emergency Services for patients in hospital.
p-ADMISSION_last_9months	Yes, No	Psych. hospitalization to stabilize symptoms.
p-PSICOTIC-ADMISSION	Yes, NoS	Psych. hospitalization for patients to stabilize psychotic symptoms
p-PSICOFARM_TREATMENT	Risperidone, Atyp. oral neuroleptic, typical inject.-neuroleptic	Patient's psychopharmacology treatments
p-SCHIZOPH_TYPE	Paranoid,Catatonic,Residual,Undifferentiated,Unorganized	Patient's Schizophrenia type
p-EEAG	Numeric [1-11]	Ranges of patient's functioning
p-ILLNESS_YEARS	Numeric	Years of illness
p-PANSSpositive	Numeric	Total score of positive symptoms
p-PANSSnegative	Numeric	Total score of negative symptoms
p-PANSS-PG	Numeric	Total score of psychopathology symptoms
p-PANSS-COMPOSED	Numeric	Total score of positive negative score
p-TSH	Numeric	Patient's TSH levels
p-T4	Numeric	Patient's T4 levels

• Hamilton Rating Scale for Depression and Anxiety (HDRS and HAM-A) [10,6]. It is used to rate the severity of caregiver depression/anxiety. The depression questionnaire (HDRS) contains 17 items pertaining to symptoms of depression experienced over the past week. Each question has between 3-5 possible responses which increase in severity. It requires about 20-30 minutes.

In the case of anxiety, the questionnaire (HAM-A) contains 14 items. The values on the scale range from zero to four: zero means that there is no anxiety, one indicates mild anxiety, two indicates moderate anxiety, three indicates severe anxiety, and four indicates very severe or grossly disabling anxiety. The total anxiety score ranges from 0 to 56. It requires about 1015 minutes.

A score of 0 to 7 in HDRS, and 0 to4 in HAM-A, is generally accepted to be within the normal range so we use dichotomic results. Scores of 20 or higher in HDRS indicate moderately severe depression and are usually required for entry into a clinical trial.

• ECFOS II: Spanish version of the Family Burden Interview Schedule (FBIS) [14]. It is designed to assess the objective and subjective burden of families of people with schizophrenia. This scale assesses family burden in eight different modules: activities of daily life, disrupt behavior restraint, expenses, caregiver's routine, concern, help, repercussions on health and assessment of general burden. Alternative responses to the scale items are distributed on a Likert-type scale, ranging from 1 (never) to 5 (every day) for frequency of occurrences and from 1 (not at all) to 4 (very much) for degree of disturbance. Assessment covered the month prior to the interviews. The questionnaire requires about 60 min.

Each module score will be on a 0-4 scale, and the total score is the sum of the different modules scores.

3   First Predictive Task - Hamilton Questionnaire

As mentioned above, the Hamilton questionnaire has two different uses: assesing *depression* and *anxiety* levels. Furthermore, in both cases the responses provided by the caregivers to the questions, can be aggregated in order to obtain a single outcome for each case. The levels are then discretized by doctors as:

- Depression: [0-5] No, [6-13] Light, [14-26] Medium, [27-39] Intense and [40-52] Extreme.
- Anxiety: [0-5] No, [6-14] Light, [15-28] Medium, [29-42] Intense and [43-56] Extreme.

Therefore, from the machine leaning perspective we can approach the problem as a standard supervised classification, and in particular we aim to obtain two classifiers accounting for the following functions:

$$f_D(P_1, \ldots, P_{15}, CG_1, \ldots, CG_{15}) \longrightarrow Depression$$
$$f_A(P_1, \ldots, P_{15}, CG_1, \ldots, CG_{15}) \longrightarrow Anxiety$$

with $values(Depression) = values(Anxiety) = \{no, light, medium, intense, extreme\}$.

In our case, decision trees are used to approximate the two classification functions. From our preliminary experiments, the results obtained with decision trees were competitive with other standard classification models and they have the added advantage of being easy to interpret by medical experts. We used the C4.5 algorithm [9] to learn the models. Figure 1 shows the trees learned over the whole dataset for both class variables (depression and anxiety). As we can observe not all the variables have been included in the tree. If we pay attention to the ones included, we can observe that they are easy and inexpensive to obtain: one simple blood analysis and some questions to the caregiver are enough to predict, from Primary Care consultations, the level of anxiety or depression for the main caregiver of a schizophrenic patient. The possibility to anticipate this burden is most important, since commonly only a few relatives are willing to be the primary caregivers of these patients, so the possibility to predict and control their depression levels is, at the same time, also beneficial for the patient.

Regarding evaluation, we use leave-one-out cross-validation and collected *accuracy* (percentage of correct predictions) and AUC[1] (area under the ROC curve). We choose this validation scheme because of the small number of available instances. Thus, 180 models are learnt, each one using 179 instances as the training set and the remaining one for validation. The results are averaged over the 180 classifiers.

For Depression prediction the C4.5 obtained 96.09% accuracy and a mean AUC of 0.96. In the case of Anxiety, it obtained 98.89% accuracy and a mean AUC of 0.98. No caregiver reached over 40 points, so the predictive models built do not handle the extreme level.

4   Second Predictive Task - ECFOS-II Questionnaire

Unlike the Hamilton questionnaire, there is no aggregation on the ECFOS-II questionnaire, so in this case the doctors must go through all the answers, analyzing them and drawing their conclusions. Furthermore, we found it difficult to get the caregiver to fill it in, sometimes due to low cooperation or to mistrust.

Our goal now is to predict the answer to each question in the ECFOS-II questionnaire from the thirty variables described in Table 1. The ECFOS-II questionnaire is divided into two modules, namely A (help to patients in daily activities) and B (help to patients in self-control), which have 10 and 7 questions respectively, all of them with two possible answers: {Yes, No}. By using a predictive model, we suggest not making an extra effort to convince the caregiver to cooperate, but just to use the obtained model to complete the gaps. Furthermore, it is even possible to detect the possibility of lies or mistakes in answering, and also to anticipate a needed treatment before visiting the consultant.

---

[1] In fact, an approximation is used because the class has 5 labels: average over the five AUCs computed by using the one-against-all methodology.

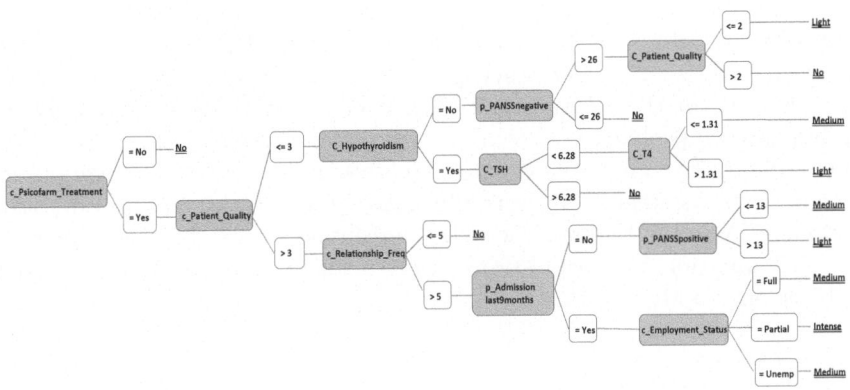

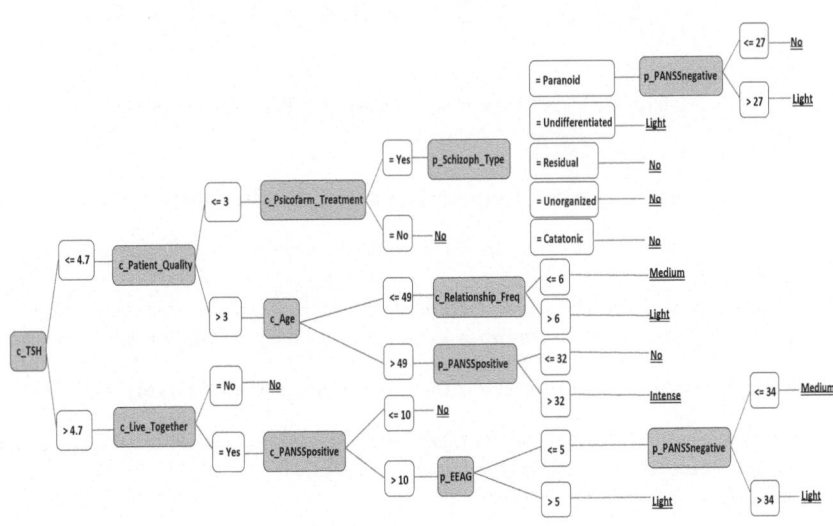

Fig. 1. Classification trees for depression (above) and anxiety (below)

Therefore, in this task we move from standard one-class supervised classification to *multi-dimensional* classification, and our goal is the inducion of the following function:

$$f(P_1, \ldots, P_{15}, CG_1, \ldots, CG_{15}) \longrightarrow (Q_{A_1}, \ldots, Q_{A_{10}}, Q_{B_1}, \ldots, Q_{B_7}),$$

or in other words, for each 30-dimensional input variable, we need to predict a binary vector of size 17, where each position in the vector corresponds to the outcome for one of the 17 questions. When class variables are binomial, the multi-dimensional problem is known as multi-label classification.

From a descriptive analysis over the 180 cases in our dataset, we can observe that, on average, a caregiver answers affirmatively to between 5 and 11 questions from Modules A and B. Figure 2 shows the percentage of caregivers who answered YES to each question, where questions 1 to 10 belong to Module A, and questions 11 to 17 belong to Module B.

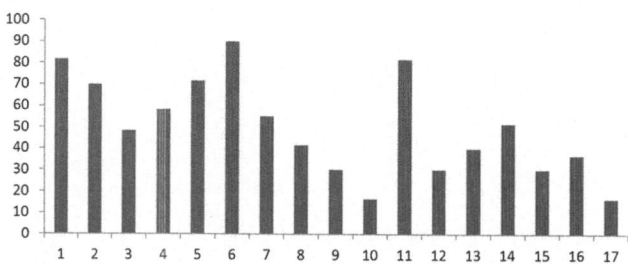

Fig. 2. %patients who answered YES to each question

The two questions most frequently answered affirmatively are:

– *Module A-6: Can the patient go to places alone on foot or by ordinary means of transport?*
– *Module B-1: Does the patient occasionally behave in an outrageous, embarrassing, annoying or inadequate manner such that you may feel ashamed or uncomfortable?*

while, the two questions most commonly answered negatively are:

– *Module A-10: Does the patient perform by him/herself standard paperwork, such as job applications, fill-in disability forms, etc.?*
– *Module B-7: Does the patient take drugs?*

The number of possible outcomes (combinations) is $2^{17} = 131072$, but, since our database only contains 180 samples, this number is delimited below 180 combinations from which the multi-label classifier learns. Moreover, we observed that among our 180 samples, there are only 59 different sets of answers to these 17 questions, which suggests that there exists some pattern in the answers, and so multi-label classification might perform well in learning and prediction.

Due to the low number of possible label-sets (59), we decided to use the multi-label classifier RAkEL[2] [13], which is a well-known model whose building procedure is based on learning from the existing sets of label values (implementation is available in [12]). Its procedure can be summarized in three well-differentiated steps:

1. Split the set of labels into disjoint subsets of size k.
2. Build a predictive model using the *label powerset* method; that is, using just one class variable in which each state refers to one of the label subsets.
3. For each test instance, use a threshold on the average prediction of all models to choose the assigned label.

The number of model label subsets it constructs is, by default, twice the number of labels: 17·2=34, as suggested in [13]. We tried to reduce this number of models in order to speed up the construction of the model, but then the classification accuracy was dramatically lower. Furthermore, modifying the size of the label subsets (3 by default) did not produce any significant change in performance. Thus, we use RAkEL with default options as setting in the Mulan API.

In order to assess the goodness of the approach, accuracy and Hamming loss (percentage of wrong predictions of labels, with respect to the total number of labels) were collected during a leave-one-out cross validation procedure.

Accuracy performance is a very restrictive goodness metric to evaluate a multi-label classifier, since one prediction is correct only when the predictions for all labels are correct. Thus, in this case one prediction on a sample is correct when the classifier correctly predicts the value of 17 labels. However, maybe due to the low number of answer combinations in the 180 answered questionnaires, the mean accuracy obtained by RAkEL is 99%, with Hamming-loss equal to 0.03%. Thus, it becomes evident that the answers to the ECFOS-II questionnaire are easily predictable, and therefore so is the caregiver burden in advance of the appearance of depression or anxiety.

5   Conclusions and Future Work

We worked with a database of 180 schizophrenia patients and the burden suffered by their family caregivers, the burden being measured through the Hamilton and ECFOS-II questionnaires. We built decision trees which can help the doctor in Primary Care consultations to predict the level of anxiety and depression in the caregivers by using variables that are easy and not very expensive to obtain. Furthermore, we used a well-known multi-label classifier, RAkEL, which was able to successfully predict the set of answers to the ECFOS-II questionnaire. By using these tools, we suggest it is possible to anticipate the treatment needed by the main caregiver of a schizophrenia patient before his/her needs or burden become more difficult to deal with. As future work, we aim to validate the

---

[2] Equivalent results where obtained configuring RAkEL with both C4.5 and k-NN classifiers.

predictive models built in this work by applying them to new real cases from Primary Care consultations, so that we can validate the models with new records and create logs of depression/anxiety treatments that are successfuly anticipated and the social and economic benefits obtained from this.

Acknowledgements. This work has been partially funded by FEDER funds and the Spanish Government (MICINN) through project TIN2010-20900-C04-03.

References

1. Angermeyer, M., Khn, L., Goldstein, J.: Gender and the course of schizophrenia: differences in treated outcomes. Schizophrenia Bulletin 16(2), 293–307 (1990)
2. Association, A.P.: DSM-IV-TR. Breviario (2002)
3. Dyck, D.G., Short, R., Vitaliano, P.P.: Predictors of burden and infectious illness in schizophrenia caregivers. Psychosom. Med. 61(4), 411–419 (1999)
4. Finkelhor, D., Gelles, R., Hotaling, G., Strauss, M.: The Dark Side of Families: Current Family Violence Research. SAGE (1983)
5. Grandón, P., Jenaro, C., Lemos, S.: Primary caregivers of schizophrenia outpatients: burden and predictor variables. Psychiatry Res. 158(3), 335–343 (2008)
6. Hamilton, M.: The assessment of anxiety states by rating. British Journal of Medical Psychology 32, 50–55 (1959)
7. McDonell, M., Short, R., Berry, C.M.: Burden in schizophrenia caregivers: Impact of family psychoeducation and awareness of patient suicidality. Family Process 42, 91–103 (2003)
8. Peralta Martin, V., Cuesta Zorita, M.: Validation of positive and negative symptom scale (panss) in a sample of Spanish schizophrenic patients. Actas Luso Esp. Neurol. Psiquiatr. Cienc. Afines 22(4), 171–177 (1994)
9. Quinlan, J.R.: C4.5: Programs for Machine Learning, 1st edn. Morgan Kaufmann Series in Machine Learning. Morgan Kaufmann (1992)
10. Ramos-Brieva, J.A., Cordero-Villafafila, A.: A new validation of the hamilton rating scale for depression. J. Psychiatr. Res. 22(1), 21–28 (1988)
11. Tsoumakas, G., Katakis, I.: Multi label classification: An overview. International Journal of Data Warehousing and Mining 3(3), 1–13 (2007)
12. Tsoumakas, G., Spyromitros-Xioufis, E., Vilcek, J., Vlahavas, I.: Mulan: A java library for multi-label learning. Journal of Machine Learning Research 12, 2411–2414 (2011)
13. Tsoumakas, G., Vlahavas, I.P.: Random k-labelsets: An ensemble method for multilabel classification. In: Kok, J.N., Koronacki, J., Lopez de Mantaras, R., Matwin, S., Mladenič, D., Skowron, A. (eds.) ECML 2007. LNCS (LNAI), vol. 4701, pp. 406–417. Springer, Heidelberg (2007)
14. Vilaplana, M., Ochoa, S., Martinez, A., Villalta, V., Martinez-Leal, R., Puigdollers, E., Salvador, L., Martorell, A., Muñoz, P.E., Haro, J.M.: Validation in Spanish population of the family objective and subjective burden interview (ECFOS-II) for relatives of patients with schizophrenia. Actas Esp. Psiquiatr. 35(6), 372–381 (2007)

Predicting Adverse Drug Events
by Analyzing Electronic Patient Records

Isak Karlsson, Jing Zhao*, Lars Asker, and Henrik Boström

Dept. of Computer and Systems Sciences, Stockholm University
Forum 100, SE-164 40 Kista, Sweden
{isak-kar,jingzhao,asker,henrik.bostrom}@dsv.su.se
http://dsv.su.se

Abstract. Diagnosis codes for adverse drug events (ADEs) are sometimes missing from electronic patient records (EPRs). This may not only
affect patient safety in the worst case, but also the number of reported
ADEs, resulting in incorrect risk estimates of prescribed drugs. Large
databases of electronic patient records (EPRs) are potentially valuable
sources of information to support the identification of ADEs. This study
investigates the use of machine learning for predicting one specific ADE
based on information extracted from EPRs, including age, gender, diagnoses and drugs. Several predictive models are developed and evaluated using different learning algorithms and feature sets. The highest
observed AUC is 0.87, obtained by the random forest algorithm. The resulting model can be used for screening EPRs that are not, but possibly
should be, assigned a diagnosis code for the ADE under consideration.
Preliminary results from using the model are presented.

Keywords: machine learning, electronic patient records, adverse drug
events.

1   Introduction

Preventable adverse drug events (ADEs) account for approximately 3.7% of all
hospital admissions worldwide and is a significant burden on the healthcare
system [1]. However, ADEs are often underreported [2]. For example, physicians
sometimes incorrectly assign diagnosis codes because they fail to identify a new
medical event as an ADE. This may not only affect patient safety, but also the
number of reported ADEs, resulting in incorrect risk estimates of prescribed
drugs. For example, an extra drug could be unnecessarily prescribed to treat
the ADE instead of solving the problem by just exchanging or even withdrawing
the responsible drug. Studies have shown an average of one unnecessary drug
per patient, including drugs with no identifiable indication or that provide little
benefit for the indication for which they were prescribed [3].

Since premarketing clinical trials normally are limited in time and in number
of patients, there is always a risk that some ADEs, including interactions with

---

* The first two authors contributed equally.

N. Peek, R. Marín Morales, and M. Peleg (Eds.): AIME 2013, LNAI 7885, pp. 125–129, 2013.

other drugs, remain undetected. To monitor such negative events, spontaneous reports have been collected, e.g., by the WHO Uppsala Monitoring Center [4]. However, such reports do not provide information on frequencies of prescribed drugs and assigned diagnoses, and they only report suspected ADEs. Large databases of electronic patient records (EPRs) can complement such spontaneous reports, allowing for detection of ADEs that have not been identified as such, by aggregating results across hundreds of thousands of patient records. Studies have shown the strength of using EPRs to detect signals that indicate ADEs [5,6]. When screening large databases of EPRs, manually identifying potential ADEs that have not been assigned appropriate diagnosis codes is, in the normal case, prevented by the cost and difficulty of the task. EPRs with previously assigned diagnosis codes for specific ADEs can be used to develop predictive models for identifying other cases that potentially should include the diagnosis code. Cases predicted to have such a code, but do not, could be considered as candidates for alerting a possibly missing code. This study exploits this idea by using machine learning for predicting one specific ADE based on information extracted from EPRs, including age, gender, diagnoses and drugs.

2   Method

2.1   Data Source

The dataset used in this study was extracted from the Stockholm EPR Corpus[1] (2009-2010) [7], which contains both structured data and clinical narratives. In this study, structured data was used to create different feature sets for model generation, and clinical narratives were used to support the manual evaluation. The diagnoses are reported using ICD-10-SE[2]. Considering the balance between a sufficiently large sample size and a not *too* severe diagnosis, which hardly would be missed, *L27.0* (*Generalized skin eruption due to drugs and medicaments*) was chosen as the diagnosis code of interest. The training set consists of 201 patients diagnosed with *L27.0* as positive examples and 261 other randomly selected patients as negative examples. From each negative example, a random diagnosis code was selected to determine a pivot time point for calculating the feature values as *before* or *not*. The deployment set consists of patients with *L30.9X*[3] (*Dermatitis, unspecified*), since an unspecific, but closely related, diagnosis code is more likely assigned when a physician fails to recognize an ADE.

Each example is represented by a (very sparse) vector with features corresponding to 1,312 different drugs, 9,863 different diagnosis codes, age and gender. Different subsets of the features, all including age and gender, were considered: (1) using only drugs (*Dr*); (2) using drugs and diagnoses (*Dr + Di*). Furthermore, the feature values were derived in two different ways: either by the presence

---

[1] This research has been approved by the Regional Ethical Review Board in Stockholm (Etikprövningsnämnden i Stockholm), permission number 2012/834-31.

[2] International Classification of Disease, Version 10, Swedish Modification.

[3] Not included in the negative random examples.

($y = \{yes, no\}$) or, to support temporality, as happened *before* the assigned diagnosis or *not* ($b = \{before, not\}$). In the first case, a value *yes* means that a certain drug or diagnosis code has been assigned to a patient at any time during the entire time span, while the value *no* means that the code is not present at all in the record. In the second case, a value *before* means that the drug or diagnosis code has been assigned at some time point before *L27.0* (or the randomly chosen code in case of a negative example, as described above), while *not* is assigned in all other cases. Hence, examples that in the second case would obtain the value *before* for some code, will be a subset of the examples that in the first case would obtain the value *yes* for the same code. Six combinations, Dr_b, Dr_y, $Dr_b + Di_y$, $Dr_y + Di_y$, $Dr_b + Di_b$ and $Dr_y + Di_b$, were investigated to evaluate which feature set results in the highest predictive performance.

2.2 Experimental Setup

To investigate the use of machine learning for predicting the selected ADE, *L27.0*, two experiments were conducted. In the first experiment, the performance of two machine learning algorithms was evaluated on the six feature sets described above using 10-fold cross validation. The selected algorithms were random forest [8], as implemented by [9], and the J-Rip rule learner [10]. The random forest algorithm was selected since it constructs highly accurate models and allows for estimates of variable importance, enabling inspection of important predictors. The rule learner was chosen as it contrasts to the opaque models induced by the random forest algorithm and instead generates somewhat less accurate models suitable for manual interpretation. The parameters of J-Rip were set to the default and the random forest was built using $1,000$ trees [9].

Potential ways of evaluating predictive models are to measure their accuracy, specificity, sensitivity and/or positive predictive value [11]. However, the area under the ROC curve (AUC) [12], which measures the probability of predicting a true positive ahead of a false positive, is often a better measure for the predictive performance of a classifier than accuracy [13], in particular when the class distributions may differ between the training and test sets. Since the class distribution in the training set by design was rather balanced, and the class distribution of the target population is unknown, AUC was found to be a suitable performance metric. In addition to looking at the predictive performance, when choosing the most suitable of the six feature sets, the variables indicated as most important by the models were also inspected.

In the second experiment, the model generated by the selected algorithm and feature set was applied to predict potentially missed diagnoses from the deployment set, none of which include *L27.0*, but the closely related *L30.9X*. These patients were ranked descendently by the probability of having *L27.0*. Since the number of patients predicted to have *L27.0* only reflects the class proportions selected in the training set, choosing the top ranked rather than all predicted to have *L27.0* were more interesting to investigate further. A medical expert was asked to inspect the narratives reported for the top ten ranked patients to find whether the evidence indicates the presence of *L27.0* or not.

3   Results

Table 1 lists the AUC obtained from the random forest and the rule learner with the six different feature sets. For all feature sets, the rule learner was outperformed by the random forest, which consequently was selected to generate the model. Although the AUC, for random forest, was hardly affected by the choice of feature set, **F1** was found most suitable since it gave the possiblity of predicting ADEs when only drugs taken *before* are available.

By applying the selected model (random forest with **F1**) on the deployment set, patients were ranked in decreasing order by the probability of having this ADE. Due to time constraints, the top ten ranked candidates were manually inspected by the medical expert, which showed that six patients' narratives supported the models' prediction indicating that *L27.0* was likely missed.

Table 1. Area under the ROC curve. F1 to F6 represent different feature sets. $Dr = drug$, $Di = diagnosis$, $b = \{before, not\}$, $y = \{yes, no\}$

Feature set	Random forest	Rule learner
F1 (Dr_b)	.86	.73
F2 (Dr_y)	.87	.77
F3 $(Dr_b + Di_y)$	.85	.58
F4 $(Dr_y + Di_y)$	.85	.62
F5 $(Dr_b + Di_b)$	.83	.57
F6 $(Dr_y + Di_b)$	.85	.58

4   Discussion

Two machine learning algorithms were applied on different feature sets to predict one specific ADE. The experimental results show that the random forest algorithm outperforms the rule learner with regard to AUC. Different feature sets were investigated, showing that increasing the dimensionality of the feature set by including patients' diagnoses, reduced the performance for both types of classifier. The decreased AUC might be due to the curse of dimensionality and the fact that disease history is not important when it comes to drug-induced skin problems. Instead of completely excluding a feature set, one way of reducing the dimensionality could be to merge specific drugs and diagnoses into families. This study concludes that the developed model may be used for detecting potential ADEs that for various reasons have been left out from the EPRs, e.g., to give alerts of a suspected ADE for which no diagnosis code has been provided.

It is interesting to note that in this study all the high-ranked patients turned out to be diagnosed with severe diseases, meaning that dermatitis might not draw enough attention compared to their underlying diseases like *multiple myeloma*. Alternatively, one could for example sample patients only from dermatology clinics instead of the entire patient population. One limitation of this study is that the target diagnosis code concerns a specific drug-induced disorder, and hence it is not clear to what extent the results can be generalized to other diagnosis codes.

This study shows that it is possible to apply machine learning algorithms for screening EPRs that are not, but probably should be, assigned a diagnosis code for the ADE under consideration. When using the models for ranking, rather than classification, a reasonable sized sample with the most likely candidates can be selected for inspection. Future research can focus on improving the the performance of predictive models by combining structured and unstructured data, and applying such models in a more general population.

Acknowledgments. This work was partly supported by the project High-Performance Data Mining for Drug Effect Detection at Stockholm University, funded by Swedish Foundation for Strategic Research under grant IIS11-0053. We would like to thank Dr. Maria Kvist for her contributions as the medical expert.

References

1. Howard, R.L., Avery, A.J., Slavenburg, S., Royal, S., Pipe, G., Lucassen, P., Pirmohamed, M.: Which drugs cause preventable admissions to hospital? A systematic review. British Journal of Clinical Pharmacology 63, 136–147 (2007)
2. Hazell, L., Shakir, S.A.: Under-reporting of adverse drug reactions: a systematic review. Drug Safet. 29(5), 385–396 (2006)
3. Steinman, M.A., Rosenthal, G.E., Landefeld, C.S., Bertenthal, D., Kaboli, P.J.: Agreement between drugs-to-avoid criteria and expert assessments of problematic prescribing. Arch. Intern. Med. 169(14), 1326–1332 (2009)
4. The Uppsala Monitoring Center, http://www.who-umc.org/
5. Hazlehurst, B., Naleway, A., Mullooly, J.: Detecting possible vaccine adverse events in clinical notes from the electronic medical record. Vaccine 27, 2077–2083 (2009)
6. Vilar, S., Harpaz, R., Santana, L., Uriarte, E., Friedman, C.: Enhancing Adverse Drug Event Detection in Electronic Health Records Using Molecular Structure Similarity: Application to Pancreatitis. PLoS ONE 7(7) (2012)
7. Dalianis, H., Hassel, M., Henriksson, A., Skeppstedt, M.: Stockholm EPR Corpus: A Clinical Database Used to Improve Health Care. In: Swedish Language Technology Conference (2012)
8. Brieman, L.: Random forests. Machine Learning 45(1), 5–32 (2001)
9. Boström, H.: Concurrent learning of large-scale random forests. In: Proceedings of Scandinavian Conference on Artificial Intelligence, pp. 20–29 (2011)
10. Witten, I.H., Frank, E.: Data Mining: Practical machine learning tools and techniques. Morgan Kaufmann (2005)
11. Bellazzi, R., Zupan, B.: Predictive data mining in clinical medicine: current issues and guidelines. International Journal of Medical Informatics 77(2), 81–97 (2008)
12. Bradley, A.: The use of the area under the ROC curve in the evaluation of machine learning algorithms. Pattern Recognition 30(7), 1145–1159 (1997)
13. Huang, J., Ling, C.X.: Using AUC and accuracy in evaluating learning algorithms. IEEE Transactions on Knowledge and Data Engineering 17(3), 299–310 (2005)

Top-Level MeSH Disease Terms Are Not Linearly Separable in Clinical Trial Abstracts

Joël Kuiper[1] and Gert van Valkenhoef[1,2]

[1] Faculty of Economics and Business, University of Groningen, Groningen,
The Netherlands
[2] Department of Epidemiology, University of Groningen,
University Medical Center Groningen, Groningen, The Netherlands

Abstract. Assessments of the efficacy and safety of medical interventions are based on systematic reviews of clinical trials. Systematic reviewing requires the screening of vast amounts of publications, which is currently done by hand. To reduce the number of publications that are screened manually, we propose the automated classification of publications by disease category using Support Vector Machines. We base our classification on the ontological structure of the Medical Subject Headings (MeSH) by treating all terms as their top-level disease category. Unfortunately the resulting classifier lacks sufficient sensitivity for use by systematic reviewers. We argue that this is partially due to the inseparability of the terminology into the disease categories and discuss how future work could address this problem.

1 Introduction

Randomized Controlled Trials (RCTs) provide the most reliable assessments of the efficacy and safety of medical interventions and as such they should inform treatment decisions [1]. This information is complicated by the massive numbers of trials that are conducted; for example, the Cochrane Library alone indexes 286,418 trials as taking place in the last decade [2]. To reduce the amount of information they need to process, decision makers often rely on systematic reviews to summarize the RCTs that concern a specific disease and/or intervention. Systematic reviewing consists of searching the literature, screening the results and summarizing the relevant evidence. In screening, whether trials are included depends on what they study, i.e. the disease, interventions and patient population. In some cases this means reducing thousands of publications to only a handful. Attempts have been made to optimize search queries to reduce the number of false positive results [3], but for a comprehensive review a broader query is required [4]. Therefore systematic reviewers maximize sensitivity and sacrifice specificity.

Accurate meta-data could reduce the number of false positives while maintaining a high sensitivity. For example, PubMed employs the Medical Subject Headings (MeSH) to provide meta-data such as anatomical terms, organisms, and diseases. However, like most meta-data initiatives it relies on the goodwill

N. Peek, R. Marín Morales, and M. Peleg (Eds.): AIME 2013, LNAI 7885, pp. 130–134, 2013.

of the authors and publishers to provide annotations. Consequently, only a fraction of publications are completely and correctly annotated. To fill these gaps in meta-data, machine learning techniques like automatic classification can be applied. Automatic classification is a type of supervised learning in which a mapping of observations to predetermined categories is built, based on a "training" set of observations for which the class is known in advance. This methodology can potentially be applied usefully to PubMed MeSH annotations: filtering by disease is an important sub-task of screening and PubMed provides a large subset of abstracts annotated with MeSH disease terms that can be used as a training set. In this paper we explore the application of automatic classification to tag abstracts with the appropriate MeSH disease terms.

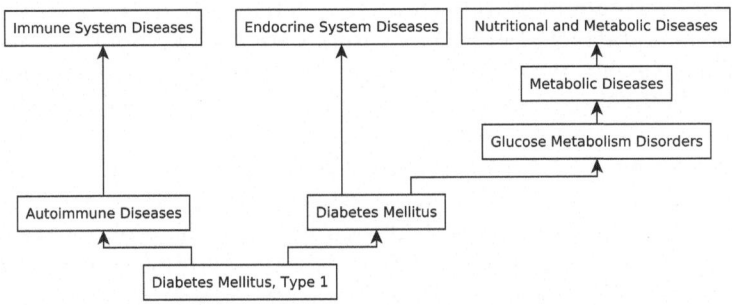

Fig. 1. *Diabetes Mellitus, Type 1* sub-graph of the MeSH disease terms

The MeSH disease terms are structured as an ontology, meaning that terms are encoded as nodes in a directed acyclic graph whose connections represent relations such as instance-of (`is-a`). For example, Diabetes Mellitus `is-a` Glucose Metabolism Disorder, which in turn `is-a` Metabolic Disease (see Fig. 1). MeSH (2013 edition) places 4308 unique disease terms in only 26 top level categories. However, since MeSH is not a strict hierarchy, most terms correspond to several top level categories; in other words the top-level categories are not mutually exclusive. *Diabetes Mellitus, Type 1*, for example, maps to the top level categories *Immune System Diseases*, *Endocrine System Diseases*, and *Nutritional and Metabolic Diseases* (see Fig. 1). This raises the question which level of description is most appropriate for applying machine learning, and how the ontological structure can be used to both simplify the classification task and aid the researcher in screening by providing familiar categorizations.

To start exploring the possibility of using the MeSH disease categories for automated classifications of RCTs, we attempt to automatically classify publications by their corresponding top level MeSH categories using Support Vector Machines (SVMs). A classifier with sufficient performance could reduce the number of false positives from literature searches and provide a starting point for more fine-grained classification of terms deeper in the ontology.

2   Methods

To obtain a representative corpus, PubMed was queried for all publications tagged with the publication type "Randomized Controlled Trial" and the MeSH term "Human". The publications' MeSH annotations were then matched against the MeSH disease terms based on exact string match. The ontological structure of MeSH was taken into account by treating all disease terms as their top level ancestor(s). This was done by first transforming the MeSH terms into the Open Biological and Biomedical Ontologies (OBO) format [5] and then extracting relationships from the resulting ontology using the OntoCAT library [6]. The disease categories *Animal Diseases, Disorders of Environmental Origin, Pathological conditions, Sings and Symptoms* and *Occupational Diseases* were excluded from the ontology because they were either irrelevant, only included very few terms, or had substantial overlap with other categories.

The title and abstract of each publication were used as input for text classification. While classification based on the full text could potentially increase the accuracy, this often is not readily available due to various licencing and technical restrictions.

To reduce dimensionality common English words were filtered from these texts and the words were stemmed using a kstem filter [7]. Each publication was treated as a bag-of-words, a representation in which the order of the words in the document is ignored. The bag-of-words representation is computationally efficient and easy to implement. Other methods for text representation might yield better performance, but often at the cost of computational efficiency and transparency.

For each of the words the Term Frequency normalized by the Inverse Document Frequency (*tf-idf* [8]) was calculated. The term frequency is the number of occurrences of a word in a document, the Inverse Document Frequency is the logarithm of the total amount of documents divided by the total occurrences of a word across all documents.

In general, classification algorithms attempt to find a mapping between labels y_i and instances x_i where $x_i \in R^n$ and $y_i \in \{-1, +1\}$. Here SVMs were used to classify the annotated publications, because they have been successful in fast large scale text classification [9,10]. SVMs attempt to perform classification by finding a maximum margin-separating hyperplane. This is done by solving the following unconstrained optimization problem:

$$\min_{w} \frac{1}{2}\mathbf{w}^T\mathbf{w} + C\sum_{i=1}^{l}\xi(\mathbf{w}; \mathbf{x}_i, y_i) \ , \tag{1}$$

with a loss function ξ and $C > 0$ as a penalty parameter. The LIBLINEAR [11] SVM implementation was used to solve the optimization in its primal form with the L2 loss function:

$$\xi(\mathbf{w}; \mathbf{x}_i, y_i) = (\max(1 - y_i\mathbf{w}^T\mathbf{x}_i, 0))^2 \tag{2}$$

The penalty factor C was varied between 0.0001 and 10 to determine the effects of introducing a softer margin. For each of the categories a binary one-vs-the-rest classifier was constructed, because publications could belong to multiple categories. Performance of the classifiers was assessed using 10-fold cross-validation with averaged specificity and sensitivity as performance measures.

3   Results

The PubMed query resulted in 404,371 publications of which the full records were retrieved in XML format (on 2012-10-29). Only 13,918 publications were annotated as a top-level disease category. When treating all terms as their top-level ancestor(s) 226,710 publications were annotated with a disease.

The specificity of the binary classifiers for each top-level disease category was consistent around 0.98 for all values of the penalty parameter C. The median sensitivity of the classifiers was 0.53 ($C = 1.0$). The classifier for *Stomatognathic Diseases* was the most sensitive (0.822, $C = 1.0$). The least sensitive classifiers were those for *Hemic and, Lymphatic Diseases* ($0.208, C = 1.0$) and *Congenital, Hereditary, and Neonatal Diseases and Abnormalities* ($0.270, C = 1.0$). Relaxing the condition for the optimal hyper-plane by decreasing the penalty factor C (i.e. introducing a soft margin) did not substantially improve the sensitivity. From this we conclude that the data on the margin were not particularly noisy, and that the data might not be linearly separable.

4   Discussion

Our classifiers had poor sensitivity (median of 0.53, whereas acceptable sensitivity would be 0.8 or higher). One explanation could be that some disease terms lack specific terminology which does not overlap with the other categories, so that the SVM fails to find a separating hyperplane. It could be that in general for medical terminology the ontological descendants of a top-level item do not sufficiently generalize that top-level item, i.e. the terminology of Diabetes and Hyperglycemia do not cluster under Metabolic Diseases. Indeed, it seems that the sensitivity of a classifier correlates with how well-defined a term is. For example, the classifier for the well-defined term *Stomatognathic Diseases* is sensitive (0.822) whereas the MeSH even suggests not to use the term *Hemic and Lymphatic Diseases* because it is too general. This raises the question for which level of description the classification problem would be easiest to solve.

To assess the separability of the data, clustering techniques could be applied. This would require the dimensionality of the data to be drastically reduced through techniques such as Latent Semantic Analysis [12] or Principal Component Analysis. Subsequent manual analysis could reveal associations between the identified clusters and MeSH disease terms. This could aid with a more classical classification task or be used as an alternative way of filtering RCTs.

However, an open question remains: whether using ontologies derived from human expertise to guide supervised classification algorithms is feasible altogether.

It could very well be that while ontologies provide familiar and accepted labels for the (human) end-user, far better categorization can be achieved without a fixed hierarchy, instead leaving the categorization up-to the algorithm at hand. Topic modelling techniques [13] such as Probabilistic Latent Semantic Analysis or Latent Dirichlet allocation, could provide techniques for finding relevant publications without the aid of a established ontology.

References

1. Evidence-Based Medicine Working Group: Evidence-based medicine. A new approach to teaching the practice of medicine. Journal of the American Medical Association 268(17), 2420–2425 (1992)
2. van Valkenhoef, G., Tervonen, T., de Brock, B., Hillege, H.: Deficiencies in the transfer and availability of clinical evidence in drug development and regulation. BMC Medical Informatics and Decision Making (2012) (in press)
3. Haynes, R.B., McKibbon, K.A., Wilczynski, N.L., Walter, S.D., Werre, S.R.: Optimal search strategies for retrieving scientifically strong studies of treatment from Medline: analytical survey. BMJ 330(7501), 1179 (2005)
4. Higgins, J., Green, S. (eds.): Cochrane Handbook for Systematic Reviews of Interventions Version 5.0.2. The Cochrane Collaboration (2009), http://www.cochrane-handbook.org (updated September 2009)
5. Smith, B., Ashburner, M., Rosse, C., Bard, J., Bug, W., Ceusters, W., Goldberg, L.J., Eilbeck, K., Ireland, A., Mungall, C.J., Leontis, N., Rocca-Serra, P., Ruttenberg, A., Sansone, S.A., Scheuermann, R.H., Shah, N., Whetzel, P.L., Lewis, S.: The OBO foundry: coordinated evolution of ontologies to support biomedical data integration. Nature Biotechnology 25(11), 1251–1255 (2007)
6. Adamusiak, T., Burdett, T., Kurbatova, N., van der Velde, K.J., Abeygunawardena, N., Antonakaki, D., Kapushesky, M., Parkinson, H., Swertz, M.A.: OntoCAT – simple ontology search and integration in java, r and REST/JavaScript. BMC Bioinformatics 12(1), 218 (2011)
7. Krovetz, R.: Viewing morphology as an inference process. In: Proceedings of the 16th Annual International ACM SIGIR Conference on Research and Development in Information Retrieval, SIGIR 1993, pp. 191–202. ACM, New York (1993)
8. Salton, G., Fox, E.A., Wu, H.: Extended boolean information retrieval. Commun. ACM 26(11), 1022–1036 (1983)
9. Joachims, T.: Text categorization with suport vector machines: Learning with many relevant features. In: Nédellec, C., Rouveirol, C. (eds.) ECML 1998. LNCS, vol. 1398, pp. 137–142. Springer, Heidelberg (1998)
10. Joachims, T.: Training linear SVMs in linear time. In: Proceedings of the 12th ACM SIGKDD International Conference on Knowledge Discovery and Data Mining, pp. 217–226 (2006)
11. Fan, R.E., Chang, K.W., Hsieh, C.J., Wang, X.R., Lin, C.J.: LIBLINEAR: A library for large linear classification. Journal of Machine Learning Research 9, 1871–1874 (2008)
12. Dumais, S.T., Furnas, G.W., Landauer, T.K., Deerwester, S., Harshman, R.: Using latent semantic analysis to improve access to textual information. In: Proceedings of the SIGCHI Conference on Human Factors in Computing Systems, CHI 1988, pp. 281–285. ACM, New York (1988)
13. Blei, D.M.: Probabilistic topic models. Communications of the ACM 55(4), 77–84 (2012)

Understanding the Co-occurrence
of Diseases Using Structure Learning

Martijn Lappenschaar, Arjen Hommersom, Joep Lagro, and Peter J.F. Lucas

Radboud University Nijmegen, The Netherlands
{mlappens,arjenh,peterl}@cs.ru.nl

Abstract. Multimorbidity, i.e., the presence of multiple diseases within one person, is a significant health-care problem for western societies: diagnosis, prognosis and treatment in the presence of of multiple diseases can be complex due to the various interactions between diseases. To better understand the co-occurrence of diseases, we propose Bayesian network structure learning methods for deriving the interactions between risk factors. In particular, we propose novel measures for structural relationships in the co-occurrence of diseases and identify the critical factors in this interaction. We illustrate these measures in the oncological area for better understanding co-occurrences of malignant tumours.

1 Introduction

Epidemiological research indicates that more than two-third of the elderly have two or more chronic diseases at the same time; the problem of managing multiple diseases, one of the most challenging issues of modern medicine, is referred to as the problem of *multimorbidity*. Its importance is rapidly increasing due to the rise in the number of elderly people. Characterisation of multimorbidity trends is usually done by specific indices. A recent systematic review [1] emphasised the heterogeneity of these indices. It also pointed out that all indices so far deal with diseases where there is a natural tendency to look for mutual influences between particular conditions, such as in cardiovascular diseases. Quite a lot less is known about disease interactions for many other diseases, even if they occur frequently. The study of interactions between these diseases offers a good starting point for the development of new methods for multimorbidity research.

A typical example is cancer, i.e. malignant tumours, the focus of the present paper. Although multimorbidity is increasingly attracting attention from oncologists, yet little is known about the interaction between cancers [2]. As cancer is becoming more and more a manageable chronic disease, and because in the ageing Western society more people are at risk for cancer, there is a growing number of patients with multiple malignancies [3]. These multiple cancers affect the survival estimate based on each tumour site, obviously because a primary tumour may have metastasised, but also because there may be multiple primary malignancies [4]. There are quite some risk factors that are implicated in the development of multiple primary malignant tumours, ranging from ageing,

N. Peek, R. Marín Morales, and M. Peleg (Eds.): AIME 2013, LNAI 7885, pp. 135–144, 2013.
© Springer-Verlag Berlin Heidelberg 2013

environmental and life-style factors, and genetic predisposition. Both for the development of clinical prediction models and the prevention of multiple malignant tumours, understanding the cause of their co-occurrence is important.

It is unlikely that a methodology investigating this will be based upon traditional statistical methods, such as logistic regression, that focus on the predictive power of specific variables for the presence or absence of one particular disease [5]. Several conceptual frameworks of multimorbidity have appeared in literature, offering distinct ways to clarify how diseases are related. Recently, we proposed a new framework of multimorbidity, based on Bayesian networks, that can be used as a basis for modelling a spectrum of multimorbidity aspects [6]. In this paper, we build upon this work by developing a new method for the identification of etiological interactions between diseases from data. In particular, we propose a number of measures that express the interaction between diseases. Furthermore, we identify the *critical factors* that relate the diseases: these factors indicate which mechanisms best explain their co-occurrence. We evaluate this approach on the most common co-occurrences of malignancies, and show that we can identify the relationships between malignancies and their critical factors.

2   Preliminaries

2.1   Statistical Measures of Association in Multimorbidity

Commonly used measures in medicine to describe associations are the relative risk (RR) and the ϕ-correlation coefficient, Pearson's correlation coefficient for binary variables. These measures have been used to investigate cancer metastasis patterns in a network-based manner, where edges in a constructed network were added because of high enough strength of RR or ϕ-correlation [7].

Let N_i be the number of patients with disease D_i, N_j the number of patients with disease D_j, N_{ij} the number of patients with both diseases D_i and D_j, and N the total number of patients. The *relative risk* of observing a pair of diseases D_i and D_j affecting the same patient is then given by

$$RR_{ij} = \frac{N_{ij}N}{N_iN_j} = \frac{P(d_i, d_j)}{P(d_i)P(d_j)} \tag{1}$$

The *ϕ-correlation coefficient* is given by:

$$\phi_{ij} = \frac{N_{ij}N - N_iN_j}{\sqrt{N_iN_j(N - N_i)(N - N_j)}} \tag{2}$$

The statistical significance of the RR depends on the sample size, the size of the prevalences involved, and the noise in the sample. Further characteristics of the RR and its use in medicine are outlined in [8]. If we evaluate the RR for a specific subpopulation by *conditioning* on a set of risk factors Q, we obtain:

$$RR_{ij}^q = \frac{N_{ij}^q N^q}{N_i^q N_j^q} = \frac{P(d_i, d_j \mid q)}{P(d_i \mid q)P(d_j \mid q)} \tag{3}$$

with N_{ij}^q the absolute prevalence of both D_i and D_j within the subpopulation of patients for which $Q = q$ holds. N^q, N_i^q, and N_j^q are defined likewise.

There are only a few situations in which multiple diseases occur together. The first possibility is that their co-occurrence is at random, i.e. exactly from what can be expected by chance. Adopting the standard probabilistic terminology, this notion is called *independent multimorbidity* [6], and it coincidences with an RR = 1. This notion coincides with earlier statistical notions e.g. random co-occurrence [9] and non-etiological associations [10]. The opposite of independent multimorbidity is called *associative multimorbidity*, which means that there is some relationship between diseases which causes the co-occurrence of the diseases to be different from expectation by chance. Typically, one is interested in a *positive* associative multimorbidity, i.e. where RR > 1.

2.2 Bayesian Networks

While independence measures provide some insight into which diseases might co-occur more frequently, they do not give much insight into the etiology as the are a number of ways these diseases can be related [6]. To model and analyse such relationships between diseases, we will use Bayesian networks, which can be used to model more complex structural relationships between disease variables in comparison to traditional regression models.

Formally, a *Bayesian network* is a tuple $\mathcal{B} = (G, X, P)$, with $G = (V, E)$ a directed acyclic graph (DAG), $X = \{X_v \mid v \in V\}$ a set of random variables indexed by V, and P a joint probability distribution of the random variables in X. In the remainder of this paper, all random variables will be binary with values *true* and *false* and we will write x for $X = true$ and $\bar{x}$ for $X = false$. P is a Bayesian network with respect to the graph G if P can be written as a product of the probability of each random variable, conditional on their parent variables:

$$P(x_1, \ldots, x_n) = \prod_{v \in V} P(x_v \mid x_{\pi(v)}) \tag{4}$$

where $\pi(v)$ is the set of parents of v (i.e. those vertices pointing directly to v via a single arc). As a convenience, we will often write v if we mean the random variable X_v that is associated to v. In Bayesian networks, the arcs between variables model dependences between variables which give rise to probabilistic conditional independence relationships. We say that set of variables X and Y are independent given variables Z if it holds that $P(X \mid Y, Z) = P(X \mid Z)$, which is denoted by $X \perp\!\!\!\perp Y \mid Z$. These independences can also be read off the graph using the well-known criterion of *d*-separation [11]. Bayesian networks can be learned from data using various methods. In this paper, we apply a *constraint-based learning method*, which uses a local statistical dependence analysis in order to build up the graph [12].

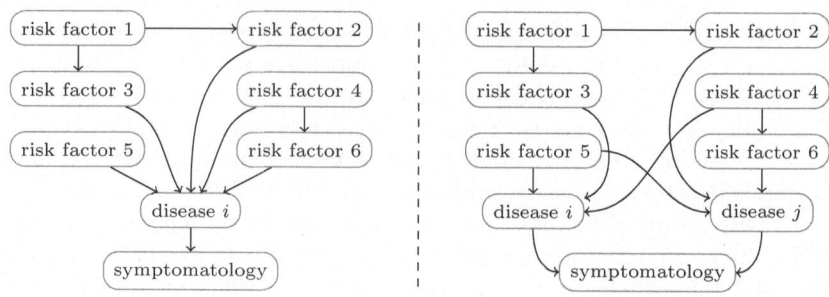

Fig. 1. Bayesian network of a single disease (left) and multiple diseases (right)

3   Models of Co-occurrence and Their Characterisation

In this section, we discuss Bayesian network structures of multimorbidity and introduce measures that describe the co-occurrence of diseases in terms of these structures.

3.1   Structural Measures of Multimorbidity

To illustrate how Bayesian network modelling can contribute to understanding the relationship between diseases, consider Fig. 1, which shows a Bayesian network of a single and a multiple disease model. In both models there is a set of risk factors present, which can be any subset of environmental, patient, genetic, and other disease related variables. Between these risk factors (in)dependency can occur. For example, in both disease models, the risk factors 2 and 3 are associated with each other through a third risk factor 1, and the risk factors 4 and 6 are directly associated. The risk factor 5 is independent from the other risk factors, however in the multiple disease model it is also a common parent of both diseases.

There are a number of characteristics considered to be relevant in multimorbidity research [6], namely whether the diseases are: (1) causally related (*direct causation model*), (2) related because of common risk factors (*heterogenic risk factor model*), or (3) the diseases are related because of risk factors that are correlated (*associated risk factor model*). Learning causal models is beyond the scope of this paper, so we will focus on characteristics of heterogenic and associated risk factors of diseases. In the example above, risk factor 5 is a common risk factor, while, for example, risk factor 3 and risk factor 6 are heterogenic risk factors. The quantitative measures that we will use in Section 4, are the number of common risk factors and the number of associated risk factor combinations that lead to associations between diseases. As these measures show the number of relationships between the most important risk factors, they given an indication of the *complexity* of the reason for co-occurrences. If both numbers are 0 and their is no direct path between the diseases, then we have the simplest type of multimorbidity, i.e. independent multimorbidity.

3.2   Critical Factors

While there can be many associations between diseases, often these diseases can be explained by only a few risk factors. For example, in Fig. 1, risk factors 1, 4, and 5 completely explain the association between the diseases. If these risks can be prevented or reduced through an intervention, both the chance of the occurrence of the individual diseases *and* the multimorbidity burden is reduced, so these are the most *critical factors* in the model. More formally, this means we are interested in sets of factors C such that, given two diseases D_i and D_j and a graph G:

1. all trails $D_i \leftarrow X_1 \leftarrow \cdots \leftarrow X_k \rightarrow \cdots \rightarrow X_n \rightarrow D_j$ in the graph G are d-separated by C, i.e. $C \cap \{X_1, \ldots, X_n\} \neq \varnothing$;
2. there is no $C' \subset C$ for which the previous condition holds.

It is easy to see that there exists such a C such that every $X \in C$ is an ancestor of both D_i and D_j. In our non-causal models, the ultimate causes are not necessarily ancestors, hence, we take any of the minimal seperating sets, which can be can be found in polynomial time [13].

Using existing techniques, it is possible to find a conditioning set Q such that $\forall q \in Q : RR_{ij}^q = 1$. If $\forall q \in Q : RR_{ij}^q = 1$, using Equation 3 this implies $\frac{P(D_i, D_j|Q)}{P(D_i|Q)P(D_j|Q)} = 1$, so therefore we have:

$$\frac{P(D_i, D_j \mid Q)}{P(D_i \mid Q)P(D_j \mid Q)} = 1 \Leftrightarrow D_i \perp\!\!\!\perp D_j \mid Q \Leftrightarrow Q \ d\text{-separates } D_i \text{ and } D_j \quad (5)$$

For example, the RR of a colorectal cancer and a respiratory cancer being a co-morbid combination is 5. If we condition on the presence of liver cancer, the RR drops to 1.3 and it remains 5 when liver cancer is not present. In this approach, no distinction can be made between direct causation and common risk factors, i.e. whether liver cancer is a common risk factor or whether it is a metastasis of a colorectal cancer that will further metastasise to the lungs. In Bayesian network structure learning, it is common practice to include background knowledge during the learning of networks, e.g. knowledge that metastatic spread of a cancer is common. Furthermore, in structure learning approaches it is possible to use model selection that gives an indication of the best possible model, which is significantly more difficult using relative risk or Pearson's correlation.

4   Experiments

4.1   Data

The Netherlands Information Network of General Practice (LINH) routinely collects patient data about diagnoses and laboratory results since 1996. Recently, these data were used to compare the occurrence of pre-existing and subsequent comorbidity among older cancer patients with older non-cancer patients in terms of odds and hazard ratios [14].

Table 1. Prevalence and co-occurrence of malignant tumours. All RRs and ϕ correlation coefficients are significant ($p < 0.05$). CD=conditional dependence.

(a) Prevelance

cancer	prevalence
skin	21.33 ‰
breast	12.11 ‰
colorectal	7.43 ‰
respiratory	6.23 ‰
prostate	5.94 ‰
bladder	2.83 ‰
liver	2.64 ‰
muscles	2.40 ‰
leukaemia	2.13 ‰
female genitals	2.02 ‰
lymphoma	1.70 ‰
cervix	1.10 ‰
stomach	1.08 ‰
kidney	1.08 ‰
pancreas	1.07 ‰
neurologic	0.91 ‰
metabolic	0.59 ‰
ureter	0.25 ‰

(b) Co-occurrence

cancer site 1	cancer site 2	p-value CD-test	RR	ϕ
pancreas	liver	7.31E-16	34	0.22
respiratory	neurologic	1.80E-15	22	0.17
respiratory	liver	2.63E-14	10	0.13
stomach	liver	7.52E-13	33	0.13
pancreas	metabolic	6.62E-10	80	0.22
leukaemia	lymphoma	6.86E-10	21	0.41
bladder	kidney	1.03E-07	27	0.28
colorectal	liver	1.09E-07	8	0.13
bladder	ureter	1.84E-07	72	0.41
skin	lymphoma	5.66E-06	5	0.12
colorectal	respiratory	4.19E-04	5	0.09
breast	respiratory	8.75E-04	3	0.14
muscles	respiratory	1.32E-03	3	0.55
colorectal	kidney	1.67E-03	7	0.37
cervix	female genitals	3.04E-03	17	0.55
bladder	respiratory	3.20E-03	7	0.16
bladder	prostate	3.21E-03	9	0.32

For a total number of approximately 150,000 patients present in this dataset we determined the presence of chronic disorders defined by O'Halloran [15]. In the remainder of this paper we will denote malignant diseases, e.g. skin cancer or breast cancer, by M_i. Remaining chronic, but benign, conditions, such as chronic liver disease or benign prostatic hypertrophy, are denoted by C_k.

Table 1 shows prevalences of the most significant comorbid combinations of malignant tumours, corrected for age and gender. A combination of two malignant tumours M_i and M_j is selected when $M_i \not\perp M_j \mid \{Age, Gender\}$, with a significance level < 0.05. For comparison, the RR and the ϕ-correlation coefficient are calculated as well.

For each malignant tumour M_i present in Table 1, the set R_i consists of all associated conditions C_k for which $M_i \not\perp C_k \mid \{Age, Gender\}$, with a significance level < 0.05, shown in Table 2. A distinction is made between disorders that are associated with the onset of a cancer, e.g. smoking, alcohol abuse, or a chronic liver disease (Table 2(a)), and disorders that are probably a consequence of a cancer, e.g. anaemia, depression, or cardiovascular disease (Table 2(b)).

Finally, we applied structure learning, using the R statistical software package bnlearn [12], for each $\{M_i, M_j, Age, Gender\} \cup R_i \cup R_j$ of each combination M_i and M_j present in Table 1. Within each structure we determined the minimum d-separation between M_i and M_j, and whether a direct association still remained between the two malignant tumours M_i and M_j. A pair of two associated risks R_k

Table 2. Chronic conditions associated with at least one of the cancers listed in Table 1, grouped by risk factors and symptomatology

(a) Associated Risks

System	Conditions
Patient	age, gender, smoking, alcohol, obesity
Digestive	oesophageal reflux, ulcer, chole-cystitis/lithiasis, viral hepatitis, chronic liver disease, irritable bowel syndrome, diverticulosis
Metabolic	diabetes mellitus, lipid disorder, hypothyroidism, hyperthyroidism, gout
Musculoskeletal	osteoporosis, rheumatoid arthritis, osteoarthritis
Neurologic	benign neurocancer, congenital anomaly
Respiratory	asthma, chronic obstructive pulmonary disease
Skin	acne, psoriasis, eczema, benign skin cancer
Urogenital	benign prostatic hypertrophy, endometriosis

(b) Associated Symptomatology

System	Conditions
Cardiovascular	hypotension, hypertension, ischemic heart disease, heart failure, arrhythmia, myocardinfarct, stroke, embolism, varicosis, flebitis
Musculoskeletal	hernia, spondylosis, tendinitis
Neurologic	headache, epilepsy, neuropathy
Psychiatric	anxiety, personality disorder, depression, organic psychosis, somatisation, neurasthenia
Blood/Renal	anaemia, purpura, renal insufficiency
Eye/Ear	macula degeneration, cataract, deafness, vertigo

and R_l can be dependent or independent when corrected for age and gender, i.e., $R_k \not\!\perp\!\!\!\perp R_l \mid \{Age, Gender\}$ or $R_k \perp\!\!\!\perp R_l \mid \{Age, Gender\}$, respectively. Dependent risk factors can be grouped into common parents and associated risks. The results are showed in Table 3.

In our results, we observe that in the majority of the cases there is no direct arc between two malignant tumours M_i and M_j if the $RR_{ij} < 10$, i.e. the association can only be explained by a set of critical factors.

Age and gender frequently act as a common parent. Therefore, they are often part of the critical factors. Only on three occasions a disease node, other than age or gender, acts as a direct common parent: chronic liver disease as common parent of pancreatic cancer and liver cancer; smoking as a common parent of respiratory cancer and bladder cancer; and benign prostate hypertrophy as a common parent of prostatic cancer and bladder cancer.

Figure 2a shows the local network structure that connects colorectal cancer and respiratory cancer. These two malignant tumours do not share a direct common parent, and there is no edge between these two nodes. However, the etiologic association can be explained by the critical factors and the elements

Table 3. Etiological measures of comorbid malignant tumours. Abbreviations: DP = directed path, RF = the number of risk factors in the local network, CP = the number of common parents, AR = the number of risk combinations that are associated, IR = the number of risk combinations that are independent.

cancer site 1	cancer site 2	DP	RF	CP	AR	IR	critical factors (min. d-separation)
pancreas	liver	yes	12	2	0	1	age, chronic liver disease
respiratory	neurologic	yes	12	0	0	4	gender
respiratory	liver	yes	15	1	3	1	age, oesophageal reflux, chr. liver disease
stomach	liver	no	10	1	4	2	age, alcohol abuse, chronic liver disease
pancreas	metabolic	yes	8	1	0	0	age
leukaemia	lymphoma	yes	3	2	0	0	age, gender
bladder	kidney	yes	10	1	1	0	age
colorectal	liver	yes	13	1	2	0	age, diverticulosis
bladder	ureter	yes	6	1	0	0	age
skin	lymphoma	no	15	1	0	3	age
colorectal	respiratory	yes	15	1	3	0	age, smoking, alcohol abuse
breast	respiratory	no	15	2	4	0	age, gender, smoking, osteoporosis
muscles	respiratory	no	13	0	3	3	asthma, arthrosis
colorectal	kidney	no	11	1	1	1	age, diverticulosis
cervix	genitals	yes	3	1	0	0	gender
bladder	respiratory	no	14	3	2	0	age, gender, smoking, benign skin tumour
bladder	prostate	no	14	3	1	0	age, gender, benign prostate hypertrophy

of directed paths, in this case: *age, smoking, alcohol abuse,* and *liver cancer.* Conditioning on these variables should lower the RR significantly. Indeed, if we condition on the facts that a patient smokes, has liver cancer, and is of age between 65 and 80, the RR observing both cancers drops from 5 to 1.8.

Figure 2b shows the local network structure that connects liver cancer and pancreatic cancer, which also appears at the top of the list in Table 1b. There is a direct association between liver cancer and pancreatic cancer. In this case, this is most likely a direct causal pathway, i.e. metastasis. The remainder of the etiology is totally explained by the direct common parents *age* and *chronic liver disease.* Colorectal cancer is associated with liver cancer, but as risk factor it is independent from pancreatic cancer.

5   Conclusions

The advantage of studying multimorbidity by Bayesian networks is that they allow modelling relationships between multiple disease variables, whereas it is also possible to learn these, to a large extent, from data. Structure learning has been applied before to medicine, for example, to predict disease related mortality [16], and also in the context of multimorbidity, e.g. in genome-wide association studies to determine genetic links between chronic diseases [17]. In

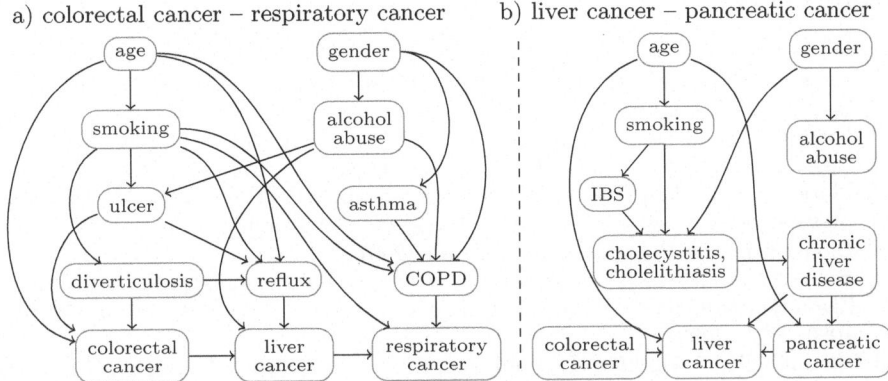

Fig. 2. Bayesian networks for comorbid combinations of cancer. Abbreviations: COPD=chronic obstructive pulmonary disease; IBS=irritable bowel syndrome.

this paper, we use these methods to explain the co-occurrence of multiple diseases in terms of their risk factors. As the types of relationships between risk factors varies, we proposed a number of novel structural measures and critical factors that lead to co-occurrences.

The results obtained are in line with knowledge known from the oncology literature. For example, long sustained exposure to chronic conditions, e.g. unhealthy lifestyles, is associated with high prevalence of breast, colorectal, respiratory and prostate cancer [18]. In the networks learned here, age and gender are often a direct parent of both malignant tumours. Other critical risk factors, e.g. smoking and alcohol abuse, are often associated by directed paths of pathophysiology to pairs of malignant tumours.

In some cases a direct edge remains in the network between the two malignant tumours. Most probable, this reflects metastasis, however direct associations found between two malignant tumours may also have another explanation, e.g. a genetic predisposition or another unknown confounder. Sometimes there a directed path of malignant tumours. This might reflect metastasis to secondary locations, e.g. *colorectal cancer → liver cancer → respiratory cancer*. The same holds for associations between risk factors, such as oesophageal reflux with diverticulosis, which may be explained by life style factors or genetics that are not present in the data.

The methodology used here shows that, even though overall relative risks between pairs of malignant tumours can be high, a direct association, e.g. metastasis, is not always the obvious reason for that. Using structure learning and concepts such as *d*-separation in Bayesian networks we identified other critical risk factors, e.g. age, gender, smoking, and alcohol abuse, in the pathogenesis of co-occurring malignant tumours. This shows that the method provides useful results for identifying critical factors of associated comorbid diseases where the role of such risk factors is less obvious.

References

1. Diederichs, C., Berger, K., Bartels, D.: The measurement of multiple chronic dis-eases - a systematic review on existing multimorbidity indices. J. Gerontol. A Biol. Sci. Med. Sci. 66, 301–311 (2011)
2. Ritchie, C.S., Kvale, E., Fisch, M.J.: Multimorbidity: An issue of growing impor-tance for oncologists. Journal of Oncology Practice 7, 371–374 (2011)
3. Mariotto, A.B., Rowland, J.H., Ries, L.A., Scoppa, S., Feuer, E.J.: Multiple cancer prevalence: A growing challenge in long-term survivorship. Cancer Epidemiology, Biomarkers and Prevention 16, 566–571 (2007)
4. Rosso, S., Angelis, R.D., Ciccolallo, L., Carrani, E., Soerjomataram, I., Grande, E., Zigon, G., Brenner, H.: Multiple tumours in survival estimates. Eur. J. Cancer 45, 1080–1094 (2009)
5. Vittinghoff, E., Glidden, D., Shiboski, S., McCulloch, C.: Regression Methods in Biostatistics: linear, logistic, survival and repeated measures models. Springer, New York (2005)
6. Lappenschaar, M., Hommersom, A., Lucas, P.: Probabilistic causal models of mul-timorbidity concepts. In: AMIA Proceedings of the 2012 Annual Symposium, Chicago, United States, pp. 475–484 (2012)
7. Chen, L., Blumm, N., Christakis, N., Barabasi, A., Deisboeck, T.: Cancer metas-tasis networks and the prediction of progression patterns. British Journal of Can-cer 101, 749–758 (2009)
8. Sistrom, C.L., Garvan, C.W.: Proportions, odds, and risk. Radiology 230, 12–19 (2004)
9. Kraemer, H.: Statistical issues in assessing comorbidity. Statistics in Medicine 14, 721–733 (1995)
10. Valderas, J., Starfield, B., Sibbald, B., Salisbury, C., Roland, M.: Defining co-morbidity: Implications for understanding health and health services. Ann. Fam. Med. 7, 357–363 (2009)
11. Pearl, J.: Probabilistic Reasoning in Intelligent Systems. Morgan Kaufmann, San Francisco (1988)
12. Scutari, M.: Learning Bayesian networks with the bnlearn R package. Journal of Statistical Software 35, 122 (2010)
13. Tian, J., Pearl, J., Paz, A.: Finding minimal d-separators. Technical report, Com-puter Science Department, Cognitive Systems Laboratory, University of California, Los Angeles, USA (1998)
14. Deckx, L., van den Akker, M., Metsemakers, J., Knottnerus, A., Schellevis, F., Buntinx, F.: Chronic diseases among older cancer survivors. Journal of Cancer Epidemiology 2012, Article ID 206414, 7 pages (2012)
15. O'Halloran, J., Miller, G., Britt, H.: Defining chronic conditions for primary care with icpc-2. Familiy Practice 21, 381–386 (2004)
16. Cooper, G.F., Aliferis, C.F., Ambrosino, R., Aronis, J., Buchanan, B.G., Caruana, R., Fine, M.J., Glymour, C., Gordon, G., Hanusa, B.H., Janosky, J.E., Meek, C., Mitchell, T., Richardson, T., Spirtes, P.: An evaluation of machine-learning methods for predicting pneumonia mortality. Artificial Intelligence in Medicine 9, 107–138 (1997)
17. Alekseyenko, A., Lytkin, N.I., Ai, J., Ding, B., Padyukov, L., Aliferis, C.F., Statnikov, A.: Causal graph-based analysis of genome-wide association data in rheumatoid arthritis. Biology Direct 6, 25–37 (2011)
18. Wei, E.K., Wolin, K.Y., Colditz, G.A.: Time course of risk factors in cancer etiology and progression. Journal of Clinical Oncology 28, 4052–4057 (2010)

Online Diagnostic System
Based on Bayesian Networks

Adam Zagorecki, Piotr Orzechowski, and Katarzyna Hołownia

Infermedica, s.c.
Plac Solny 14/3, 50-062 Wrocław, Poland
{adam.zagorecki,piotr.orzechowski,katarzyna.holownia}@infermedica.com
http://www.infermedica.com

Abstract. In this paper we present a general medical diagnostic expert system intended to serve as an educational self-diagnostic tool, openly available through the WWW. The system has been designed as an alternative to the common self-diagnosis practice among the general public of searching the Internet, finding the first disease with some matching symptoms, and treating this as a diagnosis, in contrast with the differential diagnosis offered by our system. We discuss the medical knowledge elicitation process, automated generation of Bayesian network models, and the diagnostic process. The system uses a scalable and efficient distributed reasoning engine based on multiple Bayesian networks. An analysis of over 100,000 diagnostic cases is presented. The cases are analyzed based on population characteristics such as age and gender. The results show the need for medical education and highlight the most common problems in non-emergency medical care.

Keywords: Expert systems, Bayesian networks, Computer-aided diagnosis.

1 Introduction

Ideas involving the use of a machine to help doctors in the diagnostic process were first proposed in the literature in the 1950s [1]. The first systems based on probabilistic principles were proposed in the 1960s [2], and since then the probabilistic approach has been one of the key tools for addressing the problem. With the introduction of Bayesian networks [3], they were quickly adopted to provide medical diagnosis, the most prominent early example of which is the QMR-DT system [4]. Since then a vast number of applications of Bayesian networks to the medical domain have been developed [5].

In this paper we present a general medical diagnostic expert system that we have developed, intended to serve as an educational self-diagnostic tool. The system is openly available through the WWW in two language versions: www.doktor-medi.pl in Polish for which the data discussed here was collected and an English-language version available at www.symptomate.com. The system has been designed as an alternative to the common self-diagnosis practice among

N. Peek, R. Marín Morales, and M. Peleg (Eds.): AIME 2013, LNAI 7885, pp. 145–149, 2013.

the general public of searching the Internet, finding the first disease with some matching symptoms, and pursuing this finding as a diagnosis. In contrast, our system offers differential diagnosis based on a list of symptoms provided by the user during an interactive process. The system uses a scalable and efficient distributed reasoning engine based on multiple Bayesian networks. The Bayesian network models were automatically created from a medical knowledge base developed specifically for this purpose.

Our goal was to develop and implement a system that would attempt online diagnosis with only limited information provided by the user. The setting is comparable to a patient entering the primary care doctors office the information assumed to be available is the basic facts about the patient: sex, age, height and weight. We assume that the system does not assume knowledge of the users prior health conditions; this is dictated primarily by the privacy policy.

We will also present and discuss an analysis of the results obtained from 100,000 diagnoses recorded during the first three months after the Polish-language version of the system was made available on the Internet through the WWW and mobile phone applications. A single diagnosis consists of a set of observations, some basic user data a list of symptoms that have been elicited from the user in the diagnostic process, and finally one or more suspected diseases. The diagnoses are analyzed based on population characteristics such as age and gender. In general, the results show the need for medical education and highlight the most common problems in non-emergency medical care.

2   Modelling Strategy

In our approach, we assumed that the backbone of the diagnostic BN model is a bipartite graph: a graph consisting of two layers. The disease nodes are placed in the top layer, while the symptoms nodes are in the bottom. The only links allowed are those originating from a node in the top layer to a node in the bottom layer. Additionally, to reduce the number of parameters required to specify the conditional probabilities in the nodes from the bottom layer, they are assumed to be noisy-OR models. This type of model is not a new concept in modeling diagnosis using BNs and is often referred to in the literature as BN2O [6]. We included some additional elements in the system and BN model, such as risk factors modeled as additional nodes in BN (not noisy-OR) or deterministic constraints that are partially included in the BN model and partially as additional filters (e.g. filtering out questions related to menstruation for men and for women after menopause, etc.). During the elicitation process we allow the doctors to define deterministic diagnostic rules that are intended to guide the order of questions in the diagnostic process.

The medical database comprises 150 diseases and over 600 symptoms, and the database is being continuously revised and expanded. The user interface allows the user to send feedback on the diagnosis if he or she finds it to be incorrect; this is an invaluable source of information on the systems performance and problems encountered, which the medical team attempts to rectify through the database revisions.

Although there exist specialized software tools for creation of BN, such as Bayesia, Hugin, or GeNIe, in many practical applications it would be impractical to use them because of (1) the problem of managing large networks, (2) the possibility of introducing human errors that would be difficult to identify and isolate, (3) the need for multi-user collaborative workspace. In order to facilitate knowledge elicitation for the needs of the system, we developed a web-based collaborative tool to edit the medical database.

Because of the relatively dense connectivity implied by the medical database, the state-of-the-art inference algorithms are unable to process the queries to the network in the desired time of 1 second, which we assumed to be satisfactory for the system. Our solution was to generate several BN models from the information stored in the database. The downside of this approach is that we remove probabilistic interdependencies between nodes that would belong to two different models. In order to reduce this effect, we decided to (1) reduce the number of separate BN models as much as possible, (2) allow for the same variable to appear in two or more different BN models, and (3) if possible keep densely connected subsets of nodes in one model (avoid breaking clusters).

We developed a special hierarchical aggregation algorithm that identifies the optimal number of BN models needed to achieve desired performance of the system (arbitrary query time less than 1 second). In the beginning, the algorithm creates n BNs, where n is the number of diseases in the medical data base. We assumed that each disease can only appear in one BN model, while the same symptom can appear in different BN models. Then iteratively, we combine some of the models into larger models. Since we assume that our models are BN2O it is straightforward to combine two BN2O models so that the resulting model is BN2O as well. We developed a special metric that allows us to determine the similarity between two BN2O networks based on shared symptoms and their parameters. The algorithm stops at the point when the total query time for the system of BNs exceeds a certain threshold. In practice, after each revision of the medical database the system is based on a different set of BN. Currently, the medical database is split into approximately 10 separate BNs that roughly correspond to medical specializations such as cardiology, sexual health, dentistry, etc. Any incoming query to the system is performed in parallel on all BNs the symptom nodes are instantiated (observed) in all networks. Since the disease nodes are unique, the ranking of the most likely diseases for the query is generated by simply combining the results from all BNs into a single list. In practice the system is implemented as a distributed web-service with multiple instances of BN engines based on the SMILE BN engine [7] with a load-balancing schema.

3   Results

In this section we present some analysis of the results obtained from the initial period of the system being made available for general public. The data includes

Table 1. Ten most popular diesases among male by sex and age

Age 18-30		Age 30-50		Age 50-70		Age above 70	
Male							
Discopaty	4.4	Discopaty	6.3	Discopaty		6.8	Discopaty	6.0
Anxiety	4.3	Anxiety	4.2	Prostatic Hyp.		5.8	Urge Incont.	4.6
Tension Head.	3.6	Tension Head.	3.5	Arthritis		4.0	Arthritis	4.3
Tiredness	3.0	Irritable Bowel	3.4	Irritable Bowel		3.7	Rheumat. Arth.	3.3
Irritable Bowel	2.9	Tiredness	3.0	Gallstone		3.3	Bone/Joint Tr.	3.2
Supraven. E. B	2.8	Sciatica	3.0	Rheumat. Arth.		3.1	Anxiety	2.9
Flu	2.8	Supraven. E. B	2.7	Sleep Apnea		3.1	Osteoporoza	2.8
Allergic Rhinitis	2.7	Acid Reflux	2.7	Anxiety		2.8	Irritable Bowel	2.7
Depression	2.6	Sleep Apnea	2.5	Acid Reflux		2.8	Sciatica	2.3
Migraines	2.6	Flu	2.5	Ischaem. Heart D.		2.8	Sleep Apnea	2.3
Female							
PMS	6.6	PMS	6.5	Discopaty		9.3	Discopaty	6.0
Dysmenorrhea	4.6	Discopaty	6.0	Arthritis		4.2	Arthritis	5.1
Pregnancy	4.4	Tension Head.	4.0	Rheumat. Arth.		4.1	Rheumat. Arth.	4.0
Tension Head.	3.9	Anxiety	3.7	Bone/Joint Tr.		3.7	Bone/Joint Tr.	3.6
Discopaty	3.8	Tiredness	3.5	Anxiety		3.4	Osteoporosis	3.3
Irritable Bowel	3.8	Migraines	3.4	Tension Head.		3.4	Ischaem. Heart D.	3.0
Tiredness	3.6	Irritable Bowel	3.3	Migraines		3.3	Irritable Bowel	2.9
Anxiety	3.3	Pregnancy	3.1	Irritable Bowel		3.3	Anxiety	2.7
Migraines	3.2	Dysmenorrhea	3.0	Sciatica		3.1	Acid Reflux	2.3
Gallstone	2.5	Sciatica	2.5	Depression		2.5	Migraines	2.3

100,000 diagnoses. It should be expected that some of these diagnoses are results of the users playing and testing the system, but from our experience we can expect that most of those end up as non-diagnosed cases. Some of the diagnoses can be repetitive in the sense that the user tried the system several times with slightly different answers. However, majority of the diagnoses can be assumed to be legitimate user attempts to use the system.

The Table 1 shows the diseases which were most frequently produced by the system with the percentage of their occurance. From this list we removed cases that ended in unknown diagnoses (which constituted 24.4% of all cases); however, the percentages shown in the table correspond to all cases. It is also important to remember that the system can produce more than one suspected diagnosis per user. The results demonstrate that the most popular disorders are linked to stress and an unhealthy lifestyle. Particularly interesting is the common occurrence of discopathy (which in our system is in fact a common term for a class of more specific problems), especially among younger people, in whom it can be linked to their sedentary lifestyle. It is clearly noticeable that some age-related disorders, such as Prostatic Hyperplasia or Osteoporosis, are more often diagnosed in older age groups.

4 Conclusions and Future Work

In this paper we presented an educational system for self-assessment that uses diagnostic Bayesian networks to produce a series of diagnostic questions and final diagnoses. The system has been made available to Polish-speaking Internet users. The results of 100,000 diagnoses were presented and discussed.

An interesting observation can be made regarding the nature of the problems with which users visit the website. We can speculate that the most popular diagnoses are those related to stress and an unhealthy lifestyle, especially among younger users. Diagnoses such as tension headaches, tiredness, and anxiety disorders are typically induced by stress. The leading diagnosed disease is discopathy. This may not be surprising among the older population, but among young people who spend a lot of time in front of a computer (who are likely users of the system) it is known to be a problem as well.

Because of the assumptions behind the system and the nature of the information gathered during the session with the user, it should be expected that some health conditions cannot be diagnosed by merely asking the user questions, especially those that require medical tests. This should be taken into consideration when interpreting the results obtained from the system.

Acknowledgments. The authors would like to thank Dorota Frydecka, Mateusz Palczewski, Anna Rogozińska, Katarzyna Trybucka, and Marcin Zawadzki who contributed to the creation of the medical knowledge base and Paweł Iwaszko who was responsible for the IT element. The SMILE inference engine developed at the Decision Systems Laboratory, University of Pittsburgh, is used to perform diagnostic inference (http://genie.sis.pitt.edu). The creation of the system was possible with funding provided by the Wrocław Research Center EIT+.

References

1. Ledley, R.S., Lusted, L.B.: Reasoning foundations of medical diagnosis; symbolic logic, probability, and value theory aid our understanding of how physicians reason. Science 130(3366), 9–21 (1959)
2. Warner, H.R., Toronto, A.F., Veasey, L.G., Stephenson, R.: A mathematical approach to medical diagnosis. JAMA: The Journal of the American Medical Association 177(3), 177–183 (1961)
3. Pearl, J.: Probabilistic reasoning in intelligent systems: networks of plausible inference. Morgan Kaufmann (1988)
4. Middleton, B., Shwe, M., Heckerman, D., Henrion, M., Horvitz, E., Lehmann, H., Cooper, G.: Probabilistic diagnosis using a reformulation of the INTERNIST-1/QMR knowledge base. Medicine 30, 241–255 (1991)
5. Lucas, P.: Expert knowledge and its role in learning bayesian networks in medicine: An appraisal. In: Quaglini, S., Barahona, P., Andreassen, S. (eds.) AIME 2001. LNCS (LNAI), vol. 2101, pp. 156–166. Springer, Heidelberg (2001)
6. D'Ambrosio, B.: Symbolic probabilistic inference in large BN2O networks. In: Proc. Tenth Conf. on Uncertainty in Artificial Intelligence, pp. 128–135 (1994)
7. SMILE: Structural Modeling, Inference, and Learning Engine, http://genie.sis.pitt.edu

A Probabilistic Graphical Model
for Tuning Cochlear Implants

Iñigo Bermejo[1], Francisco Javier Díez[1], Paul Govaerts[2], and Bart Vaerenberg[2,3]

[1] ETSI Informática, UNED, Juan del Rosal 16, Madrid, Spain
[2] The Eargroup, Herentalsebaan 71, B-2100 Antwerp-Deurne, Belgium
[3] Laboratory of Biomedical Physics, University of Antwerp, Belgium

Abstract. Severe and profound hearing losses can be treated with cochlear implants (CI). Given that a CI may have up to 150 tunable parameters, adjusting them is a highly complex task. For this reason, we decided to build a decision support system based on a new type of probabilistic graphical model (PGM) that we call tuning networks. Given the results of a set of audiological tests and the current status of the parameter set, the system looks for the set of changes in the parameters of the CI that will lead to the biggest improvement in the user's hearing ability. Because of the high number of variables involved in the problem we have used an object-oriented approach to build the network. The prototype has been informally evaluated comparing its advice with those of the expert and of a previous decision support system based on deterministic rules. Tuning networks can be used to adjust other electrical or mechanical devices, not only in medicine.

1 Introduction

Cochlear implants (CI) are being successfully applied to treat severe and profound hearing losses. A CI consists of a speech processor that analyzes the sound and an array of electrodes placed into the cochlea which pass an electrical signal directly to the auditory nerve.

After implantation, CIs need to be programmed or "fitted" to optimize the user's hearing capability. This is usually a challenging and time-consuming task that is typically performed by highly trained audiologists or medical doctors. CI centers and manufacturers have developed their own heuristics, usually in the form of simple "if-then" rules applied in a very flexible but individual and uncontrollable way. Recipients using incorrectly programmed CIs experience poor performance and outcomes.

One of those applications, called FOX [1], was developed by Otoconsult, an audiological clinic in Antwerp, Belgium. It is being used in several centers across Europe. FOX is based on parameterized deterministic rules, which entails some limitations, such as the difficulty to maintain the knowledge base when the number of rules increases and the inability to learn from data. The Opti-FOX project [2] was conceived to overcome these limitations. In the beginning, an approach

N. Peek, R. Marín Morales, and M. Peleg (Eds.): AIME 2013, LNAI 7885, pp. 150–155, 2013.

with supervised classification algorithms—such as the k-NN classifier—was attempted, but failed to progress due to the complexity of the problem and the small number of records available to learn from. In order to improve the results of FOX, the most promising approach seemed to build a probabilistic graphical model (PGM) because this type of model can combine expert knowledge, the power of probabilistic reasoning, and the ability to learn from data.

This paper describes briefly a new type of PGM especially tailored for tuning programmable devices and how it has been used to build a decision support system for fitting CIs.

2   Tuning Networks

A tuning network consists of an acyclic directed graph (ADG) containing chance, decision and utility nodes, and a probability distribution. As in other types of PGMs, a decision node represents a variable that is under the direct control of the decision maker, while chance nodes represent features of the system over which the decision maker has no direct control, and utility nodes represent the decision maker's preferences, measured on a numerical scale. In tuning networks, each property of the system is modeled by a relative-value node that represents a change in its value and, optionally, by an absolute-value node. In the case of a tunable parameter (for example, the sensitivity of the microphone), the relative-value node is a decision node because the programmer of the CI can increase, decrease, or keep the value of the parameter; the absolute-value node is represented as a chance node for which we have evidence, because the value of a tunable parameter is always known. We may also have evidence about the absolute-value nodes that represent measurements, such as the result of a test. Utility nodes are always relative-value nodes, as they represent the increase or decrease in the user's performance as a consequence of tuning some parameters.

An important component of tuning networks is the *tuning model*, a new canonical model based on the property of *independence of causal interaction* (ICI) [3,4,5]. Canonical models represent how a variable is probabilistically influenced by a set of parent variables [6], in general assuming a pattern of causal interaction. Their main advantage is that the number of parameters (conditional probabilities) is proportional to the number of parents, while in the general case it grows exponentially. ICI models assume that each parent produces the effect with a certain probability, independently of the values of the other parents, and the global effect is determined by a function, specific of each type of ICI model, that combines the individual effects; for example, in the noisy OR the effect is present when at least one of the causes has produced the effect.

A unique feature of the tuning model is that it assumes that every variable involved has exactly three values: increased, decreased, and not-changed, while other ICI models, such as the noisy OR and the noisy AND, assume that all variables are boolean, and other models, such as the noisy MIN and the noisy MAX impose no restriction about the number of values of each variable [5]. The tuning model assumes that a change in one of the parents causes a change in the child variable with a certain probability. When some of the parents induce an increase and others cause a decrease, the global effect depends on whether there are more increases than decreases, or vice versa, or there is a tie. It is therefore similar to a majority voting function.

Tuning networks differ from influence diagrams [7] in that they do not have a total ordering of the decisions because the order in which the parameters are tuned does not affect the result. Additionally, all the evidence is available before making the decisions, as it the in each session when programming a CI, while in influence diagrams some decision provide evidence that can be used in subsequent decisions. As a consequence, the algorithms for evaluating these two types of models are very different—see Section 3.2.

3   Construction of the Model

3.1   Model Construction

Variables in the Model. In our tuning network, the tunable parameters are those of the CI; as mentioned above, each one is represented by an absolute-value chance node and a relative-value decision node. Each electrode has several tunable parameters, e.g., the T level (the softest electrical input level detectable by the user), the M level (the electrical input level perceived as loud but comfortable), etc. Besides, the CI has a set of tunable parameters that are electrode-independent, i.e., global to the implant, such as the volume of the microphone.

The model also represents the results of a battery of different tests, such as audiometries, phoneme discrimination and speech recognition tests. Each measurement of a test is modeled with a chance node representing the current value of the test (this node receives evidence when performing the test), a chance node representing the expected change in the result of the tests given the changes in the tunable parameters, and a utility variable defining the utility function based on the other two.

Other nodes represent internal properties of the device, such as the amount of energy in the auditory nerve, which depend on the tunable parameters and in turn affect the results of the tests.

The global utility of our model is the sum of the results of all tests; therefore maximizing this utility is the same as optimizing the user's hearing ability.

The resulting model contains 202 nodes and 664 links.

Elicitation of Numerical Parameters. The probabilities and utilities have been assessed by the expert: the probabilities are subjective estimates based on his expertise while the utilities have been estimated by roughly assigning monetary value to positive and negative changes in the results of tests.

Object-Oriented Probabilistic Networks. The network, containing sets of repeated structures (such as electrodes, frequency bands and tests) was modeled following the object-oriented paradigm for PGMs as proposed by [8,9].

A class defines a structure consisting of a set of attributes and their probabilistic relations and is connected with other classes through their input parameters, namely instances of other classes. An OOPN consists of a set of instances and their causal relations.

3.2 Inference

Inference in a tuning network consists in looking for the optimal strategy, i.e., the set of changes in the tunable parameters that maximizes the global expected utility. As an exhaustive search would be computationally unaffordable, we have implemented a greedy *search and score* algorithm that examines myopically the space of possible strategies. The search is initialized by setting all policies for all decision nodes to "no change". It then iteratively looks for the single change in the strategy, i.e. a change in a decision node's policy that maximizes the global utility function.

The score for each strategy, namely the global expected utility given the strategy, is computed using an inference algorithm. Given the high number of variables in the model and its high connectivity, the cost of running exact inference algorithms is unaffordable. For that reason, we decided to use an approximate inference algorithm—namely a likelihood weighting method [10] adapted to networks with utility nodes—whose spatial and temporal complexities grow linearly with the number of nodes instead of exponentially. The main drawback of likelihood weighting is that its accuracy decreases with extremely unlikely evidence, but it still fits our needs as the observed nodes usually have no extreme probabilities.

We compared the results of this greedy algorithm—in simplified versions of our model—with those of an exact inference algorithm (variable elimination) and both returned the same optimal strategy under different evidence scenarios. The execution time of the greedy algorithm, which has been implemented to run in parallel taking advantage of multiple core processors, depends on the number of changes proposed by the optimal strategy, but in a regular desktop computer (Intel Core i5-2500 @ 3.30GHz and 8GBs of RAM) is usually under a minute.

3.3 Evaluation of the Model

We have initially built a prototype for the low-frequency electrodes, i.e., those in the range from 250 to 1000 Hz. This model has been tested on a set of cases taken from a database of real CI users. The recommendations output by our model have been compared with those of FOX, the expert system based on deterministic rules, having the expert as a judge. Given that FOX was built by this expert, it is not surprising that in general FOX's recommendations agreed with his. In many cases, also the recommendations of our model agreed with both FOX and the expert. There were, however, some cases in which our model recommended some interventions that surprised the expert, but he never deemed them non-sensical. On the contrary, he described them as "intelligent", "smart" and "worth trying".

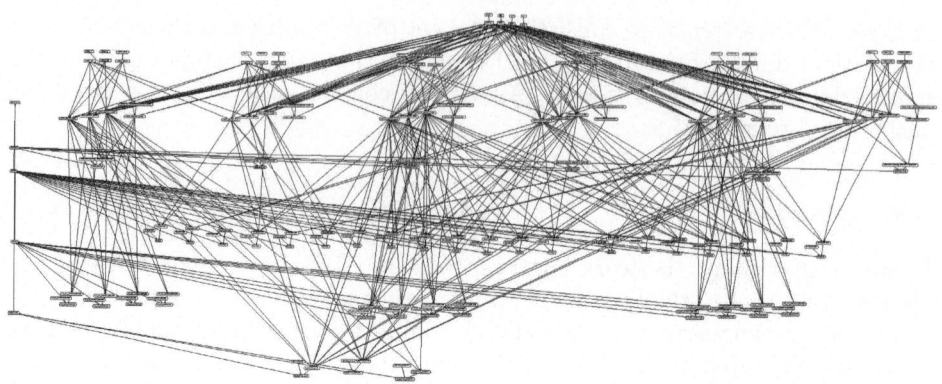

Fig. 1. Screenshot of the prototype network

On July 31, 2012 a patient at Otoconsult had a poor performance in the speech understanding tests, in spite of having an audiometry in the range of normality. The audiologists using their expertise and FOX's support, were not able to improve her abitliy to understand spoken words. However, when her implant was fitted using the advice of our prototype, her performance increased to the level of normality. Of course, this isolated result does not prove that our model outperforms FOX or the audiologists in general, but it is a promising result.

4   Conclusions and Future Work

In the context of the European project Opti-FOX, we have built a PGM for programming CIs. The development of tuning networks and our framework for OOPNs has been motivated by the needs encountered in this project, but they can be applied to adjust other electrical or mechanical devices, not only in medicine.

The advantages of our model with respect to FOX, the rule based system, are that our model is capable of complex reasoning whereas FOX only concatenates rules, that FOX is deterministic while our model handles uncertainty, and that our model will be fine-tuned by learning from data. However, FOX is still a more mature project that has been evaluated extensively and includes features that our model still lacks, such as the ability to determine the quantity by which the value of a parameter should be changed.

The most obvious next step in the project is to test the developed prototype on real CI users. Besides, we are currently working on learning the conditional probabilities from a database, in order to fine-tune the probabilities elicited by the expert. Given that our model contains unobservable variables, the usual parametric learning algorithms cannot be applied. Instead, we are using the Expectation Maximization (EM) algorithm, applied to the learning of Bayesian networks as proposed by Lauritzen [11].

Another aspect with room for improvement is the granularity of the variables. Relative-value variables were discretized into three intervals (increase, decrease, no change) to reduce the complexity of the problem. This over simplification prevents our model from accurately predicting the effect of small changes in the parameters of the CI.

Finally, the programming of a CI has a temporal aspect: it usually involves several sessions and the history of each patient is relevant. Unfortunately, the current model only considers the current values of the parameters. Turning our system into a partially-observable Markov decision process (POMDP) would allow us to model that temporal evolution and determine the optimal sequence of tests and parameter adjustments.

References

1. Govaerts, P.J., Vaerenberg, B., Ceulaer, G.D., Daemers, K., Beukelaer, C.D., Schauwers, K.: Development of a software tool using deterministic logic for the optimization of cochlear implant processor programming. Otology & Neurology 31, 908–918 (2010)
2. Szlavik, Z., Vaerenberg, B., Kowalczyk, W., Govaerts, P.: Opti-fox: towards the automatic tuning of cochlear implants. In: Proceedings of the 20th Belgian Dutch Conference on Machine Learning, pp. 79–80 (2011)
3. Heckerman, D.: Causal independence for knowledge acquisition and inference. In: Proceedings of the 9th Conference on Uncertainty in Artificial Intelligence (UAI 1993), Washington, D.C, pp. 122–127. Morgan Kaufmann, San Mateo (1993)
4. Heckerman, D., Breese, J.S.: Causal independence for probability assessment and inference using Bayesian networks. IEEE Transactions on Systems, Man and Cybernetics—Part A: Systems and Humans 26, 826–831 (1996)
5. Díez, F.J., Druzdzel, M.J.: Canonical probabilistic models for knowledge engineering. Technical Report CISIAD-06-01, UNED, Madrid, Spain (2006)
6. Pearl, J.: Probabilistic Reasoning in Intelligent Systems: Networks of Plausible Inference. Morgan Kaufmann, San Mateo (1988)
7. Howard, R.A., Matheson, J.E.: Influence diagrams. In: Howard, R.A., Matheson, J.E. (eds.) Readings on the Principles and Applications of Decision Analysis, pp. 719–762. Strategic Decisions Group, Menlo Park (1984)
8. Koller, D., Pfeffer, A.: Object-oriented Bayesian networks. In: Proceedings of the Thirteenth Conference in Artificial Intelligence (UAI 1997), pp. 302–313. Morgan Kaufmann, San Francisco (1997)
9. Bangsø, O., Wuillemin, P.H.: Top-down construction and repetetive structures representation in Bayesian networks. In: Proceedings of the Thirteenth International Florida Artificial Intelligence Research Society Conference (FLAIRS 2000), Orlando, FL, pp. 282–286 (2000)
10. Shachter, R., Peot, M.: Simulation approaches to general probabilistic inference on belief networks. In: Henrion, M., Shachter, R.D., Kanal, L.N., Lemmer, J.F. (eds.) Uncertainty in Artificial Intelligence 5, pp. 221–231. Elsevier Science Publishers, Amsterdam (1990)
11. Lauritzen, S.L.: The EM algorithm for graphical association models with missing data. Comput. Stat. Data Anal. 19(2), 191–201 (1995)

Semi-supervised Projected Clustering for Classifying GABAergic Interneurons

Luis Guerra[1], Ruth Benavides-Piccione[2], Concha Bielza[1], Víctor Robles[3], Javier DeFelipe[2], and Pedro Larrañaga[1]

[1] Computational Intelligence Group, Departamento de Inteligencia Artificial, Universidad Politécnica de Madrid (UPM), Boadilla del Monte, Madrid, Spain
l.guerra@upm.es
[2] Laboratorio Cajal de Circuitos, Centro de Tecnología Biomédica, UPM and Instituto Cajal, CSIC
[3] Departamento de Arquitectura y Tecnología de Sistemas Informáticos, UPM, Boadilla del Monte, Madrid, Spain

Abstract. A systematic classification of neuron types is a critical topic of debate in neuroscience. In this study, we propose a semi-supervised projected clustering algorithm based on finite mixture models and the expectation-maximization (EM) algorithm, that is useful for classifying neuron types. Specifically, we analyzed cortical GABAergic interneurons from different animals and cortical layers. The new algorithm, called SeSProC, is a probabilistic approach for classifying known classes and for discovering possible new groups of interneurons. Basic morphological features containing information about axonal and dendritic arborization sizes and orientations are used to characterize the interneurons. SeSProC also identifies the relevance of each feature and group separately. This article aims to present the methodological approach, reporting results for known classes and possible new groups of interneurons.

Keywords: Clustering, semi-supervised, finite mixture model, EM, projected, cortical interneurons.

1 Introduction

Neuroscience is perhaps the field of science with most interdisciplinary research approaches due to the complexity of the nervous system. In recent years, mathematical and statistical methods, and machine learning techniques have been proved to be excellent tools for analyzing different aspects of the anatomical and functional organization of the brain. A problem, which remains unsolved since the early days of the study of brain structure, is the classification of neurons. Although efforts [1] have been made in order to produce an accepted classification and terminology, experts still have differences of opinion. Solving this problem is a key milestone, not only for organizing the vast amount of data that neuroscience produces, which is fundamental for a better understanding of the structure and functions of cortical circuits, but also for helping researchers communicate with each other.

N. Peek, R. Marín Morales, and M. Peleg (Eds.): AIME 2013, LNAI 7885, pp. 156–165, 2013.

Researchers have already attempted to quantitatively classify cortical neurons using machine learning techniques. Although some adopted a supervised approach to perform this task [2, 3], most reported research was based on clustering to discern between types of neuronal data. For example, hierarchical clustering has been widely used to discover groups[1] of pyramidal cells m[4, 5] and interneurons [6, 7, 8], the main two accepted morphological types of neurons [9]. Recently, a novel, web-based interactive experiment enabled 48 worldwide experts in neuroscience to classify interneurons by visual inspection according to pre-determined criteria [10]. Thanks to this new approach, researchers were able to investigate the suitability of several anatomical terms and neuron names and concluded that supervised classification models could automatically categorize some types of interneurons in conformity with expert assignments. However, although there has for the first time been some advance in neuron naming, characterization, and classification based on community consensus, the global problem remains unsolved since experts did not reach agreement on the classification of most terms, as discussed in [10].

Thus, in this study, we propose a novel semi-supervised projected clustering method that relies on model-based clustering [11] to classify interneurons. Our classification takes basic morphological features and retrieves the known information, in the shape of data labels, from expert opinions given in [10]. Our method is able to discover possible new groups of interneurons on which the scientific community largely agrees and also identifies the relevance of each feature and group separately. Therefore, our method differs from previous approaches to this task as regards both the classification approach and how feature relevance is identified. For further details about semi-supervised learning, see [12, 13]. Different approaches related to the localized manner for identifying interesting subsets of features are reviewed in [14, 15]. More specifically, model-based clustering with embedded search of feature-relevance factors was introduced in [16] and applied to magnetic resonance spectra within a medical context in [17]. Here we present some significant results about classes of interneurons on which agreement was high in [10], and the discovery of possible new groups.

2   Materials and Methods

2.1   Data

We selected 241 three-dimensional (3D) reconstructions of interneurons from several areas and layers of the cerebral cortex of different experimental animals (mouse, rat, and monkey) and humans, from [10]. All these reconstructions were extracted from NeuroMorpho.Org [18]. From this database, we selected labeled data depending on the number of equal votes (threshold) assigned by experts in [10]. Specifically, we selected three thresholds -18, 22, and 26- used to build

---

[1] Throughout the text, group is used for clustering approaches, whereas class refers to a label in a supervised approach.

three databases: *th18*, *th22*, and *th26*. A higher threshold is assumed to mean that confidence in the labeled cells is greater.

The labeled neurons belong to four different classes: Common basket (CB), Horse-tail (HT), Large basket (LB), and Martinotti (MT). Agreement on Chandelier cells was also high, although not enough 3D reconstructed cells were available for inclusion in the analysis. Thus, there are 118 labeled cells in *th18*, distributed as 49 CB, 9 HT, 27 LB, and 33 MT; 83 labeled cells in *th22*, distributed as 24 CB, 5 HT, 29 LB, and 25 MT; and finally, 47 labeled cells in *th26*, distributed as 9 CB, 4 HT, 12 LB, and 22 MT.

We described each neuron using nine basic morphological features related to axonal and dendritic arborizations. These features were measured using Neurolucida Explorer. The specific features are: X_1 = axonal arbors (Aa) at $(0, \pi]$ (over the soma), X_2 = Aa at $(\pi, 2\pi]$ (under the soma), X_3 = dendritic arbors (Da) at $(0, \pi]$, X_4 = Da at $(\pi, 2\pi]$, X_5 = Aa < 300µm from the soma, X_6 = Aa [300µm, 600µm] from the soma, X_7 = Aa > 300µm from the soma, X_8 = Da $\leq$ 180µm from the soma, and X_9 = Da > 180µm from the soma. The aim was to simulate expert interpretation at an early stage of a visual examination, i.e. the orientation and the size of each neuron.

2.2 Method

We have created a method called semi-supervised projected model-based clustering (SeSProC) [19]. SeSProC is based on Gaussian finite mixture models; however, its input data are both labeled and unlabeled instances. It is able to classify the unlabeled instances into either known or newly discovered groups. Besides, each feature is weighted to indicate its relevance for each group.

Let the observable data $\mathcal{X} = \{\mathbf{x}_1, \ldots, \mathbf{x}_N\}$ be a set of instances, with $\mathbf{x}_i \in \Re^F, \forall i \in \{1, \ldots, N\}$. In a typical clustering problem, data are assumed to be generated from a probabilistic model given by a finite mixture of distributions with K components, and the clustering solution is gathered in the mixture using a latent variable $\mathcal{Z}$. The basic density function for an instance $\mathbf{x}_i$ is

$$p(\mathbf{x}_i \mid \Theta) = \sum_{m=1}^{K} \pi_m p(\mathbf{x}_i \mid \boldsymbol{\theta}_m),$$

where π_m is known as the mixing proportion and $\boldsymbol{\theta}_m$ is the parameter set of each component. The full parameter set of the mixture is $\Theta = \{\boldsymbol{\theta}_1, \ldots, \boldsymbol{\theta}_K, \pi_1, \ldots, \pi_K\}$. This set would be easy to find using the maximum likelihood method, if the complete-data, i.e. $\mathcal{X}$ and $\mathcal{Z}$, were known. However, $\mathcal{Z}$ is unknown and must be estimated together with the parameter set. We use the expectation-maximization (EM) [20] algorithm to calculate the expectation of the log-likelihood function with respect to the posterior distribution of the latent variable.

As SeSProC is a projected algorithm, the density function changes because the relevance of each feature for each component is also estimated to find the interesting subspaces. This information is gathered in a new latent variable $\mathcal{V}$. Defining $\rho_{mj} = p(v_{mj} = 1)$, i.e. the probability that feature j is relevant to component m, and assuming that features are conditionally independent given the component label, the new density function is

$$p(\mathbf{x}_i \mid \Theta) = \sum_{m=1}^{K} \pi_m \prod_{j=1}^{F} \Big(\rho_{mj} p(x_{ij} \mid \theta_{mj}) + (1 - \rho_{mj}) p(x_{ij} \mid \lambda_{mj}) \Big),$$

where θ_{mj} and λ_{mj} indicate the parameters for the density function if feature j is relevant and irrelevant, respectively, to component m. As before, if $\mathcal{Z}$ and $\mathcal{V}$ were known, the new complete-data log-likelihood function, with z_{im} indicating instance i's membership of component m, and v_{mj} indicating feature j's relevance to component m, would be

$$\log L(\Theta \mid \mathcal{X}, \mathcal{Z}, \mathcal{V}) = \sum_{i=1}^{N} \sum_{m=1}^{K} \Big(z_{im} \log \pi_m$$
$$+ \sum_{j=1}^{F} (z_{im} [v_{mj} (\log \rho_{mj} + \log p(x_{ij} \mid \theta_{mj}))$$
$$+ (1 - v_{mj})(\log(1 - \rho_{mj}) + \log p(x_{ij} \mid \lambda_{mj}))]) \Big).$$

As SeSProC is a semi-supervised clustering algorithm and its input contains some labeled data, $\mathcal{Z}$ is partially known. However, the unknown part of $\mathcal{Z}$ and $\mathcal{V}$ is estimated at iteration t, after the parameters from the previous iteration $t - 1$ have been fixed, by calculating the expectation of the complete-data log likelihood function using the EM algorithm, as

$$\mathbb{E}_{\mathcal{Z}, \mathcal{V} \mid \mathcal{X}, \Theta^{t-1}} [\log L(\Theta^{t-1} \mid \mathcal{X}, \mathcal{Z}, \mathcal{V})]$$
$$= \sum_{i=1}^{N} \sum_{m=1}^{K} \gamma(z_{im}) \log \pi_m$$
$$+ \sum_{i=1}^{N} \sum_{m=1}^{K} \sum_{j=1}^{F} \gamma(u_{imj})(\log \rho_{mj} + \log p(x_{ij} \mid \theta_{mj}))$$
$$+ \sum_{i=1}^{N} \sum_{m=1}^{K} \sum_{j=1}^{F} \gamma(w_{imj})(\log(1 - \rho_{mj}) + \log p(x_{ij} \mid \lambda_{mj})),$$

where $\gamma()$ is the expectation of each specific variable, with $\gamma(u_{imj}) = \gamma(z_{im}) \gamma(v_{mj})$ and $\gamma(w_{imj}) = \gamma(z_{im})(1 - \gamma(v_{mj}))$.

Number of Clusters Estimation. SeSProc also estimates the final number of clusters using a greedy forward search. The Schwartz criterion [21], also known as Bayesian information criterion (BIC), is used to compare models with different numbers of components. In the first step of the search ($s = 0$), a model with C components ($\mathcal{M}^0$) is built, C being the known labels. Then $\mathcal{M}^1$ is built with $C + 1$ components at $s = 1$ and compared with $\mathcal{M}^0$ using the BIC. The process continues, adding a component at each new step, until the convergence criterion is reached, i.e. $\mathcal{M}^s$ is better than $\mathcal{M}^{s+1}$, returning $\mathcal{M}^s$. Note that labeled instances can only belong to the C known components, whereas unlabeled instances can be members of any component $C + s$ at step s. A key aspect of this process is related to initialization. Labeled instances are used to initialize the known components, but the added components also have to be initialized. We assume that the instances that fit the components at step s of the process worst are candidates for membership of the new component added at $s + 1$, and are then used to initialize this component.

2.3 Empirical Setup

The process for obtaining input data with labeled and unlabeled instances for each class and data set was as follows: all labels of one of the known four classes were hidden to SeSProC, whereas the labels of the other three classes were unchanged. This process was designed to discriminate between unlabeled and labeled instances, since they belong to different classes of interneurons. Besides, more than one group could be found for the unlabeled instances, leading to the discovery of new groups that were unknown to the algorithm input[2].

Results were then evaluated in two respects. First, they were analyzed in terms of correctly and misclassified instances (see Section 3.1). We considered that a cell was misclassified (mc) if that cell was grouped into one of the known classes according to the labeled data. On the contrary, an instance was correctly classified (cc) if it was grouped into a completely new group, regardless of the number of new groups that were identified. We then defined accuracy as $\frac{cc}{mc+cc}$, ranging from 0 to 1. Accuracy was 1 when all unlabeled instances were grouped into new groups. We then evaluated the identified groups in terms of the newly discovered knowledge (see Section 3.2). We checked the results against a visual examination and expert opinion.

3   Results and Discussion

3.1 Discriminating Classes

Results for the discrimination of classes of interneurons on which the scientific community largely agrees are shown in Fig. 1. The evolution of the results depended on the threshold, and we find that, generally, SeSProC performance improved with a higher threshold. A higher threshold means that more experts agreed with the labels, and neurons were easier to classify.

---

[2] We base our model on the *cluster assumption* [12], which states that instances that belong to the same cluster are likely to be of the same class, whereas a class may be represented by several clusters.

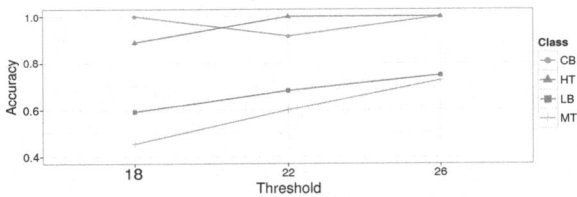

Fig. 1. Accuracy values depending on the class and the selected threshold

Results for discriminating CB cells from other classes were very accurate. For example, the 49 CB cells of *th18* were correctly discriminated from the other classes. All cells were again discriminated with *th26*, and only two (out of 24) cells were misclassified and grouped into the LB group with *th22*.

HT cells were the most distinct class of interneurons reported in this research. This was demonstrated by the good discrimination rate of HT cells from other classes, since only one out of nine neurons was misclassified with *th18*. There were no misclassified cells with *th22* and *th26*.

Discrimination of LB cells was worse than for CB and HT cells. All misclassified LB cells were confused with the CB class. This was anticipated because the shapes of some of these cells are very similar. However, many other LB cells have very different shapes, and this was identified by assigning these cells to new groups.

The discrimination of MT cells from other classes was the least accurate according to our data. With *th18*, 18 out of 33 MT cells were confused with other classes, even with the HT class. The *th18* group was conformed by a heterogeneous group of cells, which likely resemble other morphologies, but that still were considered as MT cells by the experts. However, only 6 out of 22 MT cells were misclassified with *th26*. These results revealed that the *th26* group was likely composed of cells that are morphologically distinct, i.e. those considered as representative MT cells. The discrimination rate for this class improved more than any other in the study.

Although the overall results showed an acceptable discrimination rate between the four classes of interneurons, there were some misclassified instances that were grouped into the wrong clusters. As the results of [10] show, the agreement among expert neuroscientists was rather limited. Therefore, it is far from easy to automatically discriminate cells perfectly. Regarding this point, Fig 2 shows four cells, two labeled, with at least 18 votes in [10], as CB (neurons A and C) and two as LB (neurons B and D). The discrimination between neurons A and B is visually very clear. However, differences between neurons C and D are less clear. The variability of shapes, sizes, and orientations when dealing with different populations of neurons is very high, which makes then hard to discriminate automatically based on morphological features.

To illustrate the problems related to the automatic discrimination of these classes, we performed experiments using a supervised classification approach to classify the instances. We used the naïve Bayes (NB) algorithm [22]. Although these results are out of the scope of this paper, the estimated mean accuracy

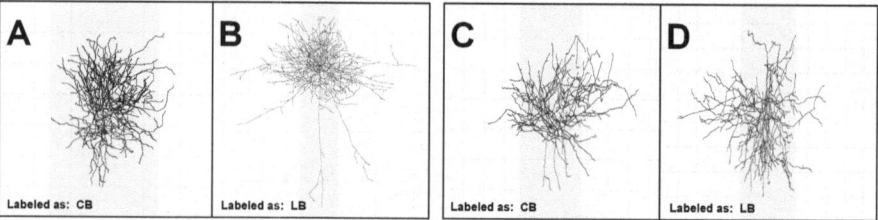

Fig. 2. Neurons A and C were labeled as CB and neurons B and D as LB by at least 18 experts in [10]. However, A and B are easier to discriminate than C and D. Note the different scales for each cell. Each square or rectangle in all figures represents 100μm.

values (using 10-fold cross-validation) ranged from 0.68 to 0.76 depending on the threshold and whether a feature subset selection process was performed before building the model. Although the approaches are not comparable, these values were lower than for our approach using SeSProC for averaged class results.

3.2   Discovering New Groups

Here we present some results illustrating the discovery of possible new groups of interneurons. Regarding CB cells, three groups were identified with *th18*. One of these groups contained 41 CB cells (see cell A in Fig. 3). The second group had three cells. The main features of these cells were that their axonal arborizations were not as dense and they had one or two descending long axonal colaterals (see cell B in Fig. 3). Finally, there were five CB cells in a third group that had very dense axonal arborizations (see cell C in Fig. 3).

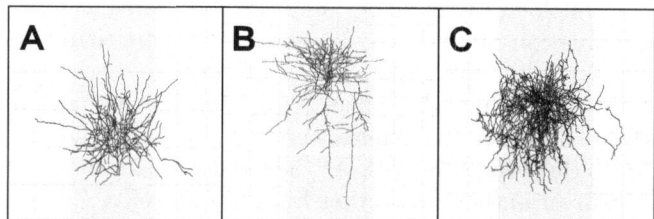

Fig. 3. Representative CB cells from each group identified by SeSProc with *th18*

Note that the population of cells changed when a different threshold was used. The eight CB cells that were grouped into B and C (see Fig. 3) with *th18* did not receive enough votes for inclusion in *th22* or *th26*. Therefore, these groups could not be identified. However, SeSProC did identify two new groups with *th26*, with five and four cells, which did not appear previously. The main difference between these groups was the size of the axonal arborizations of the neurons.

Fig. 4 shows an example of the relevance of each feature j and group m (value of ρ_{mj}, see Section 2.2) for CB groups with *th26* depending on the hidden class.

It is shown that feature relevance of the CB groups when hiding HT, LB, and MT was very similar, where features X_2 and X_8 were considered highly relevant. When CB labels were hidden in the input, SeSProC identified two previously commented groups. Features X_2, X_3, X_5, and X_6 were highly relevant for the first group, whereas features X_8 and X_9 were more relevant for the second group.

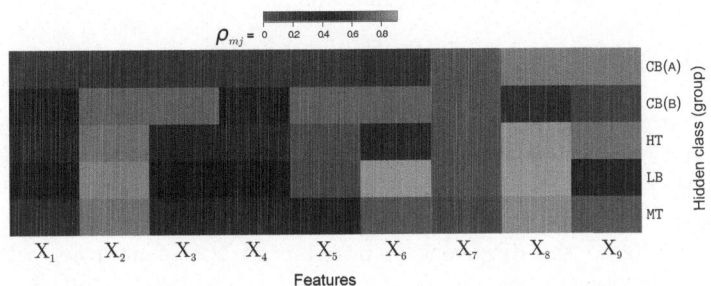

Fig. 4. Heatmap indicating the relevance of each feature (X_1-X_9) for each group (A and B) of CB cells when CB labels were hidden, and also for each group of CB cells when HT, LB, and MT labels were hidden (results for *th26*)

Regarding HT cells, only one group was identified for this type of cells regardless of the threshold. It shows the descending tight axonal arborizations that characterize this cell type.

SeSProC identified four, five, and three new groups of LB cells with *th18*, *th22*, and *th26*, respectively, revealing some interesting features after visual inspection. For example, regarding *th18*, one group contained LB cells with horizontally distributed axonal ramifications (see cell A in Fig. 5). Another group contained LB cells with a dense axonal arborization near the soma and a few descending long axonal colaterals (see cell B in Fig. 5). Finally, another two groups contained cells with sparse axonal arborizations distributed in several directions (see cells C and D in Fig. 5).

SeSProC only identified one group of MT cells with *th18* and *th22*. Two groups were identified with *th26*. The first group was mainly characterized by features

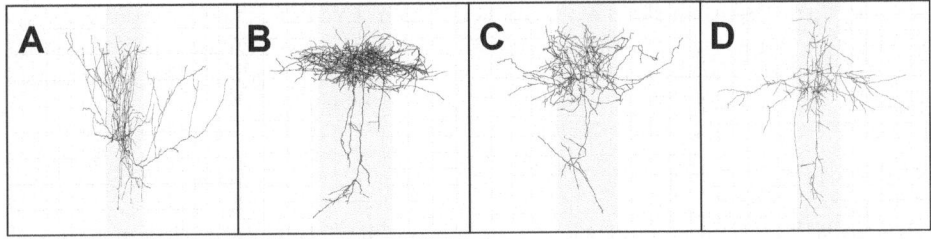

Fig. 5. Representative LB cells from each group identified by SeSProc with *th18*

describing the total cell size (X_5 to X_9), whereas features related to orientation (X_1 to X_4) were more relevant for the second group. Further analyses are necessary in order to obtain a more accurate classification for MT cells.

In summary, the fact that new groups were identified demonstrates that there is a lack in the homogeneity of the types that are defined to date. Thus, the present kind of analysis would help to advance in the understanding of the classification and characterization of neurons.

4   Conclusions

The classification of neurons is considered as one of the most challenging problems related to the study of neuronal circuits because data are scarce, experts disagree, and cells are morphologically, molecularly, and physiologically variable. We present a novel semi-supervised approach for classifying morphological neuron data, leading to the discovery of possible groups of neurons, which takes advantage of previous knowledge in the shape of data labels, and also identifies the relevance of each feature for each group.

We obtained a preliminary distinction among different classes of interneurons according to simple morphological features characterizing the size and the orientation of axonal and dendritic arbors of cells. We tackled this problem from a simple perspective regarding the morphological features since experts classify cells by visual examination. Although SeSProC outperformed a supervised classification approach, the most interesting output of our approach is related to the identification of new groups. Although preliminary results look interesting, especially for CB and LB cells, further analyses using different morphological features and labels are necessary to confirm these results.

SeSProC is open to further improvements, like the inclusion of uncertainty into labels. Instead of considering different thresholds to retrieve expert knowledge, it would be interesting to include information gathered from many experts in the shape of labels with some probability. Regarding the data, although it is generally thought that the same morphological types of neurons are found in all species, we cannot discard the possibility of inter-species variability, and further analyses are necessary in order to find representative types of neurons of particular species.

Acknowledgements. This research is partially supported by the Cajal Blue Brain Project (Spanish partner of the Blue Brain Project initiative from EPFL), the Spanish Ministry of Economy and Competitiveness TIN2010-20900-C04-04 and TIN2010-21289-C02-02 projects, and Consolider Ingenio 2010-CSD2007-00018.

References

[1] Petilla Interneuron Nomenclature Group: Petilla terminology: Nomenclature of features of GABAergic interneurons of the cerebral cortex. Nat. Rev. Neurosci. 9, 557–568 (2008)

[2] Marin, E.C., Jefferys, G., Komiyama, T., Zhu, H., Luo, L.: Representation of the glomerular olfactory map in the drosophila brain. Cell 149, 243–255 (2002)

[3] Guerra, L., McGarry, L.M., Robles, V., Bielza, C., Larrañaga, P., Yuste, R.: Comparison between supervised and unsupervised classifications of neuronal cell types: A case study. Dev. Neurobiol. 71(1), 71–82 (2011)

[4] Tsiola, A., Hamzei-Sichani, F., Peterlin, Z., Yuste, R.: Quantitative morphological classification of layer 5 neurons from mouse primary visual cortex. J. Compar. Neurol. 461, 415–428 (2003)

[5] Benavides-Piccione, R., Sichani, F.H., Yaez, I.B., DeFelipe, J., Yuste, R.: Dendritic size of pyramidal neurons differs among mouse cortical regions. Cereb. Cortex. 16, 990–1001 (2005)

[6] Cauli, B., Porter, J.T., Tsuzuki, K., Lambolez, B., Rossier, J., Quenet, B., Audinat, E.: Classification of fusiform neocortical interneurons based on unsupervised clustering. Proc. Natl. Acad. Sci. 97(11), 6144–6149 (2000)

[7] Karagiannis, A., Gallopin, T., Csaba, D., Battaglia, D., Geoffroy, H., Rossier, J., Hillman, E., et al.: Classification of NPY-expressing neocortical interneurons. J. Neurosci. 29, 3642–3659 (2009)

[8] McGarry, L.M., Packer, A., Fino, E., Nikolenko, V., Sippy, T., Yuste, R.: Quantitative classification of somatostatin-positive neocortical interneurons identifies three interneuron subtypes. Front. Neural Circuits. 4(12), 1–19 (2010)

[9] DeFelipe, J.: Cortical interneurons: From Cajal to 2001. Prog. Brain Res. 136, 215–238 (2002)

[10] DeFelipe, J., et al.: New insights in the classification and nomenclature of cortical GABAergic interneurons. Nat. Rev. Neurosci. 14(3), 202–216 (2013)

[11] McLachlan, G., Basford, K.: Mixture Models: Inference and Applications to Clustering. Marcel Dekker (1988)

[12] Chapelle, O., Schölkopf, B., Zien, A. (eds.): Semi-Supervised Learning. MIT Press (2006)

[13] Zhu, X., Goldberg, A.: Introduction to Semi-Supervised Learning. Morgan & Claypool Publishers (2009)

[14] Parsons, L., Haque, E., Liu, H.: Subspace clustering for high dimensional data: A review. ACM SIGKDD Explorations Newsletter - Special Issue on Learning From Imbalanced Datasets 6(1), 90–105 (2004)

[15] Kriegel, H., Kröger, P., Zimek, A.: Clustering high-dimensional data: A survey on subspace clustering, pattern-based clustering and correlation clustering. ACM Trans. Knowl. Discov. Data. 3(1), 1–58 (2009)

[16] Law, M.H.C., Figueiredo, M.A.T., Jain, A.K.: Simultaneous feature selection and clustering using mixture models. IEEE T. Pattern Anal. 26(9), 1154–1166 (2004)

[17] Vellido, A., Lisboa, P.J.G., Vicente, D.: Robust analysis of MRS brain tumour data using t-GTM. Neurocomputing 69(79), 754–768 (2006)

[18] Ascoli, G.A., Donohue, D.E., Halavi, M.: NeuroMorpho. Org: A central resource for neuronal morphologies. J. Neurosci. 27(35), 9247–9251 (2007)

[19] Guerra, L., Bielza, C., Robles, V., Larrañaga, P.: Semi-supervised projected model-based clustering. Data Min. Knowl. Disc. (2012) (submitted)

[20] Dempster, A., Laird, N., Rubin, D.: Maximum likelihood from incomplete data via the EM algorithm. J. R. Stat. Soc. 39(1), 1–38 (1977)

[21] Schwarz, G.: Estimating the dimension of a model. Ann. Stat. 6(2), 461–464 (1978)

[22] Minsky, M.: Steps toward artificial intelligence. In: Computers and Thought, pp. 406–450. McGraw-Hill (1961)

Cascaded Rank-Based Classifiers
for Detecting Clusters of Microcalcifications

Alessandro Bria, Claudio Marrocco, Mario Molinara, and Francesco Tortorella

DIEI, Università degli Studi di Cassino e del Lazio Meridionale, Cassino (FR), Italy
{a.bria,c.marrocco,m.molinara,tortorella}@unicas.it

Abstract. A Computer Aided Detection (CAD) system has frequently to deal with a significant skew between positive and negative class. For this reason we propose a solution based on an ensemble of classifiers structured as a "cascade" of dichotomizers where each node is robust to such skew since it is trained by a learning algorithm based on ranking instead of classification error. The proposed approach has been applied to the detection of clusters of microcalcifications in mammograms and has shown good performance in comparison with other methods well suited to deal with unbalanced problems.

Keywords: Computer aided detection, cascade of classifiers, mammography, clusters of microcalcifications.

1 Introduction

Mammography is a radiological screening technique which makes possible to detect lesions in the breast using low doses of radiation. The presence in the image of microcalcifications (μC) grouped in cluster can be an important indicator of breast cancer since they appear in 30%-50% of cases diagnosed by mammographic screenings [2]. In literature, several CAD systems have been proposed, specially using machine learning techniques based on a sliding subwindow that scans the entire image and a dichotomizer (i.e., a two-class classifier) that classifies each subwindow as positive (i.e., containing a lesion) or negative. However, when dealing with cluster detection the huge number of subwindows to be analyzed and the complexity of the classifier cause a high computational burden not easy to sustain. Therefore, in this paper an ensemble of classifiers structured as a cascade of dichotomizers with increasing complexity is proposed. This approach, which showed low computational complexity and good performance in other fields [6], allows each dichotomizer in the cascade to deal with only a part of the negative samples, thus parting the complexity of the whole problem.

However, the μC detection is also characterized by a significant asymmetry between positive and negative classes that represents a significant difficulty for every classifier. In particular, the AdaBoost dichotomizer commonly employed in the cascade structure is significantly biased by skewed class priors since it minimizes a quantity strongly related to classification error. To address this problem,

N. Peek, R. Marín Morales, and M. Peleg (Eds.): AIME 2013, LNAI 7885, pp. 166–170, 2013.
© Springer-Verlag Berlin Heidelberg 2013

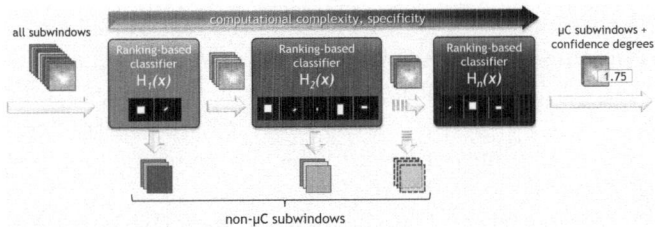

Fig. 1. A scheme of the proposed ranking-based cascade classifier

another algorithm, AsymBoost [5], has been proposed that handles the unbalanced classes through an asymmetric weight updating mechanism of the samples in the training set. AsymBoost, however, relies on a parameter k not easy to tune that should estimate how much more false negatives cost than false positives. The alternative solution presented in this paper relies on the idea that, when dealing with skewed classes, a learning algorithm that maximizes the probability of correct pairwise ranking and thus, is able to handle the asymmetric distribution of the classes without need for further parameters. On this basis, we have reformulated the learning algorithm for the node classifier in order to maximize its ranking capability rather than minimizing its classification error. Such approach was inspired by RankBoost [1], a boosting machine learning algorithm focused on ranking problems. Experiments accomplished on a full-field digital mammographic database show that the cascade approach obtains good results in comparison with other approaches presented in literature.

2   The Ranking-Based Cascade

The cascade of dichotomizers is built up as a sequence of nodes where a given subwindow passes to the next node only if the current one classifies it as containing a positive sample. Such an approach allows each dichotomizer to deal with only a part of the negative samples, thus parting the complexity of the whole problem among the classifiers. In this way, the majority of subwindows containing easily detectable background are discarded by the first stages of the cascade, while the the most confusing background configurations go through the entire cascade and are analyzed by the more specialized last stages. The detection rate D and the false positive rate F of a cascade composed by n nodes are given by $D = \prod_{i=1}^{n}(d_i), F = \prod_{i=1}^{n}(f_i)$ where d_i and f_i are the detection rate and the false positive rate of the i-th node respectively. To provide the required d_i and f_i, a *validation set* different from the training set is used since at each round a high number of negative samples is removed, thus significantly altering the original balancing between classes. For this reason, a huge *pool* of negative samples is set apart for refilling and re-balancing each set after a node is trained. Fig. 1 reports a scheme of the proposed cascade.

Let us now focus on the learning strategy of the i-th node classifier, whose structure has been inspired by RankBoost [1], a boosting machine learning algorithm suitably modified to be embedded in the cascade structure. Each node consists of a boosting-based ensemble of *weak rankings* $h_{t,i}(x)$ added in subsequent rounds $t = 1, ..., T$ and linearly combined by weights $\alpha_{t,i}$ to build the *final ranking* $H_i(x) = \sum_{t=1}^{T} \alpha_{t,i} h_{t,i}(x)$. Weak rankings are constrained to employ a single feature $f_{t,i}^r(x)$ that output a hard value determined by a threshold $\theta_{t,i}$ and equal to 0 if $f_{t,i}^r(x) \leq \theta_{t,i}$ and to 1 if $f_{t,i}^r(x) > \theta_{t,i}$.

Let us now define a *crucial pair* as a pair made by a positive sample x_1 and a negative sample x_0 and let us consider how the crucial pairs are ordered according to all possible weighted weak rankings. At each round, $h_{t,i}(x)$ and $\alpha_{t,i}$ are chosen to minimize the weighted number of misranked crucial pairs. A weight $w_{t,i}(x_0, x_1)$ is then assigned to the samples forming misranked crucial pairs and updated according the following rule:

$$w_{t+1,i}(x_0, x_1) = \frac{w_{t,i}(x_0, x_1)\exp\left(\alpha_{t,i}\left(h_{t,i}(x_0) - h_{t,i}(x_1)\right)\right)}{W_{t,i}} \tag{1}$$

where $W_{t,i}$ is a normalization factor so that $\sum_{x_0,x_1} w_{t+1,i}(x_0, x_1) = 1$. Assuming $\alpha_{t,i} > 0$, the update rule decreases the weight of crucial pairs in case of correct ranking (i.e., $h_{t,i}(x_1) = 1$ and $h_{t,i}(x_0) = 0$) and increases the weight otherwise. Finally, following [1], $\alpha_{t,i}$ is given by:

$$\alpha_{t,i} = \frac{1}{2} \ln\left(\frac{1 + r_{t,i}}{1 - r_{t,i}}\right) \tag{2}$$

where $r_{t,i} = \sum_{x_0,x_1} w_{t,i}(x_0, x_1)(h_{t,i}(x_1) - h_{t,i}(x_0))$.

3 Shaping the Cascade for Cluster Detection

The cascade approach has been suitably modeled to be applied to the detection of μC clusters. For this purpose, we have to describe the regions to be classified: since μC appear as small circular spots in the image a feature set composed by both Haar-like features and its tilted versions as proposed in [3] has been used. All features are stretched and shifted across all possible combinations on the subwindow, leading to tens of thousands of features. As a consequence, the approach presented in Sect. 2 is used during the training phase as a feature selection mechanism embedded in each node classifier. At the end of the cascade, the last node associates to each subwindow a confidence degree suitable to evaluate the possible presence of a μC. After the cascade has been applied and the likely-μC subwindows are detected a post-processing step is required to translate and merge the overlapping subwindows into likely-μC regions and a confidence degree is associated to each region by computing the mean of the confidence degrees of the subwindows belonging to that region. This value is then given as input to the clustering algorithm used to determine the clusters of μC. For this reason, we employ a sequential clustering algorithm [4] that constructs the clusters using an ordered sequence of the confidence degrees. In this way, regions with a higher confidence degree, i.e., those with the highest probability of being μC, are firstly considered by the algorithm thus leading to a better construction of the clusters.

4   Experimental Results

Experiments have been performed using a full-field digital non-public mammographic database of 198 images accurately labeled by experts. Each subwindow has a size used of 12×12 pixels, corresponding to 1.2 mm$\times$1.2 mm. Training data were extracted from 90 of the 198 images using non-overlapping subwindows, so obtaining more than 4.000 positive and about 400.000 negative samples that were equally distributed between training and validation set. To have a sufficiently wide pool, the set of negative samples was oversampled by adding subwindows partially overlapped with those already present in the set, for a total number of about 12 millions negative samples.

To verify the effectiveness of our approach we have also implemented the original Viola-Jones cascade detector based on AdaBoost [6] and the AsymBoost-based cascade [5] that is particularly performing when used with unbalanced data. The cascade detectors have been built with $d = 0.99$ and $f = 0.3$ using the same set of features. The training stage produced for our approach 12 nodes employing 417 features automatically selected from the 11.879 possible ones, while for AdaBoost and AsymBoost cascades respectively 11 and 13 nodes employing 405 and 434 features. To have also a comparison with a non-cascade boosting approach, a monolithic RankBoost detector has been implemented and trained with the same training data and feature set of the cascade detector using 100 boosting rounds. The performance of the cascade detectors and the monolithic one were evaluated on the remaining 108 images each one containing one or more clusters of μCs. The evaluation has been performed in terms of Free-response Receiver Operating Characteristics (FROC) curve, that plots the True Positive Rate versus the False Positive per image. We consider a detected cluster as true positive if it has at least 3 μC and an intersection with a labeled cluster higher than the 30%.

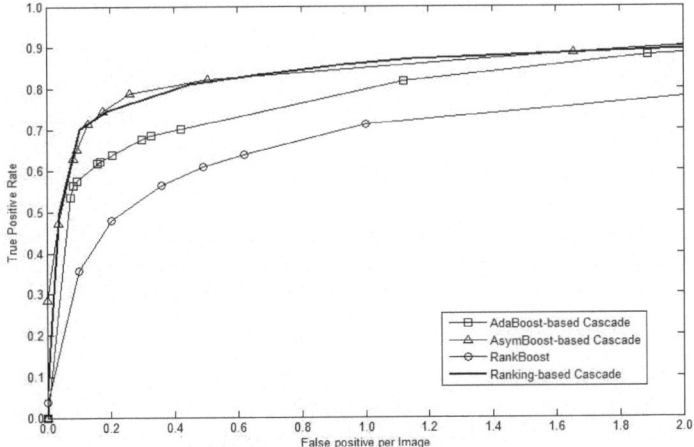

Fig. 2. The FROC curves showing the obtained results

Fig. 2 reports the FROC curves obtained for the different methods by varying the threshold on the confidence degree associated to likely-μC regions. The comparison shows that our approach significantly outperforms the monolithic RankBoost and the AdaBoost-based cascade. The AsymBoost-based cascade, instead, obtains comparable performance. However, it is worth noting that, since AsymBoost has a parameter k to be optimized, the results shown are the best obtained (with $k = 1.1$) after an optimization process. The ranking-based cascade, instead, is a nonparametric approach and this is an interesting advantage since it obtains very good performance without any parameter to be tuned.

5   Conclusions and Future Works

In this paper we have presented a new nonparametric approach to build a cascade architecture employing ranking-based classifiers to deal with highly skewed detection problems. Experiments accomplished on the detection of cluster of μC showed that the proposed method is effective when compared with other approaches. In particular, the good detection performance with respect to the monolithic RankBoost is mainly due to the detection system that is actually made of an ensemble of classifiers, each trained on a part of the available data. The difference with AdaBoost-based cascade is mainly due to the ranking-based boosting approach. AdaBoost, in fact, tries to improve its performance focusing on the most difficult samples thus implying significant possibility of overfitting that, instead, does not affect our approach. Finally, the AsymBoost cascade that is built to face an unbalanced detection problem, gives comparable performance with our method that is based on an easy-to-tune nonparametric model.

Future works will focus on the cascade structure and in particular, on an alternative architecture that should decouple the feature selection step from the classification step letting us employ learning algorithms not necessarily based on boosting.

References

1. Freund, Y., Iyer, R., Schapire, R.E., Singer, Y.: An Efficient Boosting Algorithm for Combining Preferences. J. of Mach. Learn. Res. 4, 933–969 (2003)
2. Kopans, D.B.: Breast Imaging, 3rd edn. Williams & Wilkins, Baltimore (2007)
3. Lienhart, R., Kuranov, A., Pisarevsky, V.: Empirical Analysis of Detection Cascades of Boosted Classifiers for Rapid Object Detection. In: Michaelis, B., Krell, G. (eds.) DAGM 2003. LNCS, vol. 2781, pp. 297–304. Springer, Heidelberg (2003)
4. Marrocco, C., Molinara, M., Tortorella, F.: Algorithms for Detecting Clusters of Microcalcifications in Mammograms. In: Roli, F., Vitulano, S. (eds.) ICIAP 2005. LNCS, vol. 3617, pp. 884–891. Springer, Heidelberg (2005)
5. Viola, P., Jones, M.: Fast and Robust Classification using Asymmetric AdaBoost and a Detector Cascade. Adv. in Neur. Inf. Proc. Syst. 16, 1311–1318 (2001)
6. Viola, P., Jones, M.: Robust Real-Time Face Detection. Int. J. of Comp. Vis. 57(2), 137–154 (2004)

Segmenting Neuroblastoma Tumor Images and Splitting Overlapping Cells Using Shortest Paths between Cell Contour Convex Regions

Siamak Tafavogh, Karla Felix Navarro, Daniel R. Catchpoole, and Paul J. Kennedy

Centre for Quantum Computation & Intelligent Systems,
Faculty of Engineering and Information Technology,
University of Technology, Sydney, PO Box 123, Broadway,
NSW 2007 Australia
siamak.tafavogh@student.uts.edu.au

Abstract. Neuroblastoma is one of the most fatal paediatric cancers. One of the major prognostic factors for neuroblastoma tumour is the total number of neuroblastic cells. In this paper, we develop a fully automated system for counting the total number of neuroblastic cells within the images derived from Hematoxylin and Eosin stained histological slides by considering the overlapping cells. We finally propose a novel multi-stage cell counting algorithm, in which cellular regions are extracted using an adaptive thresholding technique. Overlapping and single cells are discriminated using morphological differences. We propose a novel cell splitting algorithm to split overlapping cells into single cells using the shortest path between contours of convex regions.

Keywords: Histological image segmentation, splitting overlapping cells, neuroblastoma.

1 Introduction

Neuroblastoma Tumors (NTs) are aggressive paediatric tumours responsible for the majority of cancer deaths particularly between the ages of 0 and 4 [1]. number of neuroblastic cells is one of the most important microscopic criteria for identifying the malignancy or benignity of NTs. Identifying, analysing and counting an enormous number of cells under the microscope is an onerous task. Moreover, the mixture of overlapping and single cells within histological slides makes counting error-prone. As a result, it is critical that pathologists are assisted by a computer-based system which can count cells automatically and accurately. There are two primary challenges in developing such a system, namely, discriminating overlapping cells from single cells and splitting the overlapping cells into the single cells. These challenges arise from the fact that the process of histological slide preparation superimposes some cells on the others and thus generates overlapping cells.

Several systems for automatically counting cells have been proposed. Fatakdawala et al. [2] and Mukherjee et al. [3] employ active contour and level set algorithms for segmenting cellular regions; however, the contours of the overlapping cells produce inaccurate cell detection.

N. Peek, R. Marín Morales, and M. Peleg (Eds.): AIME 2013, LNAI 7885, pp. 171–175, 2013.

The aim of this study is to develop an accurate user interaction independent neuroblastic cell counting system that addresses the issue of overlapping cells. To accomplish this goal, we propose a cell counting algorithm consisting of three stages: 1) identifying and segmenting the cellular regions, 2) discriminating overlapping cells from single cells, and 3) splitting overlapping cells into single cells.

To validate our developed system, we compare our results with the results obtained by a pathologist. In a second experiment we compare our cell splitting algorithm with a watershed technique [4]. Finally, to evaluate the effects of using Otsu on the performance of our system, we compare it with the Kittler method [5], another robust clustering-based thresholding technique. We compute the accuracy of our system using the F-measure [6].

2   Data Acquisition and Software

The histological images used in this research were collected from the Tumour Bank of the Kid's Research Institute at The Children's Hospital at Westmead. All images have JPEG format with a size of 512×512. Twenty histological images are used for the training set and another 20 images are used for the test set. No images are in both the training and test sets. We designed our algorithm using MATLAB software (the MathWorks, Inc, Natick, MA).

3   Image Segmentation

The first step in counting the total number of neuroblastic cells in NTs is the segmentation of the cellular regions. In our system, we segment the cellular regions in three steps: pre-segmentation, segmentation and post-segmentation.

Pre-Segmentation: All the scanned histological images in our datasets are in RGB colour-space. we transform the RGB to HSV as a uniform colour-space [7]. Hue, Saturation and Value uses Euclidian distance to define the difference between colours. In HSV colour-space Hue is the luminance coordinate, Saturation is the chrominance coordinate and Value is the contrast coordinate of the pixels.

Segmentation: The colour blue distinguishes the cellular regions from other histological regions of the tissue, and we use this property to segment the cellular regions. The Otsu method is an adaptive thresholding technique that efficiently and accurately determines a different range of intensity values using the grey-level histogram of the pixels. We applied the Otus method only to the saturation coordinate of the HSV to find the optimum thresholding value of the neuroblastic regions. The thresholding value for segmenting cellular regions is 0.4824. This value is obtained empirically after applying the thresholding technique on 20 training histological images.

Post-Segmentation: The resultant cellular regions require morphological modification in preparation for further analysis. The segmented cellular regions contain numbers of isolated pixels and cells with holes or undulated contours. To improve the quality of the segmented cellular regions, we applied region filling and opening operations [8].

4   Morphological Analysis of the Cells

Single cells are usually smaller than overlapping cells, and have lower convexity due to their circular shape compared to overlapping cells. We analysed each of the cells to compute its size and convexity. %labelfig:MA To compute the size of each cell, we counted the total number of pixels within the area of the cell. We calculated the amount of cell convexity using $CR_j = \frac{CH_j}{Area_j} \; \forall j \in \{1, ..., m\}$, where CH is the cell j^{th} convex hull area, $Area$ is total number of pixels on the area of cell j^{th} and m is the total number of cells within the segmented image.

We consider a cell to be overlapping if the area of the cell is greater than the average area of all the cells within the image and CR is greater than the mean of CR of all the cells in the image. Otherwise, the cell is considered to be a single cell. The outputs of this stage are stored in two images, one containing only overlapping cells and the other containing only single cells.

5   Splitting Overlapping Cells

Our algorithm for splitting overlapping cells consists of three steps: 1) determining the convex regions of each of the overleaping cells; 2) computing the shortest path between the contour of convex regions; and 3) splitting the overlapping cells from the shortest paths.

We apply our splitting algorithm only to the obtained binary image from the morphological analysis step that contains overlapping cells. We consider the binary image as a matrix in which the row and column number of each element represents the spatial domain of the corresponding pixel within the image. To determine the convex regions for each of the overlapping cells, we create two matrices CH and A with size 512×512 (the size of the original image), in which the row and column number of each element indicates the x and y coordinates of the pixels within the original image. The matrix CH presents the coordinates of the pixels within the convex hull of the overlapping cells, and the matrix A shows the coordinates of the pixels within the area of the overlapping cells. We allocate a unique label for each cell. Thus, in CH and A we replace the value of the pixels with their corresponding label value. All the other elements of both matrices are 0. To obtain the convex regions for the overlapping cells we use $C = CH - A$. As a result of this subtraction, the mutual regions between the convex hull and the area of the cell become zero and all remaining non-zero elements indicate

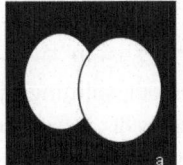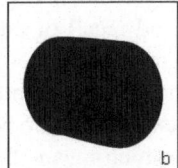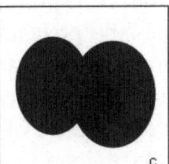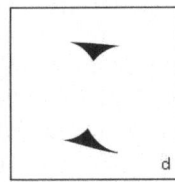

Fig. 1. a) overlapping cells, b) convex hull of the overlapping cells, c) area of the overlapping cells, d) convex regions of the overlapping cells

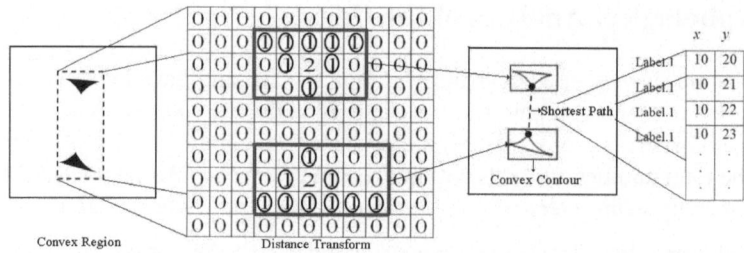

Fig. 2. Shortest path between convex regions of the overlapping cells

the convex regions. If the convex region obtained for each overlapping cell is smaller than a threshold value of 12 non-zero elements, the region is considered as noise and discarded from C. The value of the threshold was obtained empirically by tuning the 20 training images. Figure 1 indicates the convex hull, area and convex region of the overlapping cells.

To find the contour of the convex regions we, applied the distance transformation function to C. The pixels at minimum distance from the background are considered as the contour of the convex regions. We then calculate the shortest path between the contours with identical labels. The x (row number) and y (column number) coordinates of all the elements that lay in the shortest path of the two convex regions are stored in a matrix S with size $n \times 2$, where n is the elements located in the shortest paths and 2 is the x, y coordinates of the element. Figure 2 illustrates the procedure of determining the convex regions in the overlapping cell contour and their shortest paths.

Ultimately, to split the overlapping cells, we transform the value of all the pixels within the binary segmented cellular image that have the same x and y coordinates as the elements within S to zero.

6   Results

To test our developed system, 20 histological images from the test set are used, and the accuracy of our system is measured by comparison with the pathologist's results. The overall preicision, recall and F-measure for our system are 84.90%, 85.34%, 85.08% respectively.

We run two different types of experiments: 1) integrating the Kittler with our splitting algorithm, and 2) replacing our cell splitting algorithm in the system with the watershed technique. Figure 3 indicates the precision and recall of our system, Kittler plus our splitting algorithm, and Otsu plus the watershed technique. The overall F-measure of our system is 85.08%, the overall F-measure of Kittler plus our splitting algorithm is 83.02%, and the overall F-measure of Otsu plus watershed is 80.28%. The Kittler method produces more artefacts than Otsu, which means that the number of isolated pixels and regions other than cellular regions are more than the Otsu method. Also the results show that our splitting algorithm significantly improves the accuracy of the system compared to the watershed algorithm.

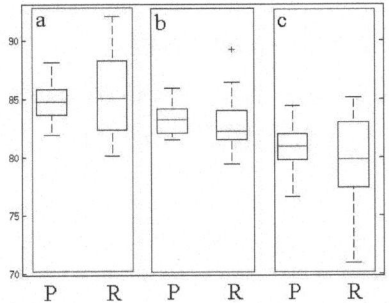

Fig. 3. a) Precision (P) and Recall (R) of our system, b) P and R of Kittler + our splitting algorithm, and c) P and R of Otsu + watershed

7   Conclusion

The number of neuroblastic cells within the Neuroblastoma Tumour is one of the major prognosis factors for pathologists, but the process of counting an enormous number of cells under the microscope is a tedious task. Moreover, the mixture of single and overlapping cells within the histological slides makes the process of counting error-prone. In this paper, we propose a user interaction independent system to assist pathologists with counting the total number of neuroblastic cells within NTs.

The advantages of our system that it is independent of user interaction, there is no over-segmentation problem in splitting the overlapping cells, the ability to split the overlapping cells at the point of overlap and heterogeneity of tumour should do does not effect the performance of the system. The overall F-measure of our system in counting the total number of neuroblastic cells is 85.04%.

References

1. Park, J., Eggert, A., Caron, H.: Neuroblastoma: Biology, Prognosis, and Treatment. Hematology/Oncology Clinics of North America 24(1), 65–86 (2010)
2. Fatakdawala, H., Xu, J., Basavanhally, A., Bhanot, G., Ganesan, S., Feldman, M., Tomaszewski, J., Madabhushi, A.: Expectation–maximization-driven geodesic active contour with overlap resolution (emagacor): Application to lymphocyte segmentation on breast cancer histopathology. IEEE Transactions on Biomedical Engineering 57(7), 1676–1689 (2010)
3. Mukherjee, D., Ray, N., Acton, S.: Level set analysis for leukocyte detection and tracking. IEEE Transactions on Image Processing 13(4), 562–572 (2004)
4. Lezoray, O., Cardot, H.: Cooperation of color pixel classification schemes and color watershed. IEEE Transactions on Image Processing 11(7), 783–789 (2002)
5. Kittler, J., Iingworth, J.: Minimum error thresholding. Pattern Recognition 19(1), 41 (1986)
6. Powers, D.: Evaluation: From precision, recall and f-factor to roc, informedness, markedness & correlation, School of Informatics and Engineering, Flinders University, Adelaide, Australia, Tech. Rep. SIE-07-001
7. Wyszecki, G., Fielder, G.: New color-matching ellipses. Journal of Optical Society of America 61(9), 1135–1152 (1971)
8. Haralick, R., Sternberg, S., Zhuang, X.: Image analysis using mathematical morphology. IEEE Transactions on Pattern Analysis and Machine Intelligence (4), 532–550 (1987)

Classification of Early-Mild Subjects with Parkinson's Disease by Using Sensor-Based Measures of Posture, Gait, and Transitions

Luca Palmerini[1], Sabato Mellone[1], Guido Avanzolini[1],
Franco Valzania[2], and Lorenzo Chiari[1]

[1] Department of Electrical, Electronic and Information Engineering,
DEI, University of Bologna,
Viale Risorgimento 2, 40136 Bologna, Italy
{luca.palmerini,sabato.mellone,guido.avanzolini,
lorenzo.chiari}@unibo.it
[2] Department of Neuroscience, University of Modena and Reggio Emilia,
via Pietro Giardini 1355, 41126 Baggiovara (MO)
f.valzania@ausl.mo.it

Abstract. Evaluation of posture, gait, turning, and different kind of transitions, are key components of the clinical evaluation of Parkinson's disease (PD). The aim of this study is to assess the feasibility of using accelerometers to classify early PD subjects (two evaluations over a 1-year follow-up) with respect to age-matched control subjects. Classifying PD subjects in an early stage would permit to obtain a tool able to follow the progression of the disease from the early phases till the last ones and to evaluate the efficacy of different treatments. Two functional tests were instrumented by a single accelerometer (quiet standing, Timed Up and Go test); such tests carry quantitative information about impairments in posture, gait, and transitions (i.e. Sit-to-Walk, and Walk-to-Sit, Turning). Satisfactory accuracies are obtained in the classification of PD subjects by using an *ad hoc* wrapper feature selection technique.

Keywords: Classification, Feature Selection, Parkinson's disease, Accelerometer.

1 Introduction

Evaluation of posture, gait, turning, and different kind of transitions, are key components of the clinical evaluation of Parkinson's disease (PD). The aim of this study is to assess the feasibility of using inertial sensors (accelerometers) to discriminate (classify) early PD subjects with respect to age-matched control subjects. Classifying PD subjects in an early stage would permit to obtain quantitative information that could be used as a decision-support system for the clinician, in a perspective of evidence-based medicine. This is the preliminary step in order to obtain a tool able to follow the progression of the disease from the early phases to the last ones and to evaluate the efficacy of different treatments. This is why in this study also

N. Peek, R. Marín Morales, and M. Peleg (Eds.): AIME 2013, LNAI 7885, pp. 176–180, 2013.
© Springer-Verlag Berlin Heidelberg 2013

a 1-year follow-up was considered: the aim was to find a method of classification that would be accurate and robust over time.

Two tests were instrumented by a single accelerometer (quiet standing - QS, instrumented Timed Up and Go test - iTUG).

Quiet standing can provide quantitative information about postural sway and postural tremor [1]. The iTUG [2-4] is the instrumented version of a simple clinical test already used by clinicians to evaluate the locomotor performance of the elderly and PD subjects; this instrumented test can provide quantitative information on possible impairments in gait and transitions (i.e., Turning, Sit-to-Walk, Walk-to-Sit).

The two tests were already considered in previous works ([1], [2]) to quantify postural [1] and locomotor [2] impairments separately with no evaluation in follow-ups.

2   Methods

We examined 20 early-mild PD subjects) and 20 healthy age-matched control subjects (CTRL, 64±6 years old, 7 males and 14 females). Thirteen PD subjects also did a 1-year follow-up. All PD subjects were examined OFF medication (Hoehn & Yahr stage ≤ 3, 62±7 years old, 12 males and 8 females. The OFF condition in PD subjects was obtained by a medication washout of at least 18 hours. Subjects wore a tri-axial accelerometer, McRoberts© Dynaport Micromod, on the lower back at L5 level. They performed QS trials [1] in 5 different conditions (eyes open/closed, dual task, standing on foam with eyes open/closed) and iTUG trials [2]. The dual task consisted in counting audibly backwards from 100 by 3s. The QS trial consisted in standing quietly for 30 seconds with arms crossed on the chest; the iTUG trial consisted of rising from a chair (Sit-to-Walk), walking 7m at preferred speed (Gait), turning around (Turning), returning and sitting down again (Walk-to-Sit).

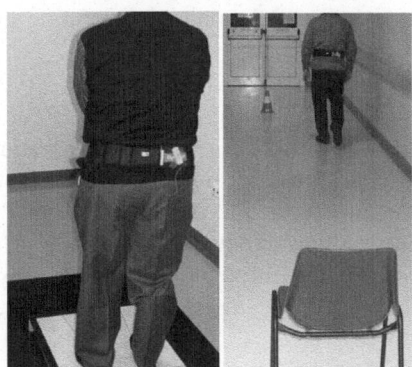

Fig. 1. Quiet Standing and Instrumented Timed Up and Go

The acceleration signals were recorded for each subject along the three orthogonal axes of the accelerometer: the first aligned with the direction of gait progression and coincident with the biomechanical anteroposterior (AP) axis of the body (front-back);

the second in the left/right direction and coincident with the biomechanical mediolateral (ML) axis of the body, and the third in the vertical direction.

Several measures were extracted from the acceleration signals.

The acceleration-derived measures extracted from QS trials quantify tremor and postural sway from quiet standing (e.g. power of high frequencies, root mean square of the signal, sway area...) [1].

The acceleration-derived measures from iTUG trials quantify duration of different components of the test, smoothness and variability of gait, range of motion during transitions (i.e. Sit-to-Walk, Walk-to-Sit), and so on [2]. The components analyzed for this study were: Sit-to-Walk, Gait, and Walk-to-Sit; Turning will be considered in following studies.

Only measures which could be considered reliable were kept for the feature selection procedure (as explained in [2]).

Finally, the total number of measures (features) which were considered is 27 (18 from QS, 9 from iTUG).

2.1   Feature Selection

Feature selection was applied in order to improve the performance of the classifiers. To select, from all the available features, a *wrapper* [5] feature selection was implemented, which was designed in [2]. To classify between the two groups we used the linear discriminant analysis (LDA) because we wanted a simple an easily interpretable classifier, to permit a clinical interpretation of the result.

In the feature selection procedure an exhaustive search among subsets of cardinality from one to three was performed. The limit of three was chosen to permit a clinical interpretation of the result (it would be difficult to associate too many features with different aspects of the disease).

Since feature selection is part of the tuning design of the classifier, it needs to be performed on the training set, in order to avoid overfitting in the final evaluation of the accuracy of the classifier [5].

The available data samples are 53: 20 CTRL subjects, 20 PD subjects on their first evaluation, and 13 PD subjects (a subset of the original 20) on their follow-up.

We randomly splitted the data in "70%-30% training-testing" by keeping the same proportion of CTRL and PD subjects in training and testing sets.

The 70%-30% rule was also applied to keep the 70% of PD subjects who had the follow-up evaluation in the training and the remaining 30% in the testing set.

Therefore, a PD subject with the follow-up had both the first evaluation sample and the follow-up sample either in the training or in the testing set. This was done in order to avoid overlapping of the datasets.

Finally, we considered 37 samples in the training set:

- 14 CTRL subjects (only first evaluation) = 14 CTRL samples
- 9 PD subjects * 2 (both first evaluation and f-up) = 18 PD samples
- 5 PD subjects (only first evaluation) = 5 PD samples

and 16 samples in the testing set:

- 6 CTRL subjects (only first evaluation) = 6 CTRL samples
- 4 PD subjects * 2 (both first evaluation and f-up) = 8 PD samples
- 2 PD subjects (only first evaluation) = 2 PD samples

The feature selection was performed in the training set with a leave-10%-out cross validation.

The classifier, built with the subset selected in the training set, was then tested in the testing set.

The LDA classifier was also tested on the same testing set with two benchmarks in order to evaluate whether the feature selection procedure that we implemented improves the performance of the selected classifier. The two benchmarks were:

- no feature selection;
- Principal Component Analysis: principal components that explained 90% of the data were selected.

3   Results and Discussion

In Table 1, the estimated misclassification rates obtained with the different FS methods are presented together with corresponding selected subsets. It can be seen that the best accuracy was achieved by the subset selected by the *wrapper* technique. Two objective features extracted from iTUG which quantify gait dynamics and smoothness, together with the total duration of the test, can discriminate with a satisfactory accuracy between early-mild PD and CTRL subjects. This was obtained with a simple classifier and few features: a possible clinical interpretation of the results is that lateral dynamics (range of motion) and vertical smoothness (reproducibility of step patterns) during gait are already impaired in early-mild PD. In addition, total duration of the iTUG test, even if it is not significantly different between CTRL and PD subjects [2] can help improving the classification. From the results it seems that iTUG is a better test with respect to QS (no features from QS were selected) in order to have an accurate classification which is also robust over

Table 1. Results of the classification with the LDA classifier

FS Method	Best Subset	Accuracy % [CI]	Sens %	Spec %
Wrapper	Total Duration of the iTUG Lateral gait dynamics during iTUG Vertical gait smoothness during iTUG	93.75 [72-99]	100	83.3
PCA	11 pcs	68.75 [44-86]	80	50
None	All Features	31.25 [84-86]	70	66.7

time. It is possible however that by considering more than three features, and/or changing classifier/FS method, accuracy could be improved by considering also QS features. The obtained accuracy would not have been obtained without feature selection; in fact considering all the features altogether would lead to a lower accuracy. This reflects the importance of performing feature selection in this kind of datasets.

It has to be noted that our relatively small sample size limits the power of our data mining perspective, as it can be seen by the large confidence intervals of the accuracies; however, separate training and testing sets were considered in order to obtain generalizable results.

4   Conclusion

The main result achieved by this work is a set of few quantitative measures, derived from a clinical test for locomotor evaluation, which can discriminate with a good accuracy between early-mild PD (both at their first evaluation and at 1-year follow-up) and CTRL motor patterns

Further experiments should be made on new subjects to validate these findings; it should also be investigated whether the presented measures remain valid for later stages of the disease and if they can track the evolution of the severity of symptoms.

Acknowledgments. The research leading to these results has received funding from the European Union - Seventh Framework Programme (FP7/2007-2013) under grant agreement n°288516 (CuPiD project). The authors wish to thank Luca Codeluppi, MD, and Valentina Fioravanti, MD, from the Department of Neuroscience, University of Modena and Reggio Emilia, Modena, Italy, for clinical supervision and assistance in data.

References

1. Palmerini, L., Rocchi, Mellone, S., Valzania, F., Chiari, L.: Feature selection for accelerometer-based posture analysis in Parkinson's disease. IEEE Transactions on Information Technology in Biomedicine 15(3), 481–490 (2011)
2. Palmerini, L., Avanzolini, G., Mellone, S., Valzania, F., Chiari, L.: Quantification of Motor Impairment in Parkinson's Disease Using an Instrumented Timed Up and Go Test. IEEE Transactions on Neural Systems and Rehabilitation Engineering (preprint, 2013)
3. Weiss, A., Herman, T., Plotnik, M., Brozgol, M., et al.: Can an accelerometer enhance the utility of the Timed Up & Go Test when evaluating patients with Parkinson's disease? Med. Eng. & Phys. 32(2), 119–125 (2010)
4. Zampieri, C., Salarian, A., Carlson-Kuhta, P., Aminian, K., et al.: The instrumented timed up and go test: potential outcome measure for disease modifying therapies in Parkinson's disease. J. of Neurol., Neurosurg. & Psychiatry 81(2), 171–176 (2009)
5. Kohavi, R., John, G.H.: Wrappers for Feature Subset Selection. Art. Intel. 97(1-2), 273–324 (1997)

False Positive Reduction in Detector Implantation

Noelia Vállez, Gloria Bueno, and Oscar Déniz

University of Castilla - La Mancha (UCLM), VISILAB Group,
ETSI Industriales, Avda. Camilo José Cela S/N, 13071 Ciudad Real, Spain
{Noelia.Vallez,Gloria.Bueno,Oscar.Deniz}@uclm.es

Abstract. The development of a detection system is normally driven to achieve good detection rates. In most cases, a good detection rate involves a number of false positive decisions. However, the false positive rate is ultimately what decides if the detection system is effective or not. Another aspect to consider in automatic detection systems is the time to analyse an image until a decision is made. Viola & Jones proposed a cascade detector that achieves good detection and false positive rates at high speed. Some authors have proposed modifications to the cascade detector in order to improve the detection rate while maintaining the same false positive rate. However, during the implantation of the system we consistently find a large number of false positive detections due to the lack of knowledge about the newly acquired images. In this work, we propose a parallel cascade detector that gradually incorporates these new false positives to achieve an acceptable false positive rate. The second cascade detector is built using the new false positive detection images and the original true positive images during the implantation period. The proposed parallel scheme reduces the false positive rate of the system at roughly the same speed.

Keywords: False Positive Reduction, Automatic Detection, Cascade of Classifiers.

1 Introduction

Several automatic detection problems based on image analysis, such as lesion detection in medicine or automatic vigilance, try to give a positive or negative decision once an image is examined. Automatic detection systems are usually developed to achieve good detection rates (the relation between the true positive (TP) detections and the system total number of events). It is well known that it may be preferable to obtain inappropriate images with false positives (FP) or false alarms than false negatives ones (FN) because the system supervisor can see and discard these false positives since they have been detected. On the other hand, false negatives are images which have been missed by the system and therefore they are not presented to the supervisor. For example, a false positive in medicine causes unnecessary worry or treatment, while a false negative

N. Peek, R. Marín Morales, and M. Peleg (Eds.): AIME 2013, LNAI 7885, pp. 181–185, 2013.
© Springer-Verlag Berlin Heidelberg 2013

gives the patient the dangerous illusion of good health. Therefore, the effort has been focused on the development of detection systems with good TP/FP rates. However, the false alarm rate is what makes the detection system useful or not.

Another factor to take into account when designing a detection system based on image analysis is the time consumed until a decision is made. The detection schema proposed by Viola-Jones is one of the most successful and widely used [1]. The Viola-Jones detector consists on a cascade of boosted classifiers based on the Haar-like features which acts as a single classifier and rapidly eliminates the negative images in the first few stages while maintaining the positive ones until the last stage (Fig. 1).

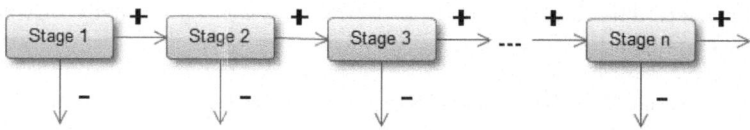

Fig. 1. Viola-Jones cascade framework

Some authors have proposed modifications to the cascade detector in order to improve the detection rate while maintaining or reducing the false positive [2–5]. However, during the implantation of the system we consistently find a large number of false positive detections due to the lack of knowledge about the newly acquired images. This problem is aggravated in the case of having small datasets for training the algorithm because the classifier does not have enough information [6]. In this work, we propose a parallel cascade detector that gradually incorporates these new false positives to achieve an acceptable false positive rate. The second cascade detector is built using the new false positive detection images and the original true positive images during the implantation period. The proposed parallel scheme reduces the false positive rate of the system at roughly the same speed. We have tested the methodology with a breast ultrasound dataset for distinguishing between images with lesions and images with normal breast tissue.

The rest of the paper is organized as follows. The parallel cascade classifier proposed and the database used are described in Section 2. Section 3 shows the results of the combined architecture. Finally, we conclude and discuss the application of the method in Section 4.

2   Methods and Materials

One alternative to reduce FPs in the implantation period is adding more stages to the original cascade. However, this solution also affects the true positive detection rate decreasing it [7].

Our method for building a parallel cascade architecture (Fig. 2) for false positive reduction in detector involves the following stages:

1. Obtain the Haar-like features [1].
2. Build the Viola-Jones cascade classifier with the training database.
3. Once the original cascade is built, use a new database with negative samples as the new instances of the system that can produce false positive detections and test the cascade with it.
4. Use the new FP detections generated and the original positive instances used in the original database to train a new Viola-Jones cascade classifier.
5. At this step, we have two cascade classifiers that can be combined and used in parallel. If a new instance arrives to the system, it will have to pass through all stages in both cascades in order to decide it is a positive finding. Otherwise, if one of the cascades discards it in one stage, the new instance is decided to be negative.

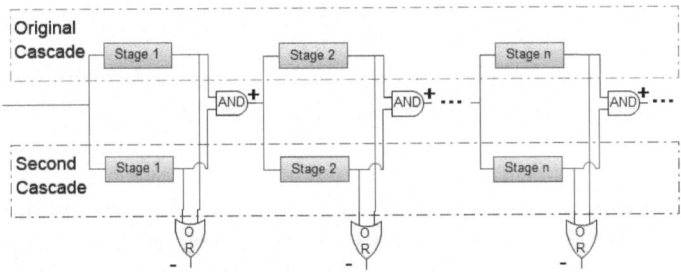

Fig. 2. Proposed parallel schema

At this point, we have to verify the independence of the two classifiers in case of the false instances to ensure an improvement in the detection system [8]. Moreover, we have to verify also the dependence between the two classifiers with the true instances to not reduce the detection rate. To check the dependence/independence of the cascade classifiers we use the Chi-squared test [9] and the Yule's Q statistic [10]. The relationship between two classifiers can be expressed in a table (Table 1).

Table 1. Relationship between two classifiers

	Classifier 1 correct	Classifier 1 wrong
Classifier 2 correct	a	b
Classifier 2 wrong	c	d

Based on the values a, b, c and d of the Table 1 the Q statistic for two classifiers can be calculated as:

$$Q = \frac{ad - bc}{ad + bc} \tag{1}$$

With the same values it is possible to calculate the χ^2 statistic:

$$\chi^2 = \frac{N(ad - bc)^2}{(a + b)(a + c)(b + d)(c + d)} \tag{2}$$

where N is the total number of elements and the χ^2 has 1 degree of freedom.

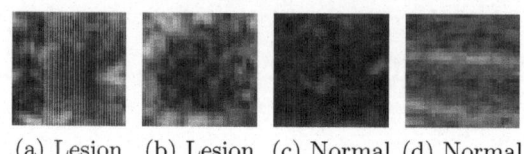

(a) Lesion   (b) Lesion   (c) Normal   (d) Normal

Fig. 3. Image samples from the breast ultrasound database used

3   Results

In order to test the proposed parallel cascade architecture, we obtained a breast ultrasound dataset for distinguishing between images with lesions and images with normal breast tissue provided by local hospitals. The dataset is composed of 37 images of lesions and other abnormalities and 500 images of breast normal tissue. The images are 30 X 30 pixels. They are all black and white images. Figure 3 shows some of them.

Firstly we train a Viola-Jones cascade with 27 of the positive images and 150 randomly selected from the negative set obtaining a cascade classifier which only fails to correctly classify one of the positive images and has a FP rate of 1%. The second cascade is built with the positive dataset and the false positive instances generated in the first cascade by another subset of 150 images from the negative dataset (21% of these second dataset). The second cascade fails on the same image as the first cascade and has a FP rate of 6%. Testing the cascade combination with the rest of the images (10 from the positive set and 300 from the negative set) we obtain a FP rate of 5.5% whereas the two classifiers obtain FP rates of 23% and 55% used alone. About the detection rate, the three classifiers correctly classify all the test images except one.

Testing the independence of the two cascades under a 5% level of significance the χ^2 is 9 for the rest of the positive instances. This value is greater than 3.84 and therefore the two cascade classifiers are dependent over the positive images. For the negative test instances, the χ^2 is 2.07 which is lower than 3.84 and we accept the independence hypothesis of the two classifiers over the negative instances. The Yule's Q statistic values are 1 and -0.27 respectively. These values indicate a large association grade between the classifiers decisions over the positive instances and a small one between the classifiers decisions over the negative instances.

4 Discussion and Conclusions

We propose in this work a parallel cascade detector for false positive reduction during the implantation of the Viola-Jones cascade. The results show an improvement of the false positive detection improving it by 15% including new information of false positives to the system for the following instances. The effectiveness of the proposed parallel combination scheme is assessed by means of the χ^2 test and the Yule's Q statistic. The system architecture can be used with other cascade classifiers and not only with the original Viola-Jones cascade to obtain better results. Moreover, this approach is compatible with different image databases and can be applied in several automatic detection problems.

Acknowledgements. The authors would like to thank the financial support from the Spanish Ministry for Economy and Competitiveness / European Regional Development Fund through the project TIN2011-24367.

References

1. Viola, P.A., Jones, M.J.: Rapid Object Detection using a Boosted Cascade of Simple Features. In: CVPR (1), pp. 511–518 (2001)
2. Lienhart, R., Maydt, J.: An extended set of Haar-like features for rapid object detection, vol. 1, pp. 900–903 (2002)
3. Sochman, J., Matas, J.: Inter-stage feature propagation in cascade building with adaboost. In: ICPR (1), pp. 236–239
4. Chen, Y.-T., Chen, C.-S.: A cascade of feed-forward classifiers for fast pedestrian detection. In: Yagi, Y., Kang, S.B., Kweon, I.S., Zha, H. (eds.) ACCV 2007, Part I. LNCS, vol. 4843, pp. 905–914. Springer, Heidelberg (2007)
5. Cheng, W.C., Jhan, D.M.: A cascade classifier using Adaboost algorithm and support vector machine for pedestrian detection. In: IEEE International Conference on Systems, Man, and Cybernetics (SMC), pp. 1430–1435 (2011)
6. Kuncheva, L.I.: Combining Pattern Classifiers Methods and Algorithms. John Wiley & Sons, Inc. (2004)
7. Castrillón, M., Déniz, O., Hernández, D., Lorenzo, J.: A comparison of face and facial feature detectors based on the Viola & Jones general object detection framework. Machine Vision and Applications 22, 481–494 (2011)
8. Kuncheva, L.I., Whitaker, C.J., Shipp, C.A.: Limits on the Majority Vote Accuracy in Classifier Fusion. Pattern Analysis and Applications 6, 22–31 (2003)
9. Agresti, A.: An introduction to categorical data analysis. John Wiley & Sons, Inc. (1996)
10. Yule, G.: On the association of attributes in statistics. Phil. Trans. 194, 257–319 (1990)

Redundant Elements in SNOMED CT Concept Definitions

Kathrin Dentler[1,2,*] and Ronald Cornet[2,3,**]

[1] Dept. of Computer Science, VU University Amsterdam, The Netherlands
[2] Dept. of Medical Informatics, Academic Medical Center,
University of Amsterdam, The Netherlands
k.dentler@vu.nl
[3] Department of Biomedical Engineering, Linköping University, Sweden

Abstract. While redundant elements in SNOMED CT concept definitions are harmless from a logical point of view, they unnecessarily make
concept definitions of typically large ontologies such as SNOMED CT
hard to construct and to maintain. In this paper, we apply a fully automated method to detect intra-axiom redundancies in SNOMED CT.
We systematically analyse the completeness and soundness of the results of our method by examining the identified redundant elements.
In absence of a gold standard, we check whether our method identifies
concepts that are likely to contain redundant elements because they become equivalent to their stated subsumer when they are replaced by a
fully defined concept with the same definition. To evaluate soundness,
we remove all identified redundancies, and test whether the logical closure is preserved by comparing the concept hierarchy to the one of the
official SNOMED CT distribution. We found that 35,010 of the 296,433
SNOMED CT concepts (12%) contain redundant elements in their definitions, and that the results of our method are sound and complete
with respect to our partial evaluation. We recommend to free the stated
form from these redundancies. In future, knowledge modellers should be
supported by being pointed to newly introduced redundancies.

Keywords: SNOMED CT, OWL 2 EL, Redundancies, Reasoning.

1 Introduction

SNOMED Clinical Terms (SNOMED CT) allows for meaning-based recording
and retrieval of clinical information, which thereby becomes (re)usable. One of
the advantages of SNOMED CT is its large size and coverage, which on the other
hand makes defining new and maintaining existing concepts a challenging task.

---

* Corresponding author.
** Remark: Ronald Cornet is a member of the Technical Committee of the Interna-
tional Health Terminology Standards Development Organization (IHTSDO), which
publishes SNOMED CT. His position at the IHTSDO, however, had no bearing on
the research study or results.

N. Peek, R. Marín Morales, and M. Peleg (Eds.): AIME 2013, LNAI 7885, pp. 186–195, 2013.
© Springer-Verlag Berlin Heidelberg 2013

Various (automated) auditing methods have been developed that can be applied to the content of controlled biomedical terminologies, amongst others to ensure the quality factor non-redundancy [16]. While such methods mostly aim at detecting equivalent concepts, also parts or elements of concept definitions, i.e. intra-axiom redundancies, are problematic. The detection of intra-axiom redundancies is required during design time. In fact, Spackman et al. reported back in 2001 that "... during the concept definition process there has been confusion among modelers about which roles need to be explicitly modeled and which ones can be left unstated. Some of this confusion arises because of uncertainty about which roles and values are inherited from supertypes" [13]. And even though redundancies are harmless from a logical point of view, they impede the maintainability of a terminology [11], [8], as they misleadingly suggest that new information has been added to a concept, while in reality, this "new" information is more general than or equivalent to information that already has been stated in the definition of the same concept or a superconcept. In this paper, we make an inventory of redundant elements in SNOMED CT concept definitions.

2   Background

2.1   SNOMED CT Concept Definitions and Rolegroups

SNOMED CT is based on the lightweight Description Logic EL^+ [1]. Its concepts are defined by conjunctions of other concepts as well as role-value pairs which are represented as exists restrictions ($\exists$), and can be either ungrouped or grouped in so-called *rolegroups* [5]. In SNOMED CT, rolegroups allow to nest or rather group existential restrictions within an existential restriction on a role named rolegroup. Concepts can be either *primitive*, i.e. specified by *necessary* conditions only (denoted by the subsumption operator $\sqsubseteq$) or *fully defined*, i.e. specified by both *necessary and sufficient* conditions (denoted by the equivalence operator $\equiv$). Example 1 presents a fully defined sample concept, which is defined by the conjunction of one concept and two rolegroups.

Example 1 (Brain stem contusion with open intracranial wound. RG stands for rolegroup).

```
Brain stem contusion with open intracranial wound ≡
    Contusion of brain with open intracranial wound ⊓
  ∃RG(∃Associated morphology.Open wound ⊓
      ∃Finding site.Intracranial structure) ⊓
  ∃RG(∃Associated morphology.Open contusion ⊓
      ∃Finding site.Brainstem structure)
```

2.2   Trivial and Non-trivial Primitive Concepts

For our evaluation, we distinguish *trivial primitive concepts*, that are primitive and subsumed by one concept only, and *non-trivial primitive concepts*, that are primitive and described by the conjunction of several concepts and optional additional exists restrictions. With regard to Example 2, we refer to the concept

Brain tissue structure as trivial primitive, and to *Structure of lobe of brain* as non-trivial primitive.

Example 2 (Structure of lobe of brain).

```
Brain tissue structure ⊑ Brain part

Structure of lobe of brain ⊑
    Brain part ⊓ Brain tissue structure
```

2.3   Redundant Elements in SNOMED CT Concept Definitions

An element that is part of a concept definition, i.e. a concept or an existential restriction, is redundant if it has been stated explicitly even though it is already implied by the definition of the same concept or a stated superconcept. Therefore, we define an element to be redundant if it is more general than or equivalent to an element that is contained in the definition of the same concept or a stated superconcept. Redundant elements can be eliminated without affecting the ontology's logical closure. For example, the concept *Brain part* in the definition of the concept *Structure of lobe of brain* in Example 2 is redundant as it subsumes the concept *Brain tissue structure*.

3   Materials and Methods

We employed the July 2012 version of SNOMED CT in Release Format 2, which was transformed to OWL with the Perl script released in the same version. The script makes use of the released concept and stated relationships tables. The latter represents the faithful representation of the information entered by modellers.

We relied on the high-performance reasoner ELK [15] to classify SNOMED CT, and to check for subsumption and equivalence relationships between concepts and roles, while Pellet [12] was used in our evaluation to explain equivalence relationships that were hard to reproduce manually. We relied on the OWL API [9] to carry out all experiments.

3.1   Method to Detect Redundant Elements in SNOMED CT Concept Definitions

We exploit the simple structure of SNOMED CT and its rolegroups to detect intra-axiom redundancies. Therefore, we adapted and extended the rules 1 to 3 of redundancy elimination for concept definitions that contain rolegroups as defined by Spackman et al. [14] (and adopted their original numbering). The rules are based on Definition 1.

Definition 1. More general or equivalent exists restriction. *An exists restriction is more general than or equivalent to another exists restriction whenever both its role and its value concept subsume or are equivalent to the respective elements in the other exists restriction.*

$$\exists R.C \sqsupseteq \exists S.D \Longleftrightarrow (R \sqsupseteq S) \text{ and } (C \sqsupseteq D)$$

All concept definitions are merely conjunctions of ungrouped or grouped exists restrictions and superconcepts. Therefore, the rules define for each of these elements whether they are redundant:

1. An ungrouped exists restriction is redundant when it is more general than or equivalent to an ungrouped exists restriction within the definition of *the same concept or a superconcept.*

   $(\exists R.C \sqcap \exists S.D \sqcap \exists T.E) \equiv (\exists S.D \sqcap \exists T.E) \iff \exists R.C \sqsupseteq \exists S.D$

2. A rolegroup is redundant when all its exists restrictions are more general than or equivalent to those contained in another rolegroup in the definition of *the same concept or a superconcept.*

   $(RG(\exists R_1.C_1 \sqcap \ldots \sqcap \exists R_n.C_n) \sqcap RG(\exists S_1.D_1 \sqcap \ldots \sqcap \exists S_m.D_m)) \equiv RG(\exists S_1.D_1 \sqcap \ldots \sqcap \exists S_m.D_m)$

   $\iff \forall i=1,\ldots,n \; \exists j=1,\ldots,m \mid \exists R_i.C_i \sqsupseteq \exists S_j.D_j$

3. An exists restriction is redundant within a rolegroup when it is more general than or equivalent to another exists restriction in *the same rolegroup.*

   $RG(\exists R.C \sqcap \exists S.D \sqcap \exists T.E) \equiv RG(\exists S.D \sqcap \exists T.E) \iff \exists R.C \sqsupseteq \exists S.D$

4. A concept is redundant when it is more general than or equivalent to one of the other concepts in the definition of *the same concept or a superconcept.*

   $(C \sqcap D) \equiv D \iff C \sqsupseteq D$

Rule 3 is an exception with regard to our redundancy definition, as it does not concern an element of a concept definition, but an element within an element. To test whether a concept is defined redundantly, these four rules are applied to a concept and all its stated superconcepts. As the rules are independent from each other, their execution order should not influence the obtained results.

3.2 Evaluation of Our Method

To evaluate the results obtained by the application of the four rules of redundancy detection, we assess the completeness and soundness of its output. In absence of a gold standard, we measure completeness by matching our findings to definitions that are likely to be redundant according to Cornet's and Abu-Hanna's method [4], and soundness by checking whether the logical closure is preserved after classifying the manipulated version of the ontology.

Completeness: Comparison of Identified Redundant Concepts to Redundant Concepts According to Cornet's and Abu-Hanna's Method.
Cornet's and Abu-Hanna's method [4] detects concepts with equivalent definitions in terminological systems represented in a description logic, to address the problems of redundancy and underspecification. Concepts that become equivalent to any superconcept when applying this method are likely to be defined redundantly [3]. Let us regard Example 3, which presents a sample group of equivalent concepts that can be detected by applying this method.

Example 3 (Group of concepts with equivalent concept definitions).

```
Finding of volume of heart sounds ⊑
    Finding of heart sounds ⊓
        ∃RG(∃Interprets.Loudness of heart sounds)

Heart sounds diminished ⊑
    Finding of volume of heart sounds ⊓
        ∃RG(∃Finding site.Heart structure)

Heart sound volume variable ⊑
    Finding of volume of heart sounds ⊓
        ∃RG(∃Finding site.Heart structure)

Heart sound inaudible ⊑
    Finding of volume of heart sounds ⊓
        ∃RG(∃Finding site.Heart structure)
```

Here, we can make two interesting observations. First, we see three concepts with definitions that obviously become equivalent when making these concepts fully defined. Second, the three concepts become equivalent to their superconcept *Finding of volume of heart sounds*, and thus, they are likely to be defined redundantly. And indeed, four steps up the concept hierarchy, we encounter their common superconcept presented in Example 4, which already contains a rolegroup that defines the *Finding site* to be the *Heart structure*.

Example 4 (Explanation for redundancy).

```
Cardiac finding ⊑
    Cardiovascular finding ⊓
        ∃RG(∃Finding site.Heart structure)
```

We evaluate the results obtained by the application of the four rules of redundancy detection by checking whether the concepts that are likely to be redundant according to Cornet and Abu-Hanna are indeed contained in the identified set of redundant concepts. In order to detect redundant definitions, we apply the approach proposed by Cornet and Abu-Hanna as follows:

1. Replace each non-trivial primitive concept by a fully defined concept with the same definition.
2. Classify the ontology.
3. For each concept in the ontology, retrieve equivalent concepts from reasoner.
4. Identify concepts that have become equivalent to any stated superconcept, as those are likely to be defined redundantly.
5. Identify and exclude indirect redundancies that emerge due to concepts being subsumed by the conjunction of concepts with equivalent definitions such as in Example 5 and wrongly identified redundancies due to the propagation of equivalence such as in Example 6.[1]

---

[1] Please note that these cases could be prevented by applying the method only on one superconcept - subconcept pair at a time instead of the entire SNOMED CT. We did not apply this method because it is not feasible even with very fast classification times.

Example 5 (Concepts without intra-axiom redundancy: Because Midwifery personnel *and* Professional midwife *have the same definitions, they become equivalent. And because* Auxiliary midwife *is being subsumed by the two of them, it also becomes equivalent.).*

```
Auxiliary midwife ⊑
    Professional midwife ⊓ Midwifery personnel

Professional midwife ⊑
    Medical, dental, veterinary/related worker ⊓
    Health visitor, nurse/midwife

Midwifery personnel ⊑
    Medical, dental, veterinary/related worker ⊓
    Health visitor, nurse/midwife
```

Please note that Cornet's and Abu-Hanna's method does not necessarily retrieve all redundant concepts. For example, a concept can refine its stated superconcept and additionally contain redundant elements. Likewise, redundant elements in fully defined concept definitions are not detected by Cornet's and Abu-Hanna's method. Therefore, the evaluation of the results of the four rules of redundancy detection can only be partial.

Example 6 (Example for wrongly identified redundancy. The concepts Pancreatic function outside reference range *and* Measurement finding outside reference range *would be equivalent if all involved concepts were fully defined.).*

```
Pancreatic function outside reference range ⊑
    Measurement finding outside reference range ⊓
    ∃RG(∃Has interpretation.Outside reference range ⊓
    ∃Interprets.Pancreatic function test)

Measurement finding outside reference range ≡
    Measurement finding ⊓
    ∃RG(∃Has interpretation.Outside reference range ⊓
    ∃Interprets.Measurement procedure)

Pancreatic function test ⊑
    Measurement procedure ⊓
    ∃RG(∃Has Method.Measurement - action)

Measurement procedure ≡
    Procedure by method ⊓
    ∃RG(∃Has Method.Measurement - action)
```

Soundness: Preservation of Logical Closure. Deleting redundant parts of concept definitions should not affect the logical closure, and therefore a change in the concept hierarchy would indicate the removal of a non-redundant part of a concept definition. Thus, we delete all identified intra-axiom redundancies and check whether the computed concept hierarchy obtained from classifying the manipulated version is the same as the one obtained from classifying the original version by bi-directional comparison of both versions to the official SNOMED CT distribution.

4   Results: Redundant Elements in Concept Definitions

Applying the four rules of redundancy detection, 35,010 of the 296,433 SNOMED CT concepts (12%) were identified to contain redundant elements in their definitions. Table 1 gives an overview of the results, only regarding the first explanation for these redundancies (the rules were applied in the same order as they are presented in this paper). 11,858 of these concepts are fully defined, and 23,152 non-trivial primitive.

Example 7 (Parenteral form thymoxamine).

```
Parenteral form thymoxamine (product) ≡
    Thymoxamine (product) ⊓
        ∃Has active ingredient.Thymoxamine (substance)

Thymoxamine (product) ⊑
    Alpha blocking vasodilator ⊓ Alpha 1 adrenergic blocking agent ⊓
        ∃Has active ingredient.Thymoxamine (substance)
```

Table 1. Detected concepts with redundant elements. The examples in column 'example' refer to the examples disseminated along the paper.

Rule	Concepts	Example and Explanation
1 (ungrouped exists restriction)	7,874	Example 7: The ungrouped exists restriction ∃*Has active ingredient.Thymoxamine (substance)* is redundant, as it is already contained in the superconcept *Thymoxamine (product)*.
2 (rolegroup)	26,599	Example 1: The first rolegroup is redundant, as it is more general than the second one, because *open wound* subsumes *open contusion*, and *Intracranial structure* subsumes *Brainstem structure*.
3 (grouped exists restriction)	6	Example 8: The exists restriction ∃*Associated morphology.-Traumatic abnormality* in the first rolegroup is redundant, as *Traumatic abnormality* subsumes *Closed traumatic abnormality*.
4 (concept)	531	Example 2: The concept *Brain part* is redundant as it subsumes the concept *Brain tissue structure*.

Example 8 (Closed skull fracture with intracranial injury).

```
Closed skull fracture with intracranial injury ≡
    Fracture of skull ⊓
        ∃RG(∃Finding site.Intracranial structure ⊓
        ∃Associated morphology.Traumatic abnormality ⊓
        ∃Associated morphology.Closed traumatic abnormality) ⊓
        ∃RG(∃Associated morphology.Fracture, closed ⊓
        ∃Finding site.Bone structure of cranium)

Explanation:
Closed traumatic abnormality ⊑ Traumatic abnormality
```

Figure 1 shows the SNOMED CT categories that the concepts with redundant elements belong to. Figure 2 depicts the distances between redundant concepts and the concepts containing the explanation for the redundancy. A distance of 0 is interesting as it makes a concept redundant with regard to its own definition. But also long distances are interesting: an element is introduced, not repeated for some concepts down the hierarchy, but then it is. The concept *Measurement of Human T-lymphotropic virus 1 recombinant glycoprotein 21 antibody and Human T-lymphotropic virus 2 recombinant glycoprotein 21 antibody* is among the concepts with the longest distance to its explanation (9 steps).

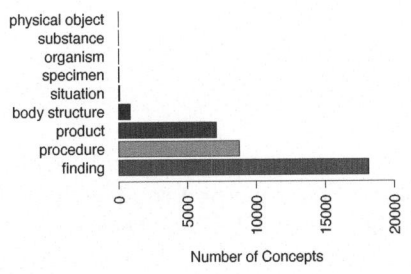

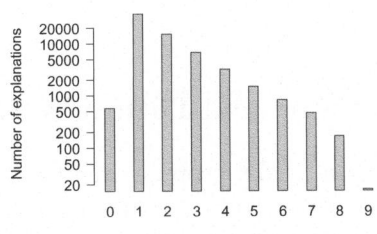

Fig. 1. SNOMED CT categories of concepts with redundancies

Fig. 2. Distances between redundant concepts and the concepts containing the explanation

An exhaustive search for all redundant elements and all explanations results in 65,336 explanations: 13,808 for rule 1, 50,680 for rule 2, 6 for rule 3 and 842 for rule 4. The maximum number of explanations is 16 for the concept *Late congenital syphilitic meningitis*. The concept with the most (6) redundant elements is *Diphtheria + tetanus + pertussis + poliomyelitis + recombinant hepatitis B virus + recombinant haemophilus influenzae type B vaccine*.

5   Evaluation

5.1   Completeness

Applying Cornet's and Abu-Hanna's method, 45,975 concept definitions with at least one other concept with a logically equivalent definition have been identified, containing a total of 12,823 non-trivial primitive concepts with definitions that are equivalent to the definition of at least one of their stated superconcepts.

12,094 of these redundancies have been confirmed to be redundant by our method to detect intra-axiom redundancies. 698 out of the 729 non-confirmed redundancies were subsumed by the conjunction of concepts, such as the concept in Example 5. For the remaining 31 non-confirmed redundancies, we successfully generated explanations with Pellet based on the manipulated version of SNOMED CT. A manual revision confirmed that all of the explanations contained further axioms that have been re-defined from being primitive to fully defined, such as the explanation given in Example 6. Therefore, the results of our method are complete with regard to Cornet's and Abu-Hanna's method.

5.2 Soundness

We generated the logical closure of both the original and the manipulated OWL versions of SNOMED CT, and compared the computed class hierarchies to the one contained in the official distribution. The OWL versions and the database table contained exactly the same set of 438,554 subclass axioms or respectively "is-a" relations.

6 Related and Future Work

In the past, most proposed methods focused at the detection of truly redundant, i.e. equivalent, concepts. Cimino has developed a method to identify multiple synonymous concepts and applied it to the 2001 UMLS Metathesaurus [2]. Grimm and Wissmann [8] provide methods to compute irredundant ontologies, and Entendre [6] makes users aware of redundancies.

The IHTSDO[2] describes methods to convert concepts into normal forms, some of which imply the elimination of redundancies, and Peng et al. [10] have proposed a method to identify redundant classifications, i.e. unnecessary, simultaneous assignments to sub- and superconcepts. The Ecco tool [7] facilitates the analysis of ontology differences by applying methods to syntactically or semantically detect effectual changes as well as ineffectual changes such as adding or deleting intra-axiom redundancies.

An interesting direction of future work would be to generalise our method. In principle, our definition of a redundant element could be operationalised directly by checking whether an element is more general than or equivalent to an element that is contained in the definition of the same concept or a stated superconcept.

7 Discussion and Conclusions

Our results show that 35,010 of all 296,433 SNOMED CT concepts (12%) are defined redundantly. These redundancies unnecessarily impede the work of knowledge modellers, and our own experience confirms that manual search for the causes of redundancies can be a tedious task. Therefore, we suggest to remove them from the stated relationships. To reach this goal, the four rules of redundancy detection would have to be applied to the entire SNOMED CT once.[3] Further redundancies should be avoided by pointing knowledge modellers to newly introduced redundancies in the definitions of the concepts they are currently working on, and explaining why these elements are redundant. As shown by Figure 2, most redundant elements are so due to nearby superconcepts, so that the explanations will most probably be intuitive. For this task, the four

---

[2] http://www.ihtsdo.org/

[3] It should be noted that applying the four rules of redundancy detection to the entire SNOMED CT is computationally expensive (ca. 6 hours on a laptop equipped with a 2.8 GHz Intel Core 2 Duo processor and 8 GB of physical memory). However, analysing only one concept is sufficiently fast to be executed as a background process.

rules of redundancy detection could be applied as a background process of terminology editing tools to the concepts that are currently being edited. In order to support these goals, we make both our tools and our results freely available[4].

References

1. Baader, F., Lutz, C., Suntisrivaraporn, B.: Is tractable reasoning in extensions of the description logic EL useful in practice? In: Proceedings of the 2005 International Workshop on Methods for Modalities, pp. 1–26 (2005)
2. Cimino, J.J.: Battling Scylla and Charybdis: the search for redundancy and ambiguity in the 2001 UMLS metathesaurus. In: Proceedings of the AMIA Symposium, pp. 120–124 (January 2001)
3. Cornet, R., Abu-Hanna, A.: Two DL-based methods for auditing medical terminological systems. In: AMIA Symposium, pp. 166–170 (January 2005)
4. Cornet, R., Abu-Hanna, A.: Auditing description-logic-based medical terminological systems by detecting equivalent concept definitions. International Journal of Medical Informatics 77(5), 336–345 (2008)
5. Cornet, R., Schulz, S.: Relationship groups in SNOMED CT. Stud. Health Technol. Inform. 31(0), 223–227 (2009)
6. Denaux, R., Thakker, D., Dimitrova, V., Cohn, A.: Entendre: Interactive Semantic Feedback for Ontology Authoring, files.ifi.uzh.ch
7. Gonçalves, R., Parsia, B., Sattler, U.: Ecco: A Hybrid Diff Tool for OWL 2 ontologies. In: Proceedings of the 9th International Workshop on OWL: Experiences and Directions (2012)
8. Grimm, S., Wissmann, J.: Elimination of redundancy in ontologies. In: Antoniou, G., Grobelnik, M., Simperl, E., Parsia, B., Plexousakis, D., De Leenheer, P., Pan, J. (eds.) ESWC 2011, Part I. LNCS, vol. 6643, pp. 260–274. Springer, Heidelberg (2011)
9. Horridge, M., Bechhofer, S.: The OWL API: A Java API for Working with OWL 2 Ontologies. In: 6th OWL Experienced and Directions Workshop (2009)
10. Peng, Y., Halper, M.H., Perl, Y., Geller, J.: Auditing the UMLS for redundant classifications. In: AMIA Symposium, pp. 612–616 (January 2002)
11. Schlobach, S., Cornet, R.: Logical support for terminological modeling. Studies in Health Technology and Informatics 107, 439–443 (2004)
12. Sirin, E., Parsia, B., Grau, B.C., Kalyanpur, A., Katz, Y.: Pellet: A practical OWL-DL reasoner. Web Semantics: Science, Services and Agents on the World Wide Web 5(2), 51–53 (2007)
13. Spackman, K.A.: Normal forms for description logic expressions of clinical concepts in SNOMED RT. In: Proceedings of the AMIA Symposium, pp. 627–631 (January 2001)
14. Spackman, K.A., Dionne, R., Mays, E., Weis, J.: Role grouping as an extension to the description logic of Ontylog, motivated by concept modeling in SNOMED. In: Proceedings of the AMIA Symposium, 712–746 (January 2002)
15. Kazakov, Y., Krötzsch, M., Simančík, F.: Concurrent Classification of $\mathcal{EL}$ Ontologies. In: Aroyo, L., Welty, C., Alani, H., Taylor, J., Bernstein, A., Kagal, L., Noy, N., Blomqvist, E. (eds.) ISWC 2011, Part I. LNCS, vol. 7031, pp. 305–320. Springer, Heidelberg (2011)
16. Zhu, X., Fan, J.-W., Baorto, D.M., Weng, C., Cimino, J.J.: A review of auditing methods applied to the content of controlled biomedical terminologies. Journal of biomedical informatics 42(3), 413–425 (2009)

---

[4] https://github.com/kathrinrin/redundancies

Medical Ontology Validation through Question Answering

Asma Ben Abacha, Marcos Da Silveira, and Cédric Pruski

Ressource Centre for Health Care Technologies (CR SANTEC),
Public Research Centre Henri Tudor,
6 avenue des Hauts-Fourneaux, L-4362 Esch-sur-Alzette, Luxembourg
{asma.benabacha,marcos.dasilveira,cedric.pruski}@tudor.lu

Abstract. Medical ontology construction is an interactive process that requires the collaboration of both ICT and medical experts. The complexity of the medical domain and the formal description languages makes this collaboration a time consuming and error-prone task. In this paper, we define an ontology validation method that hides the complexity of the formal description languages behind a question-answering game. The proposed approach differs from "classic" logical-consistency validation approaches and tackles the validation of the domain conceptualization. Reasoning techniques and verbalization methods are used to transform statements inferred from ontologies into natural language questions. The answers of the domain experts to these questions are used to validate and improve the ontology by identifying where it needs to be modified. The validation system then performs automatically the ontology updates needed to correct the detected errors.

Keywords: Ontology Validation, Natural Language Processing, Question Generation, Medical Domain, RDFS, OWL.

1 Introduction

Building and adapting medical ontologies is a complex task which requires a substantial human effort and a close collaboration between domain experts (e.g. health professionals) and ICT engineers. Even if ICT tools and automatic ontology construction techniques are mature enough to support this work [1–3], they provide only partial solutions and manual interventions from ICT experts will always be necessary if a high quality is expected. Ontologies are also the basis for numerous Clinical Decision Support Systems (CDSS) used to support medical activities therefore the quality of the underlying ontologies affects the results of using CDSSs that rely on these ontologies. In consequence, automatically built medical ontologies (including schema knowledge and individuals description) must be validated by domain experts.

However, experts from the medical domain are usually not familiar with ICT formalisms and technologies and must be assisted by knowledge engineers during the validation process, which augments the number of potential errors. If the

N. Peek, R. Marín Morales, and M. Peleg (Eds.): AIME 2013, LNAI 7885, pp. 196–205, 2013.

validation of the logical and structural aspects of the ontology like inconsistency, incompleteness or redundancy can be done automatically using dedicated tools [4], the validation of the conceptualization is more complex to do and requires relevant tools to assist the domain experts.

In this paper, we focus on how to assist Health Professionals (HP) in the validation of the conceptualization of a domain reflected in an ontology (i.e. the adequacy of the ontology with the real world) without requiring a deep knowledge in informatics. The main innovation of this research effort is to provide methods for the validation of ontologies through an interactive question-answering approach. This challenging task involves two main steps:

- The generation of questions in natural language from medical ontologies (these questions will be answered by domain experts).
- The interpretation of the information acquired from the experts to deduce if the part of the ontology that has been evaluated is valid, invalid or needs further modifications.

The remainder of the paper is structured as follows. Section 2 presents related work of the ontology validation field. Section 3 discusses existing criteria for validating ontologies and introduces an overview of our approach. Section 4 presents our method for the generation of natural language questions, while Section 5 deals with the interpretation of the provided answers. Section 6 provides a first experimental study of the approach. Section 7 wraps up with concluding remarks and outlines future work.

2 Related Work

Ontology validation is the central point of a big family of approaches interested in evaluating the structural and logical aspects of ontologies. In their work [4], vor der Bruck and Stenzhorn describe a method to validate ontologies using an automatic theorem prover and MultiNet axioms. Recently, the OOPS! system [5] has been proposed. It consists in detecting predefined anomalies or bad practices in ontologies. However, the real world representation dimension, referring to how accurately the ontology represents the domain intended for modelling, is often neglected in existing approaches for ontology validation since this has to be done manually by the experts.

In fact, few approaches addressed the validation of the domain-conceptualization side. Some of them focused on interface development to better present large amount of (structured) data without overwhelming users [6], while others used Natural Language Processing (NLP) techniques to interact with domain experts [7]. In this paper, we focus on the second type of approaches and propose a question-answering method based on NLP techniques to validate the functional aspect of the ontology as described in [8].

To our knowledge, the only work that addresses the problem of ontology validation by means of question-answering techniques is the MoKi system presented in [7]. However, the question formulation process do not integrate the fact that domain experts (e.g. in the medical domain) are not supposed to be familiar with ICT formalisms and the proposed system still require a substantial intervention of ICT experts.

3   Ontology Validation

In this section we discuss ontology validation criteria and present an overview of our approach.

3.1   Essential Validation Criteria

An ontology defines a set of representational primitives with which to model a domain of knowledge or discourse. The representational primitives are typically classes (or sets), attributes (or properties), and relationships (or relations among class members). The definitions of the representational primitives include information about their meaning and constraints on their logically consistent application [9].

Several criteria are used for the validation of ontologies, some of them address the *formal correctness* of the ontology such as [10]:

- Duplication errors: some elements of the ontology can be deduced from the others.
- Disjunction errors: defining a class as a conjunction of distinct classes.
- Consistency and coherence: check if the current definitions lead to contradictory conclusions.

Another kind of criteria tackles the closeness of the ontology to the modelled domain such as completeness. Gómez-Pérez [10] notes that it is impossible to prove the completeness of an ontology, however, it remains possible to prove the incompleteness of an element of the ontology. In this context, another important issue is the domain-level correctness of the ontology in the context of automatic ontology construction. Automated ontology construction processes are more and more required due to the huge amount of knowledge that must be modelled in some domains. For instance, in the medical field, knowledge doubles every 5 years [11] or even every 2 years [12].

In the scope of this paper we are interested in validating medical ontologies (including schema knowledge and individuals description) without relying on the method used to build them. More precisely, we focus on the domain-level correctness and target existing ontologies that have no formal errors. In this context we try to answer 4 main questions:

- Which elements need to be validated?
- How to order/rank the elements to be validated? Which validations are independent? Which ones are dependent from each other?
- How to validate these elements?
- How to make the necessary updates after each validation step?

Several criteria can be used to evaluate the quality of the domain conceptualization [13, 14]. We focus particularly on five criteria:

- The scope (or fit) of the vocabulary [13].
- The well-ness (fit) of the taxonomy (i.e. the generalization or is-a hierarchy) [13].
- The adequacy of the non-taxonomic relations (i.e. the fit of the semantic relations) [13].
- Coherence and Extensibility [14]: the ontology should be coherent in order to perform inferences that are correct w.r.t. the available definitions. It must be constructed in a manner that any concept addition cannot affect its consistency.
- Minimal Ontological commitment [14]: the ontology should have the minimum hypotheses about the real world and should not contain additional knowledge about the domain that it models.

3.2 Proposed Approach

We propose a two-fold approach to validate medical ontologies (cf. figure 1). The first step consists in generating automatically a list of natural language questions from the ontology to be validated (cf. section 4). These questions are submitted to domain experts who provide an agreement decision (Yes/No) and a textual feedback. The next step consists on interpreting expert's feedback to validate or modify the ontology (cf. section 5). The novelty of our approach is that manual interventions will be made only by HPs who will lead the ontology validation process. ICT experts will be required only when the error cannot be solved automatically. This will increase the quality of exchanges between actors and reduce errors and time consumption.

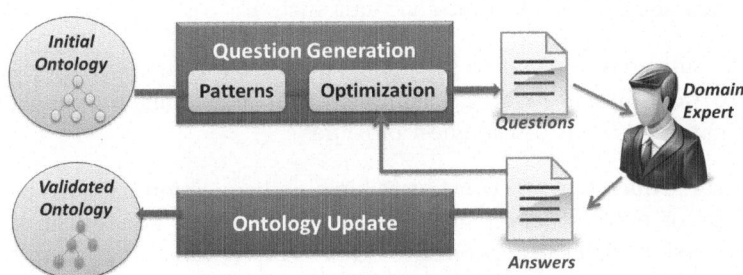

Fig. 1. Proposed Approach for Medical Ontology Validation

The proposed approach can be used to (i) validate ontologies constructed automatically from medical texts (e.g. clinical guidelines) and also (ii) to re-validate ontologies (constructed manually or automatically), since medical knowledge evolves quickly over time.

4   Question Generation from Ontologies

The aim of this step is to build relevant natural language questions from formalized knowledge in order to validate the maximum number of assertions with the minimum number of questions. Since we will use existing tools to verify the correctness of the formalism, we focus our research on validating the following types of ontology statements:

- A rdfs:subClassOf B (class A is a subclass of B)
- P rdfs:subPropertyOf Q (property P is a sub-property of Q)
- P rdfs:domain D (D is the domain class for property P)
- P rdfs:range R (R is the range class for property P)
- I rdf:type A (I is an individual of class A)
- I P J (the property P links the individuals I and J)

The proposed approach uses manually constructed patterns for each kind of ontology element as described in the following section.

4.1   Pattern-Based Method for Question Generation

We start from the hypothesis that all the elements of a medical ontology must be validated. This involves validating concepts (e.g. Substance), relations between concepts (e.g. administrated for), concept instances (e.g. activated charcoal is an instance of Manufactured Material), relations between concept instances (e.g. chest X-ray can be ordered for Chronic cough) or between concept instances and literals (e.g. "give oral activated charcoal 50g" indicates the dose of the substance to be administrated "50g"). These ontology elements provide the main keywords of the question patterns through the labels of concepts, relations and instances. Several points should be taken into account such as:

- How to build relevant natural language questions from ontology elements?
- How to take into account the complexity of answering medical questions which can be related to the question type[1]?

To answer these questions, we constructed manually question patterns associated to each type of ontological element. A question pattern consists in a regular textual expression with the appropriate "gaps" [15]. For instance, the pattern "Is DOSE of DRUG well suited for PATIENTS having DIS ?" is a textual patterns with 4 gaps: DOSE, DRUG, PATIENTS and DIS. This question pattern aims to validate a drug dose administrated to a patient having a particular disease.

Table 1 presents examples of boolean-question patterns.

---

[1] For example, as the same symptoms can refer to different medical problems w.r.t the patient age, country, etc., questions about diagnostics are expected to be more difficult than questions about complementary medical exams (e.g. Ultrasonography, Radiology).

Table 1. Examples of boolean-question patterns

Question pattern	Example of instance
Does a(n) CLASS have a(n) PROPERTY?	Does a Symptom have a Measurement Method?
	Does a Treatment have an Administration Route?
Is SUB-CLASS a type of CLASS?	Is Statistical Evidence a type of Evidence?
Is SUB-PROP a type of PROP?	Is Primary Treatment a type of Treatment?
Does a(n) CLASS1 PROPERTY a(n) CLASS2?	Does a Medical Exam diagnose a Disease?
Does INSTANCE1 PROPERTY INSTANCE2?	Does Prozac treat Schizophrenia?

4.2 Question Optimization Strategy

At this level, our main objective is how to build relevant questions from formalized knowledge in order to validate the maximum number of assertions with the minimum number of questions.

We propose an optimization strategy relying on the RDFS logical rules in order to rank the questions according to the elements that imply the more changes in the ontology. For instance, if we have the following data:

- hasSuitedAntiobioticsType *rdf:subPropertyOf* hasTreatment
- Antibiotics *rdfs:subClassOf* Treatment
- hasSuitedAntiobioticsType *rdfs:range* Antibiotics

and the expert invalidates "Antibiotics *rdfs:subClassOf* Treatment", than the property hasSuitedAntiobioticsType cannot be declared as a sub-property of hasTreatment because the hasSuitedAntibioticType relation has not a common range with the property hasTreatment which leads to a formal error w.r.t to RDFS entailment rules.

We consider all RDFS entailment rules[2]. Table 2 presents some inversed forms of these rules in order to show the impact of invalidating each one of the target ontology statements.

Table 2. Examples of ontology update rules w.r.t. invalidated elements

NOT A rdfs:subClassOf B	⇒ NOT A rdfs:subClassOf C s.t. C rdfs:subClassOf B
NOT P rdfs:domain A	⇒ NOT P rdf:subPropertyOf Q s.t. Q rdfs:domain A
NOT I rdf:type A	⇒ NOT <I, P, J> s.t. P rdfs:domain A
	NOT <J, P, I> s.t. P rdfs:range A

---

[2] http://www.w3.org/TR/rdf-mt/#RDFSRules

Thus, questions could be ranked in a manner that allows to delete some of the remaining questions if one of the RDFS entailment rules apply. This leads to the following validation order:

1. A rdfs:subClassOf B
2. P rdfs:domain D and P rdfs:range R
3. P rdfs:subPropertyOf Q
4. I rdf:type A
5. I P J

5   Feedback Interpretation and Ontology Validation

The second step of our approach is the exploitation of experts' feedback to validate or modify the target ontology. The ontology to be validated may contain concepts, individuals and relations defined between concepts or individuals.

Feedback consists in two main parts: an assertion on the correctness of the target knowledge and a free textual explanation if provided. In the scope of this paper we take into account ontologies that are formally-valid (with no inconsistencies) and focus on the validation of domain conceptualization. In this context, "Yes" answers will have no impact on the ontology. The ontology will be modified on the "No" answers provided by the domain experts. Invalidating an ontology element will have different impacts according to the element type as we have discussed in section 4.2.

We use the same RDFS entailment rules to update the ontology. The ontology item invalidated by the expert and the inferred invalidations are deleted from the ontology as well as the questions that were associated to them.

6   Experiments and Discussion

We tested our approach on three different medical ontologies[3]:

- Caries Ontology (CO)[4]
- Disease-Treatment Ontology (DTO)[5]
- Mental Diseases Ontology (MDO)[6]

In a first step, we studied the number of generated questions according to the number of ontology elements to be validated. Table 3 presents the number of questions w.r.t. the number of classes, properties and instances of each ontology (DTO, MDO and CO) without question optimization.

---

[3] In this paper, we work on medical ontologies in English but our approach can be applied to other languages.

[4] CO was developed manually by an expert in the dentistry at CRP Henri Tudor.

[5] We constructed an OWL translation of the ontology proposed by Khoo et al. [16].

[6] http://mental-functioning-ontology.googlecode.com/svn-history/r19/trunk/ontology/MD.owl

Table 3. The number of Ontology Elements (OE) and the number of generated questions for different medical ontologies without optimization

Ontology	Class Number	Property Number	Instance Number	Total Number of OE	Question Number
DTO	49	148	0	197	165
MDO	149	76	18	243	243
CO	26	266	13	305	290

The number of generated questions depends on the ontology size and shows the importance of implementing adequate questions ranking and optimization strategies, in particular for large ontologies. In our experiments, our optimization method works better in case of ontologies with many instances.

For the CO ontology, this strategy helps minimizing the number of submitted questions from 290 to 283 questions with only 4 NO answers. For the MDO ontology, our method allows asking 239 questions instead of 243 with only 2 NO answers. In case of ontologies with more NO answers (i.e. more invalid elements), the number of deleted questions will increase.

For the DTO ontology, there is no available instances and in the same time there was not "NO answers" given by the expert, so the initial number of questions was conserved. The ontologies used in these experiments were constructed manually and semi-automatically. More experiments should be conducted on automatically constructed ontologies in order to evaluate more accurately the benefits of question optimization.

In the case of ontologies with few invalid elements (few NO answers), we are currently working on presentation-level optimizations to reduce the time needed to answer the questions by the experts. In particular, we study two main presentations: question factorization according to an ontology element (concept, relation or individual) and logical chaining (A hasRelation1With B, B hasRelation2With C, etc.). These representations can help medical experts to reduce the time needed to understand and answer the questions.

These experiments also showed the need to add other specific types of questions and answers in order to acquire missing information and to enrich the ontology when necessary. For instance, an answer to a question can be YES for one group of patient (e.g. Infant) and NO for another group or under a specific condition (e.g. co-morbidity). Our validation approach can also lead to the isolation of a concept or of a branch of the ontology. We are working on improving our system by adding for the expert the possibility to precise a contextual element or condition that clarifies ambiguous situations. We also work on integrating factual questions in our system in order to add missing information to the ontology. Figure 2 presents our method to exploit factual questions in order to enrich the ontology. Future work will also include the development and the evaluation of our approach when considering more complex OWL semantics (instead of only RDFS).

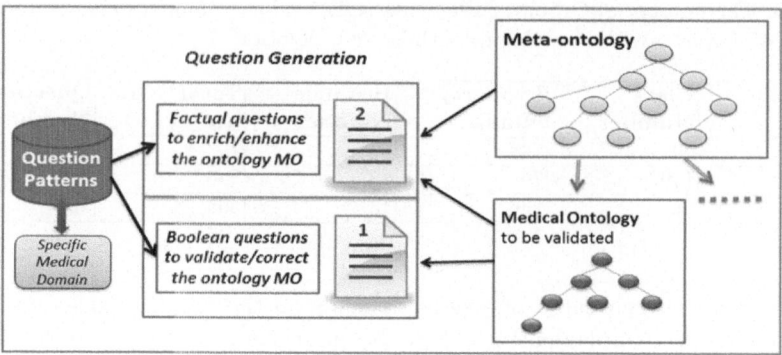

Fig. 2. Improving Question Generation

7   Conclusion

With the rise of automatic ontology construction methods, the problematic of ontology validation interests more and more research efforts, but mostly at a formal level. In this paper, we tackled the problem of ontology validation from a conceptual and a semantic point of view. We proposed a different approach based on question answering to ease the communication between the domain experts and the ontology validation system. Natural language questions are generated from the medical ontology to be validated and presented to domain experts. The acquired answers are then used to update/correct the ontology. The main contribution of this work is the combination natural language processing techniques and logical reasoning in order to support the ontology validation task. This combination provides the means for a non ICT expert (i.e. someone that do not have a deep knowledge in the ontology representation formalism) to validate the elements of the ontology. We continue to work on the optimization of the number of questions and some preliminary outcomes are presented in this paper. We plan to improve our Question Generation module by adding more optimization strategies and question types. Another enhancement could be to model specific domain knowledge as logical (domain-level) rules in order to decrease the number of ontology elements that need to be validated. Future work will also include the development of relevant heuristics for the selection of a small set of relevant questions from big ontologies.

References

1. Liu, K., Hogan, W.R., Crowley, R.S.: Natural language processing methods and systems for biomedical ontology learning. Journal of Biomedical Informatics 44(1), 163–179 (2011)
2. Navigli, R., Velardi, P.: From glossaries to ontologies: Extracting semantic structure from textual definitions. In: Proceedings of the 2008 Conference on Ontology Learning and Population: Bridging the Gap between Text and Knowledge, pp. 71–87. IOS Press, Amsterdam (2008)

3. Ruiz-Martínez, J.M., Valencia-García, R., Fernández-Breis, J.T., Sánchez, F.G., Martínez-Béjar, R.: Ontology learning from biomedical natural language documents using umls. Expert Systems with Applications 38(10), 12365–12378 (2011)
4. vor der Bruck, T., Stenzhorn, H.: Logical Ontology Validation Using an Automatic Theorem Prover. In: Proceedings of the 2010 Conference on ECAI 2010: 19th European Conference on Artificial Intelligence, pp. 491–496. IOS Press (2010)
5. Poveda-Villalón, M., Suárez-Figueroa, M.C., Gómez-Pérez, A.: Validating Ontologies with OOPS! In: ten Teije, A., Völker, J., Handschuh, S., Stuckenschmidt, H., d'Acquin, M., Nikolov, A., Aussenac-Gilles, N., Hernandez, N. (eds.) EKAW 2012. LNCS, vol. 7603, pp. 267–281. Springer, Heidelberg (2012)
6. Pohl, M., Wiltner, S., Rind, A., Aigner, W., Miksch, S., Turic, T., Drexler, F.: Patient development at a glance: An evaluation of a medical data visualization. In: Campos, P., Graham, N., Jorge, J., Nunes, N., Palanque, P., Winckler, M. (eds.) INTERACT 2011, Part IV. LNCS, vol. 6949, pp. 292–299. Springer, Heidelberg (2011)
7. Pammer, V.: Automatic Support for Ontology Evaluation Review of Entailed Statements and Assertional Effects for OWL Ontologies. PhD thesis, Graz University of Technology (March 2010)
8. Gangemi, A., Catenacci, C., Ciaramita, M., Lehmann, J.: Modelling Ontology Evaluation and Validation. In: Sure, Y., Domingue, J. (eds.) ESWC 2006. LNCS, vol. 4011, pp. 140–154. Springer, Heidelberg (2006)
9. Gruber, T.: Ontology. In: Encyclopedia of Database Systems (2008)
10. Gómez-Pérez, A.: Ontology evaluation. In: Handbook on Ontologies, pp. 251–274 (2004)
11. Engelbrecht, R.: Expert systems for medicine—functions and developments. Zentralbl Gynakol 119(9), 428–434 (1997)
12. Hotvedt, M.O.: Continuing medical education: actually learning rather than simply listening. JAMA 275(21), 1637–1638 (1996)
13. Porzel, R., Malaka, R.: A Task-based Approach for Ontology Evaluation. In: Procceding of ECAI 2004, Workshop Ontology Learning and Population, Valencia, Spain (August 2004)
14. Gruber, T.R.: A translation approach to portable ontology specifications. Knowledge Acquisition 5(2), 199–220 (1993)
15. Hearst, M.: Automatic acquisition of hyponyms from large text corpora. In: Proceedings of the 14th International Conference on Computational Linguistics (COLING 1992), pp. 539–545 (1992)
16. Khoo, C.S., Na, J.C., Wang, V.W., Chan, S.: Developing an ontology for encoding disease treatment information in medical abstracts. DESIDOC Journal of Library & Information Technology 31(2) (2011)

Lexical Characterization and Analysis of the BioPortal Ontologies

Manuel Quesada-Martínez[1], Jesualdo Tomás Fernández-Breis[1],
and Robert Stevens[2]

[1] Departamento de Informática y Sistemas
Facultad de Informática, Universidad de Murcia
CP 30100, Murcia, Spain
manuel.quesada@um.es, jfernand@um.es
[2] School of Computer Science, University of Manchester, UK
robert.stevens@manchester.ac.uk

Abstract. The increasing interest of the biomedical community in ontologies can be exemplified by the availability of hundreds of biomedical ontologies and controlled vocabularies, and by the international recommendations and efforts that suggest ontologies should play a critical role in the achievement of semantic interoperability in healthcare. However, many of the available biomedical ontologies are rich in human understandable labels, but are less rich in machine processable axioms, so their effectiveness for supporting advanced data analysis processes is limited. In this context, developing methods for analysing the labels and deriving axioms from them would contribute to make biomedical ontologies more useful. In fact, our recent work revealed that exploiting the regularities and structure of the labels could contribute to that axiomatic enrichment.

In this paper, we present an approach for analysing and characterising biomedical ontologies from a lexical perspective, that is, by analysing the structure and content of the labels. This study has several goals: (1) characterization of the ontologies by the patterns found in their labels; (2) identifying which ones would be more appropriate for applying enrichment processes based on the labels; (3) inspecting how ontology re-use is being addressed for patterns found in more than one ontology.

Our analysis method has been applied to BioPortal, which is likely to be the most popular repository of biomedical ontologies, containing more than two hundred resources. We have found that there is a high redundancy in the labels of the ontologies; it would be interesting to exploit the content and structure of the labels of many of them and that it seems that re-use is not always performed as it should be.

Keywords: Biomedical ontologies, OWL, Ontology Engineering, Bioinformatics.

1 Introduction

Many biomedical ontologies have now been developed, stimulated by the increasing importance of biomedical ontologies in the scientific community. In fact,

N. Peek, R. Marín Morales, and M. Peleg (Eds.): AIME 2013, LNAI 7885, pp. 206–215, 2013.
© Springer-Verlag Berlin Heidelberg 2013

important challenges like semantic interoperability in healthcare consider ontologies fundamental as stated in the SemanticHealth final report [2] and SemanticHealthNet (`http://www.semantichealthnet.eu`). Many of these ontologies have not been created by ontology engineers, but by domain experts. This should help the veracity of the domain knowledge, but not necessarily the engineering of the ontology.

BioPortal [4] is likely to be the most important repository of biomedical ontologies, and contains more than three hundred biomedical ontologies and controlled vocabularies so far and such knowledge resources come from a variety of ontology builders. Consequently, the analysis and characterization of the properties of BioPortal ontologies becomes relevant in order to allow users and developers of biomedical ontologies to know what they can expect from such ontologies.

Many Bioportal ontologies are related to the OBO Foundry (`http://www.obofoundry.org`). The OBO Foundry has developed a series of criteria that developers of biomedical ontologies should use to contribute to the development of an orthogonal collection of biomedical ontologies (`http://obofoundry.org/crit.shtml`). Such a collection of ontologies should benefit from the re-use of the content produced in already existing ontologies and be human and machine friendly. On the humans side, the OBO Foundry proposes to use a systematic naming convention, thus ontologies should have meaningful labels and be well documented. However, as shown in [7], this is not a specific property of OBO ontologies, but found in many available ontologies. On the machine side, ontologies should be machine processable and labels are not very useful for this. The benefit we can expect from the machine processing of the ontologies depends on the axiomatic richness of the ontologies and on other factors related to the quality of the ontology, discussion which is out of the scope of the present paper. However, according to our experience with biomedical ontologies, such richness is limited. Many such ontologies are no more than plain taxonomies and controlled vocabularies, so they have a lower degree of axiomatisation.

Thus, methods for the axiomatic enrichment of biomedical ontologies would permit ontologies to be computationally more powerful. Given that biomedical ontologies are supposed to be rich in labels, our working hypothesis is that the content and structure of such labels can be useful information for supporting the axiomatic enrichment. By structure of the labels we mean the regularities that can be found in the groups of words that form such labels.

The richness of the labels means that the corresponding texts may be encoding biomedical domain knowledge. Consequently, their study should be useful for deriving domain knowledge and enriching the axiomatic definition of the ontology classes. For example, the expression *negative regulation* stands for the prevention or reduction of, generally, a biological process. This linguistic expression appears in several biomedical ontologies. On the one hand, the lack of axioms would only permit machine to exploit the labels but not the biological meaning of the concept. On the other hand, it is not guaranteed that all the ontologies in which *negative regulation* is found share the axioms, if any, for this concept.

In previous work [6], we showed that the labels of the classes of relevant biomedical ontologies like GO [1] or SNOMED-CT (http://www.ihtsdo.org/snomed-ct/) were suitable for application of the enrichment process proposed in [3]. In the current paper, a systematic analysis of the labels of BioPortal ontologies is performed, whose objectives are: (1) characterising the ontologies by their labels; (2) identifying which ontologies are more suitable for applying enrichment processes; (3) analysing whether ontology content is re-used in an appropriate way in existing biomedical ontologies. Such a study will provide new insights about biomedical ontologies and will drive our research on the enrichment of such ontologies.

2   Methods

2.1   Representation and Extraction of Lexical Patterns

Our basic assumption is that groups of words that appear in many labels are likely to encode some domain meaning. We call such groups of words (or tokens) lexical patterns. In our approach, a lexical pattern has some basic descriptors associated, like its content, length (number of tokens), or frequency in an ontology. We are going to illustrate these concepts using the *Vaccine Ontology* (http://bioportal.bioontology.org/ontologies/49452). Its lexical pattern of length one *virus* appears in 25.57% of the labels. On the other hand, the lexical pattern *preparation of* has length 2 and it appears in 14.34% of the labels. Other examples are *canine*, *Rhinotracheitis-Virus*, *protein vaccine*, *Modified Live virus* and so on.

When analysing the labels of a particular ontology, we are also interested in knowing which lexical patterns correspond to the full label of a class, and which ones are contained in the labels of external ontologies. If a lexical pattern corresponds to a full label of a class, it might be encoding the meaning of a domain concept and there should be a relation between this class and the other labels in which the pattern is found. Moreover, the axioms extracted from such lexical pattern might be used as templates for creating the axioms for those related classes. If a lexical pattern is found in the labels of external ontologies, this might indicate that some content and axioms might be re-used and shared.

For instance, the lexical pattern *virus* is not a class despite it is a relevant concept in an ontology about vaccines. Besides, *virus* has been found as the full label of classes in another 4 BioPortal ontologies. This fact does not mean that these concepts are equivalent, but at least they should be considered by a domain expert to be re-used when the need for a 'virus' class arises. Something similar occurs with the lexical pattern *canine* which is not a class but could be defined and linked with labels that contain it to indicate that these vaccines are focused on canines. We cannot only re-use classes but also properties. For instance, the lexical pattern *encoding* of the Vaccine Ontology is an object property of the Bone Dysplasia Ontology (http://purl.org/skeletome/bonedysplasia#encoding).

Our method represents the groups of tokens found in the labels of an ontology as a graph, which is built as the ontology is processed. For each class we extract its label, which is split using blank as delimiter. After this, each token is a node of the graph, and each arrow represents that the tokens appear consecutively and in that order in a label. We also store additional information for each node like the position in the label (e.g., the same word could appear several times in the same label) and the URI of the class to speed up further analyses. Once the ontology labels are represented in the graph, we apply our algorithm to identify lexical patterns within the ontology. Finding a lexical pattern of length N requires to navigate through N edges starting from an initial node. We can obtain the whole set of lexical patterns within an ontology by repeating the process in all the nodes of the graph. Despite we considered options like n-gram or high performance graph databases, the complexity of the links between our tokens and the need for a fast answer given the size of many biomedical ontologies led us to develop this graph representation.

Figure 1 shows the representation of three labels using our representation. Underlined boxes represent initial nodes; solid white boxes stand for the final node of labels; and solid gray boxes are neither initial nor final nodes. In any case, a node can play different roles at the same time such as *canine*, which is an initial and intermediate node. The arrows represent edges and the numbers refer to the identification of the labels where it appears. If we analyse this figure, the pattern *canine distemper virus* (length 3) can be found. The node *virus* has input arrows from labels 1, 2 and 3. This means that it is contained in these three labels. The arrow between *distemper* and *virus* is labelled 1,3, and this means that both words appear consecutively in these two labels being a lexical pattern of length two and with two repetitions. Consequently, *distemper virus* is a lexical pattern that appears in labels 1, 3 but not in 2.

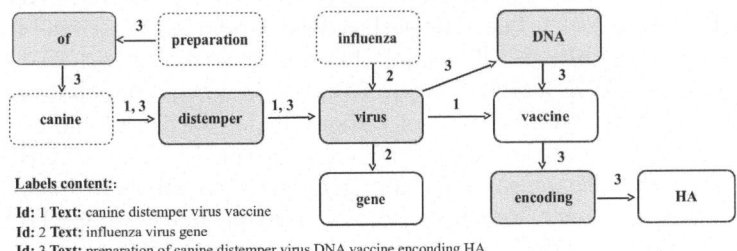

Fig. 1. Graph representation of the content of three labels

Once the graph is built, we filter out some groups of words. On the one hand, groups of words which consist only of stop-words, that is, words without meaning, are filtered. Every word group must reach a *coverage* threshold, which is the minimum percentage of labels in which a group of words must appear to be considered a lexical pattern in a particular analysis process. This enables different analyses demands to be performed and to adjust the result set to different goals of the ontology designer. Our method does not need to rebuild the graph for each change in the coverage threshold.

2.2   Shared Lexical Patterns

Once the set of lexical patterns for a given ontology has been obtained, we could look for such patterns in the labels of external ones. In our context, this means that it should be likely to find common lexical patterns in different ontologies. However, finding matches would not mean that the corresponding classes are equivalent or refer to the same domain knowledge, though the inspection of such alignments could be interesting for the designer. In our method, we identify an *exact match* when a lexical pattern and the label of an external ontology are the same. It is worth pointing out that the lexical patterns could or not being a class in the input ontology. Finding such shared lexical patterns and, even more importantly, such shared classes is relevant for the enrichment of the ontologies since existing axioms in external ontologies could be re-used in the source ontology.

Furthermore, we propose the inspection of IRIs for the *exact matches* to check if they refer to the same concepts. For instance, the lexical pattern *protein* is found as a class with the same IRI http://purl.obolibrary.org/obo/CHEBI_36080 in *CHEBI, microRNA Ontology, Gene Expression Ontology* and *Regulation of Gene Expression Ontology*. That might be a sign of good re-use. In other cases we could not assume this fact. For instance, the lexical pattern *influenza* has been found as a class in 7 external ontologies with 7 different IRIs. Knowing if they refer to seven different concepts is beyond the scope of this work, but it might be a sign of a lack of re-use.

3   Results

We have analysed the BioPortal ontologies publicly accessible in OWL and OBO format in December 2012. The analysis has been supported by a home-made software tool called OntoEnrich [5]. Since this tool only works with OWL ontologies, we used the OWL Syntax Converter (http://owl.cs.manchester.ac.uk/converter/) to get OWL versions of the ontologies only available in OBO format. In this way, our base contained 286 ontologies (177 OWL, 109 OBO). Given that 44 had no labels, we automatically generated the labels from the IRIs. 70 ontologies were not processed because of importing inaccessible OWL files or failure in the OBO to OWL conversion.

We have analyzed the labels of the ontologies for different coverage values: from 1% to 5% with increments of 1. Here we show the results with the coverage set to 1%, but the complete set is available at http:\miuras.inf.um.es/aime. For each ontology, we obtained a series of metrics, the main ones being:

- *Number of labels*: number of labels in an ontology.
- *Number of lexical patterns*: number of lexical patterns found in the ontology.
- *Classes affected by lexical patterns*:number and percentage of classes in which lexical patterns are found.
- *Classes affected by matches*: number and percentage of classes for which exact matches are found.
- *Repetition of words*: percentage of repeated words in the ontology labels.

3.1   Global Characterization of BioPortal Ontologies

Table 1 shows the summary of the characterization of the 216 ontologies analyzed, whose main findings are described next.

- Labels: 90% of the classes have labels. This value suggests that the BioPortal ontologies are rich in labels, so their analysis might be interesting. Besides, 68.5% of the words used in labels are repeated and this is a sign of regularity. The mean of repeated labels is 0.90% which is a good result, but the maximum value of 31%, which means that almost 1 out of 3 classes share a full label. This ratio is greater than 5% for 7 ontologies.
- Lexical patterns: With a coverage of 1%, the mean number of lexical patterns is 63, the highest being 555 repetitions in the *Ontology of Data Mining*. The mean percentage of classes for which patterns are found is 56%. This means that many BioPortal ontologies may have regularities in their labels.
- Matches in external ontologies: The mean number of external matches per ontology is 124.7. This means that many patterns of each ontology are found many times in other BioPortal ontologies as full labels of classes. The mean number of external matches per lexical pattern is 44% and the percentage of classes that are covered by lexical patterns with external matches is 46% so these classes contain knowledge that exists in other resources, making the possibility of reusing content from external ontologies evident.

3.2   Cluster Analysis

We have applied agglomerative hierarchical clustering to the percentage of classes with patterns with coverage 1%. The analysis of the dendrogram suggested the existence of three main groups of ontologies. Then, we applied k-means (k=3) to get a representation of the three groups and to get each ontology associated

Table 1. Summary of data for different analysed variables

		Min.	1st Qu.	Median	Mean	3rd Qu.	Max.
Number of classes		3	132	339	5 678	1 544	286 400
Number of labels		1	98	290	5 130	1 285	232 300
Repeated Words in labels	%	50.00	61.32	68.25	68.50	76.05	97.59
Repeated labels	%	0	0	0	0.9085	0.2740	31.86
Number of Lexical Patterns		0	10	42	63.6	85	555
Classes covered by LPs	%	0	36.62	63.33	56.67	80.80	100
Number of external matches per ontology		0	18	68	124.7	122	1 298
Number of external matches per LP	%	0	25.29	45.05	44.47	64.10	100,00
Classes covered by LPs with external matches	%	0	20	46.02	43.66	67.19	100

Table 2. Centroid of the clusters

Variable	Cluster1	Cluster2	Cluster3
%ClassesWithPatterns	82.25	48.84	7.87
Ontologies	87	76	53

with one of the three clusters obtained, whose centroids have the values shown in Table 2.

The cluster analysis splits the base of ontologies in three differentiated groups. Cluster 1 includes the ontologies for which most of the classes of the ontology have lexical patterns associated. The ontologies of this cluster are the most suitable for applying enrichment methods by exploiting the lexical patterns, and they represent 40% of the ontologies analyzed. Cluster 2 includes the ontologies for which around half of the classes of the ontology have associated lexical patterns. We cannot say these ontologies could not benefit from the application of enrichment methods, but they could be assigned a lower priority. This cluster includes 35% of the ontologies, which means that 75% of the BioPortal ontologies analyzed could benefit from enrichment processes. Finally, Cluster 3 includes those ontologies whose classes do not have many patterns associated. Consequently, they seem to be not very interesting for the enrichment based on the exploitation of the lexical patterns. This group has 25% of the ontologies analyzed. This cluster also includes the ontologies for which patterns have not been found with coverage 1%. The members of each cluster are listed at http:\miuras.inf.um.es/aime.

3.3   Cluster Analysis of the OBO Foundry Ontologies

As mentioned in the introduction, the OBO Foundry defined a series of principles for building biomedical ontologies, among which using rich labels and a systematic naming convention are relevant for this work. If ontology builders follow such principles, the structure and content of the labels should be descriptive about the meaning of the concept. We have analysed which OBO Foundry ontologies are associated with each cluster. It should be noted that, at the time of writing, there are not many ontologies recognized as OBO Foundry members, but more that are candidate to be OBO Foundry ontologies. For an ontology to be a member, the OBO Foundry must have checked that they have been developed by following different criteria.

The OBO Foundry member ontologies are: Gene Ontology, CHEBI, Phenotypic quality, Protein Ontology, Xenopus anatomy and development and Zebrafish anatomy and development. The Gene Ontology appears in Cluster1, CHEBI in Cluster3, the Phenotypic quality ontology could not be processed and the other three ontologies appear in Cluster2. These results are in line with our expectations. Given that CHEBI is oriented to types of chemical entities and given its size it is likely that the patterns found do not appear in at least 1% of the classes. The results of using the lowest coverage (around 0%) show 16 out of the most frequent 20 lexical patterns have a frequency below 1%.

The analysis of the candidate ontologies reveals that 33 ontologies belong to Cluster1, 32 to Cluster2 and 10 to Cluster3. This means that 86% of the ontologies analysed are in Cluster1 or 2, what can be interpreted as these ontologies follow the guideline for labels.

3.4   Analysis of Lexical Patterns

Table 3 describes the set of patterns obtained with 1% of coverage considering the whole set of analyzed ontologies. It should be pointed out that 31% (4011) of the patterns appear in more than one ontology. We have analyzed the impact of using coverages 2%, 3%, 4% and 5% in the results obtained. Figure 2 shows the percentage of lexical patterns found for each coverage value, considering the total number of patterns found using such coverages. It can be seen that the 5% of coverage hardly ever find lexical patterns (mean= 8.92 patterns) and that many ontologies follow similar distributions of percentage of lexical patterns.

Table 3. Numerical metrics about the precise analysis of the lexical patterns

Lexical Patterns		Length			Frequency		
Total	Unique	Min.	Mean	Max.	Min.	Mean	Max.
13 805	9 494	1,0	1,841	12,0	2,0	115,6	5660,0

The coverage is a frequency threshold, so increasing its value means that the least frequent patterns would be removed. We have also analyzed the impact of the coverage in the distribution of ontologies after applying the clustering. The expected result was a reduction in ontologies in Cluster1 since we are removing patterns and, therefore, less classes are affected. The number of ontologies in Cluster2 remains relatively stable, while the number of ontologies drops from 87 to 28 in Cluster1. However, the number of ontologies in each group is quite similar for 3%, 4% and 5%. This means that many ontologies present many regularities with frequency lower than 3%. The same result has been found for the OBO Foundry ontologies. Two member ontologies move from Cluster2 to Cluster3 with coverage 5%. For such coverage, the distribution of ontologies is: Cluster1 (8), Cluster2 (32) and Cluster3 (35).

3.5   Analysis of Re-use of Concepts

We have studied the external matches found in terms of reusability. As mentioned, if both source and target classes of an external match for a given pattern share the same IRI, this would be a sign of good re-use. We have then analysed whether such IRI sharing happened in the external matches. The mean value of external matches is 3.357 and the number of IRIs is 2.651, so around 79% of the source and target classes have different IRIs. For instance, the lexical pattern *human* appears in 5 ontologies using 5 different IRIs, and *infection* appears in 9 ontologies using 9 IRIs too. We have not inspected whether the corresponding classes have equivalence axioms linking the different IRIs.

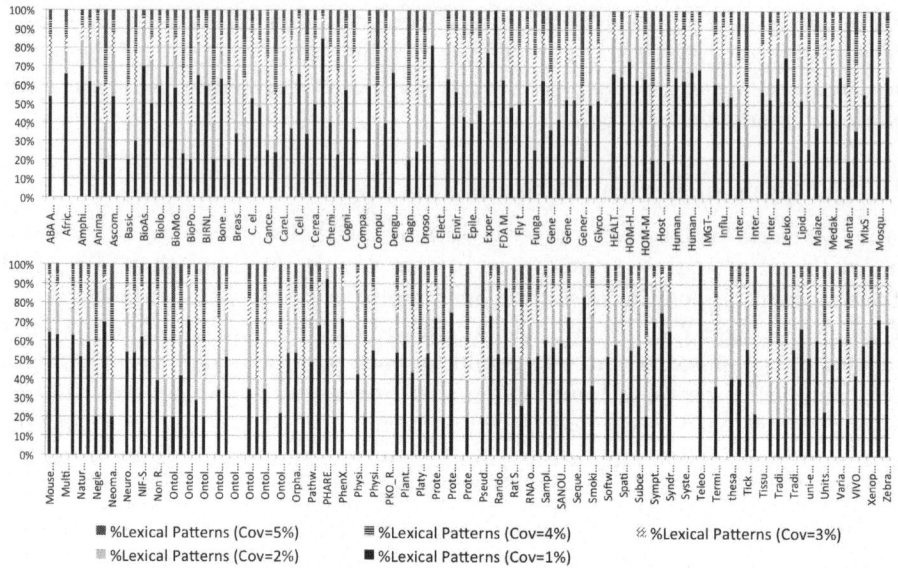

Fig. 2. Percentage of lexical patterns found for different coverages (1%, 2%, 3%, 4% and 5%), considering the total number of lexical patterns found using such coverages

4   Conclusions and Further Work

Important challenges in healthcare, like the achievement of semantic interoperability of healthcare records, require the use of good, useful ontologies for different purposes. Bioportal ontologies contain many ontologies rich in text content but not so rich in axiomatic content. The axiomatic enrichment of such ontologies could be done by exploiting the content and structure of the labels. In this paper, we have analysed the labels of Bioportal ontologies and we have been able to classify them in terms of suitability for applying enrichment processes. From our results, we suspect that re-use is not used by the biomedical ontologies builders as much as they should, although we should perform a more detailed analysis of the external matches. We think we could develop an ontology-dependent metric to get an appropriate coverage threshold. The regularities in labels of some ontologies might happen in a particular areas of the ontology. This might be the case of highly modularized ontologies with several independent modules, in which regularities in the labels within each module. Those patterns might be filtered out with a coverage of 1%, but our method and our OntoEnrich tool permit to adjust the coverage to the user needs. In this work, the re-use of concepts has been analyzed from a lexical perspective. Bioportal stores mappings between the Bioportal ontologies and we plan to compare such mappings with our external matches to improve our knowledge about re-use in biomedical ontologies. As a result of this work, we know more about the lexical properties of Bioportal ontologies, which will permit us to develop effective axiomatic enrichment processes.

Acknowledgements. This project has been possible thanks to the Spanish Ministry of Science and Innovation through grant TIN2010-21388-C02-02 and fellowship BES-2011-046192 (Manuel Quesada-Martínez), and co-funded by FEDER.

References

1. Consortium, G.O.: Gene Ontology: tool for the unification of biology. Nature Genetics 23, 25–29 (2000)
2. European Commission. Semantic interoperability for better health and safer healthcare. deployment and research roadmap for Europe (2009) ISBN-13 : 978-92-79-11139-6
3. Fernandez-Breis, J.T., Iannone, L., Palmisano, I., Rector, A.L., Stevens, R.: Enriching the gene ontology via the dissection of labels using the ontology pre-processor language. In: Cimiano, P., Pinto, H.S. (eds.) EKAW 2010. LNCS, vol. 6317, pp. 59–73. Springer, Heidelberg (2010)
4. Noy, N.F., Shah, N.H., Whetzel, P.L., Dai, B., Dorf, M., Griffith, N., Jonquet, C., Rubin, D.L., Storey, M.-A.D., Chute, C.G., Musen, M.A.: BioPortal: ontologies and integrated data resources at the click of a mouse. Nucleic Acids Research 37(Web-Server-Issue), 170–173 (2009)
5. Quesada-Martínez, M., Fernández-Breis, J.T., Stevens, R.: Enrichment of owl ontologies: a method for defining axioms from labels. In: Proceedings of the First International Workshop on Capturing and Refining Knowledge in the Medical Domain (K-MED 2012), Galway, Ireland, pp. 1–10 (2012)
6. Quesada-Martínez, M., Fernández-Breis, J.T., Stevens, R.: Extraction and analysis of the structure of labels in biomedical ontologies. In: Proceedings of the 2nd International Workshop on Managing Interoperability and Complexity in Health Systems, MIXHS 2012, pp. 7–16. ACM, New York (2012)
7. Third, A.: "Hidden semantics": what can we learn from the names in an ontology? In: 7th International Conference on Natural Language Generation (2012)

Ontology-Based Reengineering of the SNOMED CT Context Model

Catalina Martínez-Costa[1,*] and Stefan Schulz[1,2]

[1] Institute of Medical Informatics, Statistics and Documentation,
Medical University of Graz, Austria
[2] Institute of Medical Biometry and Medical Informatics,
Freiburg University Medical Center, Germany
{catalina.martinez,stefan.schulz}@medunigraz.at

Abstract. SNOMED CT is a terminology system partially built on formal-ontological principles. Although its on-going redesign efforts increasingly consider principles of formal ontology, SNOMED CT's top-level categories and relations still reflect the legacy of its predecessors rather than formal ontological principles. This is apparent in its *Context Model*, which blends characteristics of information models with characteristics of ontologies. We propose a reengineering of the SNOMED CT Context Model formulated with ontology design patterns based on the BioTopLite upper ontology. Our analysis yields a clear division between clinical situations in a strict sense and information artefacts that denote clinical situations.

Keywords: Ontologies, SNOMED CT, Electronic Health Record.

1   Introduction

SNOMED CT [1] is a large medical terminology system, partially built on formal-ontological principles. It has around 311,000 representational units (SNOMED CT concepts) embedded in a comprehensive multi-hierarchical taxonomy and enriched by DL (description logics) axioms. A large part of its content originated from the UK coding system CTV3, in which single codes often represent a complex clinical situations and epistemic states. SNOMED CT groups these terms into a separate hierarchy, called Context Model, with the root *Situation with explicit context*. Examples are *Family history of smoking*, *Diabetic foot at risk*, *Heart failure confirmed*, etc.

In theory, systems that represent the meaning of domain terms (terminologies / ontologies) should be kept separate from systems that place that meaning in a situational or epistemic context (information models) [2]. In practice, both approaches tend to overlap, which produces a plurality of syntactically and terminologically different possibilities to encode the same piece of information, which constitutes a severe barrier to semantic interoperability [3]. In [4], we found evidence that also many concepts in the SNOMED CT *Finding* and *Disorder* hierarchies reflect clinical situations. In this work, we will investigate whether the SNOMED CT hierarchy *Situation with*

---

* Corresponding author.

N. Peek, R. Marín Morales, and M. Peleg (Eds.): AIME 2013, LNAI 7885, pp. 216–220, 2013.

explicit context can be interpreted as a hierarchy of clinical situations according to our definition. We will also explore whether the logic EL++ is appropriate to capture the meaning of this content, or whether a more expressive language is needed. We propose ontology design patterns that allow the creation of a redesigned model.

2   Methods

2.1   The SNOMED CT Context Model

According to [5], a SNOMED CT concept includes context if its name explicitly represents information that might otherwise be represented by another less context-rich concept. Context elements typically alter the meaning in such a way that the resulting concept is no longer a child of the original one. E.g., *Tonsillectomy planned* is not placed under *Tonsillectomy*, but linked to it via '**associated procedure**'.

Ideally, epistemic and contextual aspects of clinical documentation are represented in information models only. However, SNOMED CT was designed to be usable without being embedded in any specific information model. Its *Situation with explicit context* hierarchy therefore plays the role of a simplified information model, which uses dedicated relations and constraints such as '**associated finding**', '**finding context**', etc. Accordingly for instance, the concept *Heart failure excluded* (*situation*) is represented in the DL interpretation of the SNOMED CT syntax [6] as:

'*Heart failure excluded* (*situation*)' subclassOf '*No cardiac failure* (*situation*)' and
   RoleGroup some (('**associated finding**' some '*Heart failure* ') and
      ('**finding context**' some '*Known absent* ') and
      ('**temporal context**' some '*Current of specified* ') and
      ('**subject relationship context**' some '*Subject of record* ')) $\qquad$ (1)

If the opposite is meant, *viz.* that the heart failure is *present*, the value of '**finding context**' changes to '*Known present*'. In the same concept three types of information are merged: (i) epistemic information such as *Known absent, Suspected*, or *Changed,* (ii) other contextual information like temporal reference (*Current, Past*) or subject relationship (*Subject of record, Person in the family*), and (iii) the reference to the clinical concept proper (*Heart failure, Tonsillectomy*). The problem in this representation (EL++) is that the clinical concept is related via an existential restriction (some). According to DL semantics, it implies that for every instance of '*Heart failure excluded*' some instance of '*Heart failure*' exists, a clearly unintended entailment. There are other cases, such as *Suspected heart failure*, in which we are not referring directly to a situation in which heart failure is clearly present or absent, but to the state of knowledge of the author of this statement. This justified our decision to categorize this type of SNOMED concepts under the BioTopLite[1] category *Information Object*.

2.2   The *Clinical Situation* Interpretation

Recently, we provided a logical formalization for SNOMED CT findings and disorders using the *Clinical Situation* concept. According to this, **a clinical situation is a**

---
[1] BioTopLite. http://purl.org/biotop/biotoplite.owl

temporal part (phase) of a person's life in which some clinical condition is present in that person at all points in time. This interpretation has been shown more suitable, especially in the context of the ICD-SNOMED CT harmonization activities [2]. It means that all these concepts should be understood as situations that are defined in terms of some clinical condition using the relation 'has condition' (which corresponds to the 'role group' relation in SNOMED CT). In BioTopLite[1], the class *Condition* is defined as the disjunction of disposition, material object and process. The following table reflects our current analysis of the ontological categories of SNOMED CT, restricted to findings and disorders, as well as to related situations.

Original SNOMED hierarchies	*Reinterpretation based on the BioTopLite ontology*
Clinical finding (finding)	'*Clinical situation*' and **'has Condition'** some '*Clinical condition*'
Situation with explicit context (situation)	'*Clinical situation*' and **'has Condition'** some '*Clinical condition*'
	'*Information entity*' and **'is about situation'** only *ClinicalSituation* and **'has information object attribute'** some '*Information object attribute*'

Sometimes SNOMED CT concepts indirectly refer to clinical situations by stating some information about them, such as *suspected* or *at risk*. These concepts are categorized as information entities that refer to the clinical situation via the relation 'is about situation'. We here use the universal restriction (only) to avoid asserting the existence of an entity the existence of which cannot be guaranteed. This is an acceptable approximation, as second-order statements are not permitted in DL.

3   Results

The application of the previous patterns requires the use of more expressivity than the provided by the present SNOMED CT description logic representation, due to the use of negation and the universal restriction (only). Here, we apply the previous patterns to some of the most frequent design patterns found in the context model. As default we assume that the values from the context model 'subject relationship context' and 'temporal context' are '*Subject of record*' and '*Current or specified*', respectively.

Clinical finding present (situation): A clinical finding present is characterized by the qualifier value '*known present*'. As we consider concepts in the finding hierarchy as situations, we here simply equate the situation concept with the finding concept:

Original SNOMED CT representation
'*Has a sore throat (situation)*' **equivalentTo** '*Clinical finding present (situation)*' and **'role group'** some ('**associated finding**' some '*Sore throat symptom (finding)*' and '**finding context**' some '*Known present*' and '**temporal context**' some '*Current*' and '**subject of record**' some '*Subject or record*')
Modified SNOMED CT representation
'*Has a sore throat (situation)*' **equivalentTo** '*Sore throat symptom (finding)*'

Clinical finding absent (situation): It has as finding context value *'known absent'*. We have reinterpreted it as a clinical situation that does not have any situation having that condition. At the beginning, we applied this pattern maintaining the original taxonomy, but this lead to numerous wrong inferences. Therefore, we removed the original parents and obtained the inverted hierarchy.

Original SNOMED CT representation
'Absence of stress (situation)' equivalentTo *'Clinical finding absent (situation)'* and **'role group'** some (**'associated finding'** some *'Feeling stressed (finding)'* and **'finding context'** some *'Known absent'* and **'temporal context'** some *'Current or specified'* and **'subject of record'** some *'Subject or record'*)
Modified SNOMED CT representation
'Absence of stress (situation)' equivalentTo ClinicalSituation and <u>not</u> (**'has processual part'** some *'Feeling stressed (finding)'*)

History of clinical finding in subject (situation): The history of a clinical finding defines the temporal context as *'Past'*. We refer to the past history of some condition, which does not need not to be present during all patients' past life, but at least once.

Original SNOMED CT representation
'History of antepartum hemorrhage (situation)' equivalentTo *'History of disorder (situation)'* and *'History of pregnancy (situation)'* and **'role group'** some (**'associated finding'** some *'Antepartum hemorrhage (disorder)'* and **'finding context'** some *'Known present'* and **'temporal context'** some *'In the past'* and **'subject of record'** some *'Subject or record'*)
Modified SNOMED CT representation
'History of antepartum hemorrhage (situation)' equivalentTo *'Information item'* and **'is about situation'** <u>only</u> (*'Biological life'* and **'has processual part'** some *'Antepartum hemorrhage (disorder)'*)

Suspected clinical finding (situation): A suspected clinical finding includes the finding context value *'Suspected'*. We have defined it as an information entity that refers to a possible situation defined by a condition and the epistemic attribute *'Suspected'* qualifies the information entity.

Original SNOMED CT representation
'Suspected lung cancer (situation)' equivalentTo *'Suspected malignancy (situation)'* and *'Suspected respiratory disease (situation)'* and **'role group'** some (**'associated finding'** some *'Malignant tumor of lung (disorder)'* and **'finding context'** some *'Suspected'* and **'temporal context'** some *'Current or specified'* and **'subject of record'** some *'Subject or record'*)
Modified SNOMED CT representation
'Suspected lung cancer (situation)' equivalentTo *'Information item'* and **'has information object attribute'** some Suspected and **'is about situation'** <u>only</u> *'Malignant tumor of lung (disorder)'*

4   Conclusions

The binding of terminologies and ontologies to clinical information models brings up the challenge of linking information objects that are about types / concepts being not necessarily instantiated [7], where the use of universal restriction ('only') was advocated as an approximate solution. The EU Network of Excellence *SemanticHealthNet*[2] targets the so-called boundary problem, including a maximum of stakeholders representing semantic (quasi-) standards (EN 13606, HL7, openEHR, IHTSDO, WHO). This study is part of this project endeavour, in which approaches that use information models and terminologies together should become interoperable with approaches that favour single codes for complex statements, such as supported by the SNOMED CT Context Model, or the content model of the upcoming ICD-11[3].

Our ontological analysis of the different representational patterns that occur in the SNOMED CT Context Model has shown that this hierarchy contains two kinds of concepts. Only one kind corresponds to what we had introduced as *Clinical situation* proper. The other kind corresponds to information entities that refer to types (not necessarily tokens) of clinical situations. Here, we have suggested ontology design patterns for some of the most frequent ones found in the context model. Their formalization as described requires more expressivity than the one supported by the EL profile. We are currently implementing some of them; and our first results suggest that the shift from OWL-EL to OWL-DL has no devastating consequences on reasoning performance. However, more scaling test will have to be performed.

Acknowledgments. This work has been funded by the SemanticHealthNet Network of Excellence within the EU 7th FP, Call: FP7-ICT- 2011-7, agreement no.: 288408.

References

1. IHTSDO (Intern. Health Terminology Standards Development Organisation). SNOMED CT, http://www.ihtsdo.org/snomed-ct (last accessed: March 2013)
2. Schulz, S., Schober, D., Daniel, C., Jaulent, M.C.: Bridging the semantics gap between terminologies, ontologies, and information models. Stud. Health Technol. Inform. 160(pt. 2), 1000–1004 (2010)
3. Stroetmann, V.N., Kalra, D., Lewalle, P., et al.: Semantic Interoperability for better health and safer healthcare - Deployment and Research Roadmap for Europe. SemanticHEALTH Report: European Communities (2009)
4. Schulz, S., Rector, A., Rodrigues, J.M., Spackman, K.: Competing Interpretations of Disorder Codes in SNOMED CT and ICD. In: Proc. of AMIA 2012 Symp., pp. 819–827 (2012)
5. International Health Terminology Standards Development. SNOMED CT® Technical Implementation Guide. Copenhagen, Denmark (July 2012)
6. Spackman, K.A., Dionne, R., Mays, E., Weis, J.: Role grouping as an extension to the description logic of Ontylog, motivated by concept modeling in SNOMED. In: Proc. AMIA Symp., pp. 712–716 (2002)
7. Schulz, S., Stenzhorn, H., Boeker, M., Smith, B.: Strengths and limitations of formal ontologies in the biomedical domain. Rev. Electron Comun. Inf. Inov. Saude 3(1), 31–45 (2009)

---

[2] SemanticHealthNet. http://www.semantichealthnet.eu/

[3] ICD-11. http://www.who.int/classifications/icd/revision/contentmodel/en/index.html

Using a Cross-Language Approach to Acquire New Mappings between Two Biomedical Terminologies

Fleur Mougin[1] and Natalia Grabar[2]

[1] LESIM, INSERM U897, ISPED, University Bordeaux Segalen, France
fleur.mougin@isped.u-bordeaux2.fr
[2] STL, UMR 8163, CNRS, University Lille 3, France
natalia.grabar@univ-lille3.fr

Abstract. The exploitation of clinical reports for generating alerts especially relies on the alignment of the dedicated terminologies, i.e., MedDRA (exploited in the pharmacovigilance area) and SNOMED International (exploited recently in France for encoding clinical documents). In this frame, we propose a cross-language approach for acquiring automatically alignments between terms from MedDRA and SNOMED International. We had the hypothesis that using additional languages could be helpful to complement the mappings obtained between French terms. Our approach is based on a lexical method for aligning MedDRA terms to those from SNOMED International. The concomitant use of multiple languages resulted in several hundreds of new alignments and successfully validated or disambiguated some of these alignments.

Keywords: biomedical terminologies, mapping, cross-language methods.

1 Introduction

The semantic interoperability among the communicating systems involves the exploitation of terminological resources. However, the alignment[1] between some terminologies is not always available, despite the intensive research studies already performed. Indeed, the pairs of terminologies relevant to a given medical field may not be treated yet. For instance, when we look for the alignment between MedDRA (exploited in the pharmacovigilance area) and SNOMED International (exploited recently in France for the encoding of clinical documents), we can find nearly nothing. It is noteworthy that through the UMLS®, the current mapping between MedDRA and SNOMED International is only 31%, which seriously impedes the situation.

This study falls within the French project RAVEL (Retrieval And Visualization in ELectronic health records) in which it is necessary to link pharmacovigilance databases to information present in clinical patient documents. In this frame, we propose a lexical approach, which exploits cross-language knowledge, for acquiring automatically alignments between terms from MedDRA and SNOMED International.

---

[1] In this paper, we use equally the terms "alignment" and "mapping".

N. Peek, R. Marín Morales, and M. Peleg (Eds.): AIME 2013, LNAI 7885, pp. 221–226, 2013.
© Springer-Verlag Berlin Heidelberg 2013

2   Background

MedDRA. The Medical Dictionary for Regulatory Activities[2] (MedDRA) has been designed for the encoding of adverse drug reactions chemically induced by drugs. It contains a large set of terms which are hierarchically structured. The 15.1 version of MedDRA used in this study is available in French, English and Spanish.

SNMI. The Systematized NOmenclature of MEDicine International[3] (SNMI) is a multi-axial terminology providing a very large coverage of the biomedical domain. This terminology is composed of concepts organized hierarchically. The English version of SNMI is included in the UMLS and the Spanish one can be created from the Spanish version of SNOMED CT (also in the UMLS). The French version of SNMI is made available by the national Agency of Shared Health Information Systems[4].

UMLS. The Unified Medical Language System® (UMLS) [1] includes two sources of semantic information: the Metathesaurus® and the Semantic Network. The former integrates over 150 terminologies, including MedDRA and SNMI. The version used in this study (2012AA) contains more than two million concepts which correspond to clusters of terms (and codes) coming from the different terminologies. The Semantic Network is a much smaller network of 133 semantic types organized in a tree structure. These semantic types have been aggregated into fifteen coarser semantic groups [2], which represent subdomains of biomedicine (e.g., **Anatomy**). Each Metathesaurus concept has a unique identifier (CUI) and is assigned at least one semantic type.

Related Works. The mapping between terminologies and ontologies is an active research area independently of the application domain. The ontology alignment evaluation initiative[5] gathers a great number of researchers around this topic. In the biomedical area, researchers work also on the alignment of several terminologies. First of all, the existence of the UMLS and its intensive international exploitation testify about it [3]. However, few works have addressed the mapping between MedDRA and other resources, such as SNOMED CT. Four experiences in English aimed at improving the current alignment of these two terminologies by exploiting hierarchical relations [4,5] or simple synonyms and a decomposition of MedDRA terms [6,7]. We are not aware about existing works on the alignment between MedDRA and SNMI.

A few works have studied the alignment of terminologies in a cross-language context. For instance, multilingual resources such as WordNet or UMLS may be exploited in such a way [8,9]. Thus, the existing alignment in one language, which can be more complete than in other languages, may be exploited to sort out the alignment between terms from other languages. With this approach, the implicit information becomes explicit for other languages. Another example of the cross-language alignment exploits parallel corpora [10] in order to build bilingual dictionaries. In this work, the assumption is that if two words are mutual translations, then their more frequent collocates are likely to be mutual translations as well.

---

[2] https://meddramsso.com/
[3] http://www.ihtsdo.org
[4] http://esante.gouv.fr/snomed/snomed/
[5] Ontology alignment evaluation initiative, from:
   http://oaei.ontologymatching.org

In our work, we propose to exploit the cross-language context differently. We aim at generating novel alignments independently in three languages (French, English and Spanish). We then study the complementarity of the resulting alignments.

3   Methods

Step 1: generating mappings. We designed a lexical approach, which aligns Med-DRA to SNMI terms. First, all these English, French and Spanish terms were segmented into words and then normalized according to: punctuation {*Atrioventricular block, complete*; *Atrioventricular block complete*}, variation of word order {*Edema Quincke's*; *Quincke's edema*}, stopwords {*Mycoplasma hominis pelvic inflammatory disease*; *Pelvic inflammatory disease due to Mycoplasma hominis*}, inflectional {*Cough decreased*; *Decreased coughing*} and derived {*Colon perforation*; *Perforation of colon*} forms, but also synonyms {*Angioleiomyoma*; *Angiomyoma*}. With this approach, we exploited several resources in each language (Table 1), in addition to the terms to be aligned: stopword lists, morphological and synonymy resources.

Table 1. Number of terms in MedDRA and SNMI and then in the lexical resources

	English	French	Spanish
MedDRA	72,867	66,092	65,435
SNMI	164,069	150,689	162,699
Stopwords	183	70	209
Morphological resources	90,583	155,468	17,520
Synonyms	101,805	14,914	35,214

Step 2: filtering mappings. The UMLS semantic groups (SGs) propose a partition of the UMLS concepts. We exploited this information for filtering out wrong mappings. We thus compared the SGs to which belong the UMLS concepts of MedDRA and SNMI terms. If they were not the same, we considered the proposed mapping as wrong and eliminated it. For example, a mapping was found between *Body mass index* (MedDRA) appearing in the UMLS concept *Body mass index procedure* (C0005893) and *Body mass index* (SNMI) part of the UMLS concept *Body mass index* (C1305855). This mapping was automatically removed because these two concepts belong to distinct SGs: **Procedures** and **Physiology**, respectively.

Step 3: comparing mappings between languages. We computed the number of alignments which are common between the different languages. We had the hypotheses that cross-language mappings could be helpful for multiple aspects: (1) enrichment: the alignments generated in other languages are exploited to complete the alignments acquired in French; (2) validation: an exact mapping (i.e., a mapping 1-1) found in multiple languages is more likely to be correct; (3) disambiguation: if a mapping 1-N is obtained in a given language while only one of these pairs is encountered in another language, this allows to eliminate the pair(s) which are found in only one language. We calculated the number of mappings, which satisfied our hypotheses.

4   Results

4.1   Mapping Results

We distinguished three situations among the resulting alignments (Table 2):

- The aligned terms are part of distinct UMLS concepts, themselves belonging to distinct SGs. An example is the pair *Uroporphyrin / Uroporphyrins*. These terms are respectively part of the UMLS concepts C0202193 and C0042093, which belong to the SG **Procedures** and **Chemicals & Drugs**, respectively. Such alignments are automatically removed from the newly generated mappings;
- The aligned terms are clustered in a unique UMLS concept. For example, *Rash acneiform* and *Acneform eruptions* are part of the UMLS concept C0175167. In this situation, the generated alignments can be automatically considered as correct;
- The aligned terms are included in distinct UMLS concepts belonging to a unique SG. One such pair is *May-Hegglin anomaly / May Hegglin syndrome*. These terms are respectively clustered in the UMLS concepts C0340978 and C0272184, both belonging to the SG **Disorders**. Such alignments need to be evaluated manually.

Table 2. Number of generated mappings in each language

	Distinct SGs	Same UMLS concept	New	Total
English	493	3,230	1,135	4,858
French	250	1,506	1,400	3,156
Spanish	148	3,006	351	3,505

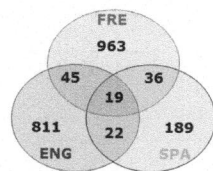

Fig. 1. Comparison of new mappings generated in English, French and Spanish

4.2   Comparing Mappings According to the Languages

Regardless of the languages, our approach results in 2,085 distinct new mappings between MedDRA and SNMI (Fig. 1). The mappings specific to a unique language complete those obtained in the two other languages. Few mappings overlap between the three languages. Indeed, only 6.2% of mappings found between MedDRA and SNMI terms involve more than one language. An example is the mapping between the MedDRA terms *Infection due to Mycobacterium fortuitum* (FRE: *Infection à Mycobacterium fortuitum*, SPA: *Infección por Mycobacterium fortuitum*) and the SNMI terms *Mycobacterium fortuitum infection* (FRE: *Infection à Mycobacterium fortuitum*, SPA: *Infección por mycobacterium fortuitum*), which are respectively part of the UMLS concepts C0275711 and C0877567. This low overlap is however helpful to validate 77 exact mappings and to disambiguate 42 mappings 1-N, which were found between MedDRA and SNMI terms. The previous example illustrates the "validation aspect". The MedDRA term *Familial tremor* can illustrate the "disambiguation aspect". It was mapped to the following SNMI terms in English: *Essential tremor*, *Persistent tremor* and *Congenital trembles* and in French: *Tremblement grossier* (i.e., *Coarse Tremor*) and *Tremblement essentiel* (i.e., *Essential tremor*). By combining the mappings generated in each language, we can conclude that the mapping between the MedDRA term *Familial tremor* and the SNMI term *Essential tremor* is the best one.

5   Discussion

Overall, the approach presented in this paper provided more than eleven thousands mappings between MedDRA and SNMI terms. 47.7% to 85.8% of these mappings were deemed correct automatically because they belong to a unique UMLS concept. More than two thousands of the remaining mappings are entirely new (because they are part of distinct UMLS concepts). Regarding our hypotheses, the complementarity of the results obtained in each language confirms the interest of using a cross-language approach for mapping purposes. Conversely, the overlap of new mappings according to the languages is very low. We assume this is due in part to the fact that the aligned terms remain specific in each language. We remind that this overlap was however useful to mutually validate or disambiguate some of the generated mappings.

For future works, we would like to exploit the compositional structure of MedDRA terms, as done in previous studies [6,7], for improving the mapping between MedDRA (which has complex and compositional terms) and SNMI (which has syntactically more simple terms). Finally, a manual validation of new mappings should be performed by medical experts.

Acknowledgments. The authors acknowledge the support of the French ANR and the DGA, under grant Tecsan (ANR-11-TECS-012).

References

1. Lindberg, D.A., Humphreys, B.L., McCray, A.T.: The Unified Medical Language System. Methods Inf. Med. 32(4), 281–291 (1993)
2. Bodenreider, O., McCray, A.T.: Exploring semantic groups through visual approaches. J. Biomed. Inform. 36(6), 414–432 (2003)
3. Fung, K.W., Bodenreider, O.: Utilizing the UMLS for semantic mapping between terminologies. In: AMIA Annu. Symp. Proc., pp. 266–270 (2005)
4. Bodenreider, O.: Using SNOMED CT in combination with MedDRA for reporting signal detection and adverse drug reactions reporting. In: AMIA Annu. Symp. Proc., pp. 45–49 (2009)
5. Alecu, I., Bousquet, C., Mougin, F., Jaulent, M.-C.: Mapping of the WHO-ART terminology on SNOMED CT to improve grouping of related adverse drug reactions. Stud. Health Technol. Inform., 833–838 (2006)
6. Nadkarni, P.M., Darer, J.D.: Determining correspondences between high-frequency MedDRA concepts and SNOMED: A case study. BMC Med. Inform. Decis. Mak. 10, 66 (2010)

7. Mougin, F., Dupuch, M., Grabar, N.: Improving the mapping between medDRA and SNOMED CT. In: Peleg, M., Lavrač, N., Combi, C. (eds.) AIME 2011. LNCS, vol. 6747, pp. 220–224. Springer, Heidelberg (2011)
8. Malaisé, V., Isaac, A., Gazendam, L., Instituut, T., Brugman, H.: Anchoring dutch cultural heritage thesauri to WordNet: Two case studies. In: Proc. of the Workshop on Language Technology for Cultural Heritage Data, pp. 57–64 (2007)
9. Merabti, T., Soualmia, L.F., Grosjean, J., Palombi, O., Müller, J.-M., Darmoni, S.J.: Translating the foundational model of anatomy into French using knowledge-based and lexical methods. BMC Med. Inform. Decis. Mak. 11(1), 65 (2011)
10. Och, F.J., Ney, H.: Improved statistical alignment models. In: Proc. of the 38th Annual Meeting on Association for Computational Linguistics, pp. 440–447. Association for Computational Linguistics, Stroudsburg (2000)

Clinical Time Series Prediction
with a Hierarchical Dynamical System

Zitao Liu and Milos Hauskrecht

Department of Computer Science, University of Pittsburgh, Pittsburgh, PA, USA
{ztliu,milos}@cs.pitt.edu

Abstract. In this work we develop and test a novel hierarchical framework for modeling and learning multivariate clinical time series data. Our framework combines two modeling approaches: Linear Dynamical Systems (LDS) and Gaussian Processes (GP), and is capable to model and work with time series of varied length and with irregularly sampled observations. We test our framework on the problem of learning clinical time series data from the complete blood count panel, and show that our framework outperforms alternative time series models in terms of its predictive accuracy.

Keywords: Time Series, Gaussian Processes, Linear Dynamical System.

1 Introduction

The problem of modeling of clinical time series comes with a number of challenges [1]. First, time series for the different patients admitted to hospital are hard to align; they start at different times with respect to the disease, and they may vary in length depending on the span of patient's hospitalization. Second, observations corresponding to the different laboratory tests are collected at different times, and the time elapsed between two consecutive observations may vary. The challenge is to build models and algorithms that are both accurate and flexible enough to represent such time series.

We propose and develop (1) a hierarchical dynamical system model to represent the clinical time series data, and (2) algorithms that can (a) learn the model efficiently from observational data, and (b) support predictive inferences. Our model is built by combining two machine learning frameworks used frequently for modeling dynamical systems in statistical machine learning: the Linear Dynamical System (LDS) [2] and the Gaussian Process (GP) model [3]. LDS, or Kalman filter [2] is the most frequently used approach for modeling dynamical systems in practice. The model comes with numerous computational advantages and well-understood algorithms for both model learning and model inference. The model defines a state-space process with linear transitions between two consecutive states taken at discrete time points. Hence it assumes some predefined and fixed time discretization. However, observations in clinical time series are often spaced irregularly in time. To address this problem we extend the linear dynamical system with a secondary (lower-level) Gaussian process defined over time

N. Peek, R. Marín Morales, and M. Peleg (Eds.): AIME 2013, LNAI 7885, pp. 227–237, 2013.

windows, instead of fixed-time points. The parameters of the Gaussian process are controlled by the higher-level LDS. The advantage of the Gaussian process is that observations are treated as the function of time and can be defined for an arbitrary observation sequence. This extension gives us the flexibility needed to model time series with observations sampled unevenly in time.

We experiment with and test the new model on clinical time series prediction problem. More specifically, we define, build and run the model for six common blood tests from the complete blood count panel. Our results show that the model leads to a more accurate predictive performance than existing time series models. In addition, we show our model is more robust and performs well when the number of patients and observations used to train the model is small.

Our paper is organized as follows. In Section 2, we review the basics of linear dynamical systems and Gaussian process models. In Section 3 we describe the time series prediction problem we want to solve and present the new hierarchical framework that combines the two models. We present experimental results that consist of predicting future values for six common lab tests and compare our method to alternative modeling approaches in Section 4. In Section 5, we summarize the work and outline future model extensions.

2   Background

2.1   Linear Dynamical System (LDS)

The Linear Dynamical System (LDS) is a classic and widely used real-valued time series model. An LDS on variables $\mathbf{z}_{1:T}$, $\mathbf{y}_{1:T}$ is defined using the following two equations:

$$\mathbf{z}_t = A\mathbf{z}_{t-1} + \mathbf{e}_t; \qquad \mathbf{y}_t = C\mathbf{z}_t + \mathbf{v}_t \tag{1}$$

where $t \in \{1, \ldots, T\}$ is the discrete time index; $\mathbf{z}_1$ is the initial state distribution with mean $\boldsymbol{\pi}_1$ and covariance matrix V_1, $\mathbf{z}_1 \sim \mathcal{N}(\boldsymbol{\pi}_1, V_1)$, $\mathbf{z}_t$ are the hidden states defining the process that are generated with the help of the transition matrix A with the independent zero mean noise $\mathbf{e}_t$, $\mathbf{e}_t \sim \mathcal{N}(\mathbf{0}, Q)$; and $\mathbf{y}_t$ are the observations generated by the emission matrix C and independent variant noise $\mathbf{v}_t \sim \mathcal{N}(\mathbf{0}, R)$. The LDS is characterized by the state transition probability $p(\mathbf{z}_t|\mathbf{z}_{t-1})$, where $p(\mathbf{z}_t|\mathbf{z}_{t-1}) = \mathcal{N}(A\mathbf{z}_{t-1}, Q)$, and the state-observation probability $p(\mathbf{y}_t|\mathbf{z}_t) = \mathcal{N}(C\mathbf{z}_t, R)$. The complete set of the LDS parameters is $\Lambda = \{A, C, Q, R, \boldsymbol{\pi}_1, V_1\}$. The parameters can be learned from the observed data sequences using the Expectation-Maximization (EM) algorithm.

The advantage of the linear dynamical model is its simplicity. The disadvantages are its linearity which may prevent one from modeling more complex time series data, and the fact that the model is a discrete-time model with observations and predictions restricted to fixed time intervals.

2.2   Gaussian Process (GP) Regression

The Gaussian process is a nonparametric nonlinear Bayesian model popular in statistical machine learning [3]. The GP is best viewed as an extension of the multivariate Gaussian to infinite-sized collections of real-valued variables defining the distribution over random functions. A GP is represented by the mean function $m(\mathbf{x}) = \mathbb{E}[f(\mathbf{x})]$and the covariance function $K(\mathbf{x}, \mathbf{x}') = \mathbb{E}[(f(\mathbf{x}) - m(\mathbf{x}))(f(\mathbf{x}') - m(\mathbf{x}'))]$, where $f(\mathbf{x})$ is the real-valued process. Since GP represents a Gaussian distribution over functions, it can be used to estimate the values of function f at an arbitrary position x_*. This application is referred to as Gaussian Process Regression [3]. The GP regression equations are:

$$\bar{f}_* = K(x_*, \mathbf{x}) \left[K(\mathbf{x}, \mathbf{x}) + \sigma^2 I \right]^{-1} \mathbf{y} \qquad (2)$$

$$Cov(f_*) = K(x_*, x_*) - K(x_*, \mathbf{x}) \left[K(\mathbf{x}, \mathbf{x}) + \sigma^2 I \right]^{-1} K(x_*, \mathbf{x}) \qquad (3)$$

where I is the identity matrix, $\mathbf{x}$ is the input vector and $\mathbf{y}$ is the output or target vector, $\bar{f}_*$ is the posterior function mean and $Cov(f_*)$ is the posterior covariance. With the right choice of the covariance function, the associated prediction uncertainty increases in regions away from observations, while it shrinks when it is close to observed data.

2.3   Gaussian Process Time Series Models

In time series modeling Gaussian processes are used primarily to capture the nonlinear dynamics and nonlinear relations among states and observations [4]. Briefly, the models assume that there exists a sequence of latent variables $\mathbf{z}_t$ that evolve over time through a Markovian process specified by a Gaussian process f and the observations $\mathbf{y}_t$ are generated by another Gaussian process u from corresponding latent variables: $\mathbf{z}_t = f(\mathbf{z}_{t-1}) + \mathbf{e}_t$; $\mathbf{y}_t = u(\mathbf{z}_t) + \mathbf{v}_t$. The notation $\mathbf{z}_t$, $\mathbf{y}_t$, $\mathbf{e}_t$, $\mathbf{v}_t$ is the same as the notation used in the previous section for LDS. Briefly, the LDS assumes linear dependencies among latent states and observations, while the Gaussian-process-based model replaces the linear dependences with more general non-linear functions f and u represented by Gaussian processes.

The existing GP-based dynamical models [5–8] come with a number of limitations. First, all of the existing models set GP's mean function to zero, which severely limits the functions one can represent. Second, similarly to LDS, they assume the observations are obtained at the same (regularly sampled) times, which is not true in the real world. Discretizing irregular sampled time series may introduce unnecessary inaccuracy and hence lower the model's accuracy and performance.

In this paper, we address the shortcomings of these methods by defining a hierarchical dynamical system that splits the process into a sequence of dependent local Gaussian processes and by using the LDS to capture the dependences between these local GPs. This is unlike [9] where local GPs are independent to each other. The local GPs' dependences naturally account for the transitions of mean functions and the irregular samples are handled by the local GPs.

3   Hierarchical Dynamical System

3.1   Problem Description

We define the time series prediction/regression function for clinical time series as: $g : \mathbf{Y}_{\text{obs}} \times t \to \hat{\mathbf{y}}$, where $\mathbf{Y}_{\text{obs}}$ is a sequence of past observation-time pairs $\mathbf{Y}_{\text{obs}} = (\mathbf{y}_i, t_i)_{i=1}^{n}$, such that, $0 < t_i < t_{i+1}$, $\mathbf{y}_i$ is a p-dimensional observation vector made at time (t_i), and n is the number of past observations; and $t > t_n$ is the time at which we would like to predict the observation $\hat{\mathbf{y}}$.

Typically, the prediction function assumes that the values (observations) are given at regularly sampled discrete-time points, which means $t_{i+1} - t_i = L$, where L is a constant reflecting the data-sampling interval. However, in this work we assume our observations are sampled irregularly from some process which is more general and more common in real-life settings. For example, in the clinical domain, observations that correspond to lab test values for a patient during his or her hospital period are often recorded irregularly due to the different patients' health conditions or the different sample-collection times.

3.2   Hierarchical Dynamical System (HDS)

In this section, we develop a two-layer hierarchical dynamical model that lets us represent the entire time series information in a more flexible manner. The key structure of the model is shown in Figure 1. Briefly, the model consists of two hierarchically related processes: the Gaussian process and the linear dynamical system. The Gaussian process is restricted to a time window of a finite duration and it is used to represent time series and its changes for shorter time spans. Longer-term process changes are modeled and controlled by the linear dynamical process. In the first layer, which is shown in a dashed line box, we transform the entire irregular time series data into m windows $\{w_i\}_1^m$ using a predefined window size and a predefined overlap size. Each window w_i in Figure 1 relates observations $\{y_i^1, y_i^2, \ldots, y_i^{N_i}\}$ using the same window-specific GP and N_i is the number of observations in window w_i. Hence, instead of using a single GP we capture the variation in the entire time series by using many different window-specific Gaussian processes. We denote the GP for window w_i as GP_i.

The sequence of window-specific GP_is (more precisely their parameters) is linked together using the higher-level LDS (in layer 2). That is, the LDS represents the dynamics and changes of parameters γ_i defining individual GP_i. We assume the different GP_i share the same covariance function parameter Θ. The parameters γ_i that define the mean of the window-specific GP_i are unobserved (hidden). In the learning phase, we estimate γ_i measurements $\{y_i^1, y_i^2, \ldots, y_i^{N_i}\}$ observed in window w_i. Meanwhile, in the prediction phase, γ_i is controlled by the LDS and evolves in time. The LDS is defined as:

$$\mathbf{z}_t = A\mathbf{z}_{t-1} + \mathbf{e}_t; \gamma_t = C\mathbf{z}_t + \mathbf{v}_t \tag{4}$$

where parameters $\{\gamma_i\}$ act like observations, and $\mathbf{e}_t$ and $\mathbf{v}_t$ are zero-mean normally distributed random variables with covariance matrices Q and R

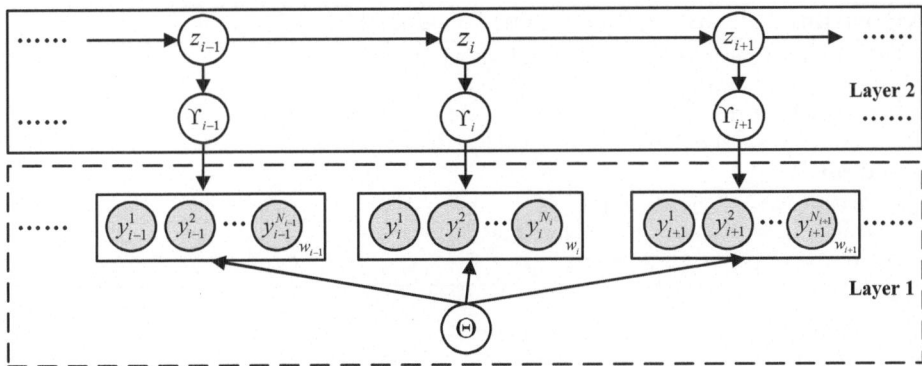

Fig. 1. Graphical illustration of our hierarchical dynamical model combining the Gaussian process and the linear dynamical system

respectively. Similarly to regular LDS introduced earlier in Section 2.1, π_1 and V_1 are the initial state mean and variance.

3.3 Learning

The parameters of our hierarchical dynamical model are learnt in the two steps. In step 1 we learn the covariance function Θ. In step 2, we first estimate parameters $\{\gamma_i\}$ and then use them to learn the parameters of linear dynamical System in layer 2.

Step 1. Since GPs share the same covariance function, we use the entire time series data to make the estimation of the parameters Θ in the covariance function. We set Θ by maximizing the likelihood and seek the partial derivatives of the likelihood with respect to each parameter θ_i in Θ.

$$\frac{\partial}{\partial \theta_i} \log p(\mathbf{Y}|\Theta) = -\frac{1}{2}\mathrm{Tr}\left[K^{-1}\frac{\partial K}{\partial \theta_i}\right] + \frac{1}{2}\mathbf{Y}^T K^{-1}\frac{\partial K}{\partial \theta_i}K^{-1}\mathbf{Y} \tag{5}$$

where K is covariance matrix for all training data.

Step 2. We first estimate all parameters $\{\gamma_i\}$ representing the means of window-specific GPs from observations in windows $\{w_i\}$. In general, there are many different ways to estimate $\{\gamma_i\}$. Let h be a function used for estimating the mean of the Gaussian process from observations $\{y_i^j\}$. Examples of h can be $min, max, mean$ functions that return the minimum, maximum or mean observed value in the window. In our model, we use the value of the most recent observation in each window to estimate $\{\gamma_i\}$, that is, $\gamma_i = h(\{y_i^j\}) = y_i^{N_i}$. Once we get $\{\gamma_i\}$, we treat values of different $\{\gamma_i\}$ as the observations for the LDS (layer 2) in our hierarchical dynamical system. To learn the parameters of the LDS, we use the Expectation-Maximization(EM) learning algorithm to [10] iteratively re-estimate the parameters $\Lambda = \{A, C, Q, R, \pi_1, V_1\}$ defining the LDS [11]. The learning algorithm is summarized in Algorithm 1.

Algorithm 1. Learning Hierarchical Dynamical Model

Do initialization and split the data into windows.
// learn Θ, $\Theta = (\theta_1, \ldots, \theta_d)$
for $i = 1$ **to** d **do**
  Get θ_i by any gradient based optimizer based on Eq.5
end for
// learn $\{A, C, Q, R, \pi_1, V_1\}$
Learning LDS from the EM algorithm. See [11]
return $\Omega = \{\Theta, A, C, Q, R, \pi_1, V_1\}$

3.4 Prediction

Once the hierarchical dynamical system is learned from the training data we would like to use it to support time series prediction on future time series. Given the initial observations $\mathbf{Y}_{obs}$ and an arbitrary time index t modeling a sequence of future times, our objective is to predict $\hat{y}$ at time t.

To support the prediction inference, we need the following steps:

Step 1. Split $\mathbf{Y}_{obs}$ and t into windows.

Step 2. For windows that do not contain t, compute γs through mean estimation function h and feed them into Kalman Filter algorithms(See $Kalman\_Filter$ in Appendix A.1) to infer the most recent hidden state $\mathbf{z}_k$ where k is the index of the last window that does not contain t.

Step 3. Get $\boldsymbol{\gamma}_{k+1} = CA\mathbf{z}_k$ from $\mathbf{z}_{k+1} = A\mathbf{z}_k$ and $\boldsymbol{\gamma}_{k+1} = C\mathbf{z}_{k+1}$.

Step 4. If t is in window $k+1$ use observations $(\mathbf{y}_{k+1}, t_{k+1})$ in window $k+1$ and $\boldsymbol{\gamma}_{k+1}$ to make the prediction, where $\hat{y} = \boldsymbol{\gamma}_{k+1} + K(t, t_{k+1})K^{-1}(t_{k+1}, t_{k+1})(\mathbf{y}_{k+1} - \boldsymbol{\gamma}_{k+1})$; otherwise find out the window index i where t belongs to. The prediction at t is $\hat{y} = CA^{i-k}\mathbf{z}_k$.

The prediction algorithm is summarized in Algorithm 2.

Algorithm 2. Prediction with the Hierarchical Dynamical System

---

Split $\mathbf{Y}_{obs}$ and t into windows.
Find all k windows that do not contain t.
Estimate $\{\gamma_i\}_{i=1}^{k}$ using mean estimation function h in these k windows.
// Compute z_k by $Kalman\_Filter$ algorithm.(See Appendix A.1)
$\mathbf{z}_k = Kalman\_Filter(\{\gamma_i\}_{i=1}^{k}, A, C, R, Q, \pi_1, V_1)$
if t is in window $k + 1$ **then**
  $\boldsymbol{\gamma}_{k+1} = C\mathbf{z}_{k+1} = CA\mathbf{z}_k$
  // Observations in window $k + 1$ are $(\mathbf{y}_{k+1}, t_{k+1})$
  $\hat{\mathbf{y}} = \boldsymbol{\gamma}_{k+1} + K(t, t_{k+1})K^{-1}(t_{k+1}, t_{k+1})(\mathbf{y}_{k+1} - \boldsymbol{\gamma}_{k+1})$
else
  $\hat{\mathbf{y}} = CA^{i-k}\mathbf{z}_k$
end if
return $\hat{\mathbf{y}}$

---

4   Experimental Results

We have tested our approach on time series data obtained from electronic health records of approximately 4,500 post-surgical cardiac patients stored in PCP database [12–14]. To test the performance of our prediction model, we randomly selected 1000 patients with the *Complete Blood Count*(CBC) panel test[1] whose hospitalization is longer than 10 days. We selected six tests from the CBC panel to learn the time series models, and applied them to time series prediction tasks. The six tests, their means and standard deviations are listed below:

- *White Blood Cell* (WBC) a count of the total number of white blood cells in a person's sample of blood. Mean: $11.98(\times 10^9)$; standard deviation: 6.06.
- *Mean Corpuscular Hemoglobin* (MCH) is a calculation of the average amount of oxygen-carrying hemoglobin inside a red blood cell. Mean: 33.87(pg); standard deviation: 0.81.
- *Mean Corpuscular Hemoglobin Concentration* (MCHC) is a calculation of the average concentration of hemoglobin inside a red cell. Mean: 30.53(g/dL); standard deviation: 1.81.
- *Mean Corpuscular Volume* (MCV) is a measurement of the average size of patient's red blood cell. Mean: 90.12(fL); standard deviation: 4.56.
- *Platelet* (PLT) count is the number of platelets in a given volume of blood. Mean: $201.15(\times 10^9)$; standard deviation: 126.01.
- *Red cell Distribution Width* (RDW) is a calculation of the variation in the size of red blood cells. Mean: 16.68(%); standard deviation: 2.64.

To evaluate the performance of our hierarchical dynamical system (HDS-GPLDS) approach we used the five-fold cross validation approach to split the examples into the training and testing sets, such that 200 examples formed the test data, and 800 training examples were used to vary the size of the training set from 100 to 800 in increments of 100 examples and reported the average results. Since the CBC panel is typically ordered once or just a few times a day, we used the default Gaussian process window size of seven days. The covariance function is the combination of the mean reverting and the periodic functions([15]). The mean reverting function forces the process to approach the long term mean, but at the same time permits temporary deviations from the mean corresponding to episodic events or complications. The periodic function can capture the fluctuation within the short period of time and keep the variation of different values within a reasonable range. The covariance function is defined as:

$$K(\mathbf{t}, \mathbf{t'}) = \sigma_1 \exp(\alpha_1 |\mathbf{t} - \mathbf{t'}|) + \sigma_2 \exp(\alpha_2 \sin^2 \left[\frac{\omega}{2\pi}(\mathbf{t} - \mathbf{t'}) \right]) \qquad (6)$$

where $\Theta = (\sigma_1, \alpha_1, \sigma_2, \alpha_2, \omega)$ are the parameters optimized from the data.

---

[1] CBC test is used as a broad screening test to check for such disorders as anemia, infection, and many other diseases.

We compared the HDS-GPLDS predictions to four other methods:

- Linear dynamical system (LDS) trained on the entire time series with a three-hour period discretization. We applied Gaussian process interpolation to fill the missing values [16].
- Window-based linear dynamical system(WLDS). This model is different from the LDS model. It splits the time series first into windows the same way as HDS-GPLDS and, after that, it trains an LDS using the last observation in each window.
- Standard Gaussian Process regression (GP) with covariance function defined in Eq. 6.
- Nonlinear dynamical system using GPIL algorithm for inference and learning with the Gaussian kernel covariance function for both the transition and observation models [8].

We evaluated and compared the performances of the different methods by calculating the Root Mean Square Error (RMSE) on the test predictions. More specifically, the RMSE is defined as follows:

$$RMSE = \left[n^{-1} \sum_{i=1}^{n} |y_i - \hat{y}_i|^2 \right]^{1/2}$$

where y_i is the true value, $\hat{y}_i$ is the predicted value and n is the number of data points. The results of RMSE on the six lab tests from the CBC panel (for gradually increasing training and test data sets as described above) are summarized in Figure 2.

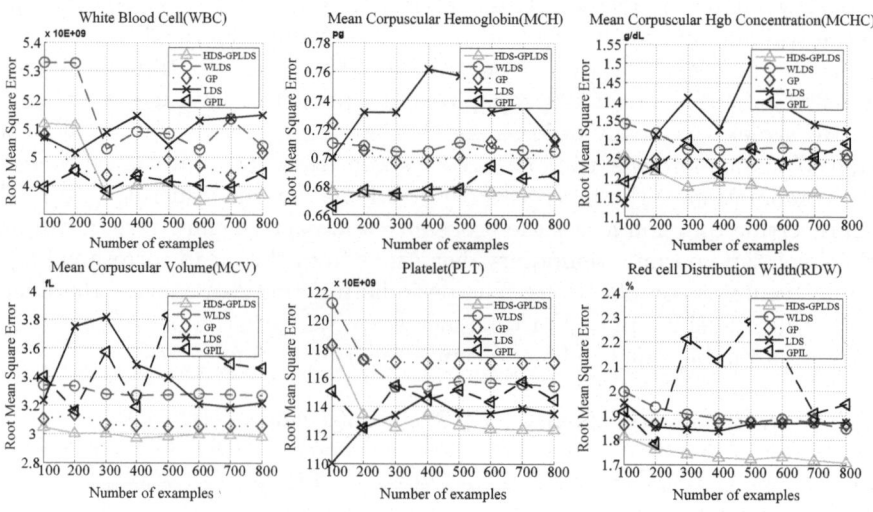

Fig. 2. Root Mean Square Error (RMSE) on CBC test samples

4.1   Discussion

The results of our experiments (Figure 2) show that our hierarchical dynamical system (HDS-GPLDS) outperforms all other methods in terms of prediction errors on all six CBC lab tests. One of the advantages of our method is that its prediction error is small even when it is trained on a small number of patients and observations. In the following we discuss the obtained results in more depth.

First, by comparing HDS-GPLDS, GP and LDS, GPIL, we can see that methods with continuous functions (HDS-GPLDS, GP) are much stable than discretized methods (LDS, GPIL). Their performances are gradually improved with the increase of training examples. The reason is that the discretized methods do require any discretization or interpolations for the irregular sampled dataset, which may bring inaccuracy in the training and prediction phases.

Second, HDS-GPLDS/GP outperform WLDS/LDS. The reasons are (1) the values from patients' tests are always around a normal range plus some variation. The combination of the mean-reverting and periodic functions captures this phenomenon: the mean reverting function forces the predicted values within a normal range and the periodic function allows the fluctuation and variation flexibility. However, WLDS and LDS cannot capture these variations due to the linearity embodied in their linear models. (2) WLDS and LDS solve the multi-step prediction problem by constructing a single model from past observations and predict future values iteratively. Since they use predictions from the past, both are very susceptible to the error accumulation: errors generated in the history are propagated into future predictions. In contrast to this the HDS-GPLDS/GP make the multi-step predictions directly and hence do not suffer this problem.

Third, comparing to other methods, HDS-GPLDS does not require a large number of training examples, and it can still perform well for small training data sizes. In contrast to this, error rates for other methods are initially high and they are decreased by a large amount when more examples are used to train them. Stable performance on small training data is very important in practice.

Fourth, comparing GP and HDS-GPLDS, we can see that the HDS-GPLDS is much better than the GP approach. The results show that a single constant mean is not enough in the complex time series setting. The evolution of mean variables in the consequent windows is modeled by a linear dynamical system, which expresses a stronger descriptive ability. During the prediction phase, the predicted mean is used by the GP to make a more accurate prediction.

5   Conclusion

In this work, we have presented a novel two-layer hierarchical dynamical system for multi-step time series prediction. Comparing with the traditional linear state space systems and modern Gaussian process regression, this novel system is (1) more robustness to irregular sampling; (2) more robust for small training data sizes; (3) more accurate in making the long-term multi-step predictions. Experimental results on real world clinical data from electronic health records systems demonstrated that our prediction model achieves errors that are statistically significantly lower than errors of other state of the art approaches. The limitation of out current work is the analysis of univariate time-series model. In the future, we plan to study and model dependences among multiple time series, as well as, extensions to switching-state [17] and controlled [18, 19] dynamical systems.

Acknowledgments. This work was supported by grants 1R01LM010019-01A1 and 1R01GM088224-01 from the NIH. Its content is solely the responsibility of the authors and does not necessarily represent the official views of the NIH.

References

1. Combi, C., Keravnou-Papailiou, E., Shahar, Y.: Temporal information systems in medicine. Springer Publishing Company (2010) (Incorporated)
2. Kalman, R.: Mathematical description of linear dynamical systems. Journal of the Society for Industrial & Applied Mathematics, Series A: Control 1, 152–192 (1963)
3. Rasmussen, C., Williams, C.: Gaussian processes for machine learning, vol. 1. MIT Press, Cambridge (2006)
4. Rasmussen, C., Kuss, M., et al.: Gaussian processes in reinforcement learning. Advances in Neural Information Processing Systems 16 (2004)
5. Deisenroth, M., Huber, M., Hanebeck, U.: Analytic moment-based gaussian process filtering. In: Proceedings of the 26th ICML, pp. 225–232. ACM (2009)
6. Wang, J., Fleet, D., Hertzmann, A.: Gaussian process dynamical models for human motion. IEEE Transactions on PAMI 30, 283–298 (2008)
7. Ko, J., Fox, D.: Learning gp-bayes filters via gaussian process latent variable models. Autonomous Robots 30, 3–23 (2011)
8. Turner, R., Deisenroth, M., Rasmussen, C.: State-space inference and learning with gaussian processes. In: Proceedings of 13th AISTATS, vol. 9, pp. 868–875 (2010)
9. Nguyen-tuong, D., Peters, J.: Local gaussian process regression for real time online model learning and control. In: Advances in NIPS (2008)
10. Dempster, A.P., Laird, N.M., Rubin, D.B.: Maximum likelihood from incomplete data via the em algorithm. Journal of the Royal Statistical Society. Series B (Methodological), 1–38 (1977)
11. Ghahramani, Z., Hinton, G.: Parameter estimation for linear dynamical systems. Technical Report CRG-TR-96-2, University of Totronto (1996)
12. Hauskrecht, M., Valko, M., Batal, I., Clermont, G., Visweswaran, S., Cooper, G.: Conditional outlier detection for clinical alerting. In: AMIA Annual Symposium Proceedings, vol. 2010, pp. 286–290. AMIA (2010)
13. Hauskrecht, M., Batal, I., Valko, M., Visweswaran, S., Cooper, G.F., Clermont, G.: Outlier detection for patient monitoring and alerting. Journal of Biomedical Informatics 46(1), 47–55 (2013)
14. Valko, M., Hauskrecht, M.: Feature importance analysis for patient management decisions. In: 13th International Congress on Medical Informatics, NIH Public Access, pp. 861–865 (2010)
15. Bibbona, E., Panfilo, G., Tavella, P.: The ornstein–uhlenbeck process as a model of a low pass filtered white noise. Metrologia 45, S117 (2008)
16. Gibbs, M., MacKay, D.: Efficient implementation of gaussian processes (1997)

17. Kim, C.J.: Dynamic linear models with markov-switching. Journal of Econometrics 60, 1–22 (1994)
18. Hauskrecht, M., Fraser, H.: Modeling treatment of ischemic heart disease with partially observable markov decision processes. In: Proceedings of the AMIA Symposium, pp. 538–542. American Medical Informatics Association (1998)
19. Kveton, B., Hauskrecht, M.: Solving factored mdps with exponential-family transition models. In: 16th International Conference on Automated Planning and Scheduling, pp. 114–120 (2006)

Extraction, Analysis, and Visualization of Temporal Association Rules from Interval-Based Clinical Data

Carlo Combi and Alberto Sabaini

Department of Computer Science
University of Verona, Italy
{carlo.combi,alberto.sabaini}@univr.it

Abstract. Temporal association rules have been recently applied to interval-based temporal clinical data, to discover complex temporal relationships. In this paper, we first propose a refinement of the Data-Mining algorithm proposed by Sacchi et al. (2007) for the extraction of temporal association rules, improving the algorithm complexity in case of anti-monotonous rule support. Then, we address the non-trivial problem of displaying and visually analyzing this kind of data, through the use of an OLAP-based multidimensional model, and by proposing a visualization solution explicitly dealing with temporal association rules.

1 Introduction

With the rapid increase of stored clinical data, the interest in the discovery of hidden information has exploded in the last decade. This discovery has mainly been focused on data classification, data clustering and relationship finding. One important problem that arises during the discovery process is treating data with temporal dimensions [4]: indeed, a large number of data analysis problems deals with the interpretation of time-varying data, and focuses on the interpretation of time intervals where one or more time series assume a behavior of interest. Temporal association rules have been recently applied to interval-based temporal clinical data, to discover complex temporal relationships among data [1,5]: as an example, a temporal association rule mined from a clinical database could be expressed as *if there is an increase of the heart rate and an overlapping steady state of systolic pressure, then usually a decrease of diastolic pressure follows.* The complexity of the underlying mining algorithms has to be suitably studied both from a theoretical point of view and from a more experimental real-world perspective, as usually such rules are mined on huge amount of clinical data. Moreover, a still open research issue regards how to provide the discovered temporal association rules to physicians, in order to allow them to focus on the most interesting and important discovered associations.

According to this scenario, the main goal of this paper is to propose a new OLAP-based methodology for the extraction, analysis, and visualization of temporal clinical association rules. Indeed, OLAP and related datawarehouse methodologies provide some sound models to store, manage, and analyze huge amounts

N. Peek, R. Marín Morales, and M. Peleg (Eds.): AIME 2013, LNAI 7885, pp. 238–247, 2013.

of (even clinical) data according to a multidimensional data view [3]. More precisely, in this paper, we first propose a refinement of the algorithm proposed by Sacchi et al. (2007) for the extraction of temporal association rules, improving the algorithm efficiency in case of anti-monotonous rule support. Then, we address the non-trivial problem of displaying and visually analyzing temporal association rules, through the use of a multidimensional model, and by proposing a new visualization solution explicitly dealing with temporal association rules. Throughout the paper, we will focus on the hemodialysis domain, where huge amounts of data are acquired during hemodialysis treatments and need to be mined, to assess the quality of the provided care. This paper is structured as follow: in Section 2 we formally define temporal association rules; in Section 3 we describe the extensions of the algorithm proposed in [5]; in Section 4 we describe our approach for the visualization of temporal rules; in Section 5 we draw some conclusions and discuss possible future work.

2   Background

In the following we will introduce basic concepts related to temporal association rules, by extending and generalizing the approach described in [5]. A temporal fact f represents a class of episodes of the same type: e.g., temporal fact highSBP represents the set of episodes when the considered patient had high systolic blood pressure. Each episode e is associated to the interval when the episode holds. By $e.start$, $e.end$ we denote the starting and ending point of the interval associated to e, respectively. We denote as E_f the set of episodes of a temporal fact f.

A *temporal association rule* (TAR) is a temporal pattern that exists between episodes of *temporal facts* belonging to a reference set *FoI* (Facts of Interest). To specify a TAR it is necessary to introduce the concept of temporal *precedence*: by $\preceq$ we denote relation *precedes* between two intervals a and b: $a \preceq b \iff a.start \leq b.start \wedge a.end \leq b.end$.

Definition 1. *(Temporal Association Rule (TAR)). A TAR is an implication of the form* $\{a_1, \ldots, a_n\} \xrightarrow{p} c$, *where* $\{a_1, \ldots, a_n\} \subset FoI, c \in FoI$ *with* $c \notin \{a_1, \ldots, a_n\}$, *and* $p = \langle LS, GAP, RS \rangle$ *is the parameter set determining the relation between the antecedent and the consequent.*

To determine an occurrence of the antecedent, there must exist a non empty intersection between all the episodes e_i corresponding to facts a_i, respectively. More specifically, we say that a (composite) antecedent occurrence has interval $[maxStart, minEnd]$, where [5]: $maxStart \stackrel{def}{=} \max(e_i.start \mid 1 \leq i \leq n)$, $minEnd \stackrel{def}{=} \min(e_i.end \mid 1 \leq i \leq n)$.

Set p is composed by the following parameters: (i) *Left Shift (LS):* maximum distance allowed between *maxStart* and *c.start*; (ii) *Gap (GAP):* maximum distance allowed between *minEnd* and *c.start*; (iii) *Right Shift (RS):* maximum distance allowed between *minEnd* and *c.end*.

Definition 2. *(Occurrence of a TAR). An episode set* $\{e_1, \ldots, e_n, e_c\}$ *is an occurrence of a TAR* $\{a_1, \ldots, a_n\} \xrightarrow{p} c$, *with* $p = \langle LS, GAP, RS \rangle$, *if (i)* $\{e_1, \ldots, e_n\}$ *is an antecedent occurrence and* e_c *is a consequent episode; (ii) the antecedent occurrence precedes the consequent episode, i.e.,* $[maxStart, minEnd] \preceq c$; *(iii) all the quantitative constraints imposed by* p *are satisfied.*

TARs are considered in the final result of the temporal mining only if some quantitative features of their occurrence sets are above some fixed thresholds. In [5], temporal support and confidence are introduced and used to this end: the *temporal support* of a TAR r is the ratio between the rule time span RTS and the overall time span TSO containing the mined episodes: $supp(r) \stackrel{def}{=} \frac{RTS(r)}{TSO_{FoI}}$. $RTS(r)$ corresponds to the overall time span of the rule and is evaluated as the sum of durations of minimal intervals each containing both the antecedent episodes and the consequent one of a TAR occurrence. The *temporal confidence* of a TAR r, denoted as $conf(r)$ is the ratio between the number of antecedent occurrences part of a rule occurrence r ($NARTS$), and the number of antecedent occurrences within the mined episodes (NAT): $conf(r) \stackrel{def}{=} \frac{NARTS(r)}{NAT(r)}$.

3   Discovering TARs

In this section we describe the extensions to the mining algorithm proposed in [5]. Informally, the algorithm looks for unitary rules, i.e., having a single temporal fact in both antecedent and consequent. Then it tries to enlarge the antecedent by combining previously mined rules with the same consequent. The existing algorithm does it by executing a series of steps: among them, the *Candidate Generation* step is very time consuming, as it must consider any possible combination of facts to build a new antecedent.

The new features we will add to the mining algorithm may be summarized in the following steps: 1. we redefine the concept of rule occurrence; 2. then, we introduce a new strategy for measuring the temporal support.

The basic motivation for both the mentioned steps is that we have to reconsider the property of anti-monotonicity we assume in Apriori-like algorithms: anti-monotonicity may be defined in our context as "if a set of episodes is frequent, then all of its subsets must be frequent as well". This important property allows one to build possible antecedents in a faster way, as antecedents can be extended only with temporal facts that have been already proven to be frequent (i.e., part of other antecedents). As in [5], by computing the temporal support considering for each rule occurrence the minimal interval containing both the antecedent episodes and the consequent one (i.e., considering an extended convex "union" of intervals), while expressing quantitative constraints with respect to the intersection of episode intervals, it could be that the property of anti-monotonicity does not hold. This leads to two implications:

– for *unitary* TARs, the adopted notion of occurrence effectively limits the temporal span of the single antecedent episode with respect to the interval of the consequent episode.

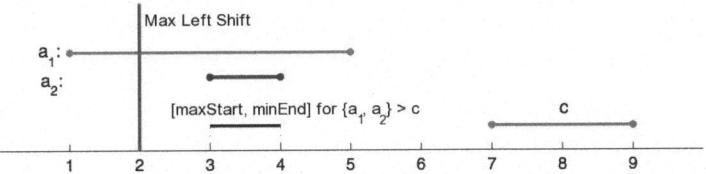

Fig. 1. An example of frequent TAR, $\{a_1, a_2\} \rightarrow c$, not discovered by the algorithm with parameters set to $LS = 5, RS = +\infty, GAP = +\infty$

- for *non-unitary* TARs, no limitations are directly imposed to the start or the end of antecedent episodes, because the precedence constraint and the quantitative parameters are expressed with respect to the intersection of the corresponding intervals. So, episodes may participate in the antecedent of a TAR occurrence and potentially begin and/or end arbitrarily back and/or forward in time with respect to the time points induced by quantitative constraints.

Therefore the model admits TARs as those represented in Figure 1, which, however, the mining procedure is not able to detect: in this case, having $LS = 5, RS = +\infty, GAP = +\infty$ (which means that the consequent may start at most 5 seconds after the earliest start of one of the antecedents), the episode a_1 begins too early and, thus, TAR $a_1 \rightarrow c$ will be not detected. Having only TAR $a_2 \rightarrow c$, the mining algorithm will not try to combine these two antecedents and will not detect the TAR $\{a_1, a_2\} \rightarrow c$. It is worth noting that this non anti-monotonicity is heavily depending on the fixed quantitative parameters, which need to be finely tuned to extract all the interesting TARs.

To avoid the non anti-monotonicity issue, we propose here a *restricted* version of the original model with anti-monotonous temporal support: this restriction will also lead to a more efficient mining algorithm. Furthermore, we introduce a stronger precedence constraint, called *total precedence constraint*: the goal is to give the user the capability of excluding rules, where one episode of the antecedent ends after the consequent.

In order to simplify the tuning of the quantitative parameters and to ensure that the temporal support is anti-monotonic, we consider only two parameters and the corresponding constraints: 1. LS_d: the maximum allowed (always positive) difference between $c.start$ and the minimum starting point ($minStart$) of episodes, being part of the antecedent occurrence; 2. GAP_d: the maximum allowed (always positive) difference between $c.start$ and $minEnd$. Parameter LS_d explicitly limits the starting point of any episode of the antecedent occurrence. Parameter GAP_d, instead, combines RS and GAP, as it relates the end of the antecedent occurrence to the start of the consequent episode. GAP_d is an upper limit for both.

It is now possible to reformulate the definition of occurrence of a TAR as follows.

Definition 3. *(Occurrence of a TAR). A set of episodes $\{e_1, \ldots, e_n, e_c\}$ is an occurrence of TAR $\{a_1, \ldots, a_n\} \xrightarrow{p} c$, with $p = \langle LS_d, GAP_d \rangle$ if $\forall i \in [1, n]$ $e_i \in E_{a_i} \wedge e_c \in E_c$ and all the following requirements are verified: 1. there is an* *antecedent occurrence (i.e., intersecting episodes preceding the consequent) 2. all the quantitative constraints imposed by p are met: $(e_c.start - minStart) \leq LS_d$ and $(e_c.start - minEnd) \leq GAP_d$.*

Finally, we introduce a different measure for the temporal support, suitable for the control of the algorithm. In this case we consider as the start of the TAR occurrence, the time point where *all episodes are holding* (i.e., the start of the antecedent occurrence), while the end of the occurrence is given by the end of the consequent episode (rather than considering as start of the occurrence the minimum start of considered episodes, and as the end the maximum end of episodes). The new proposed algorithm, given the anti-monotonicity for the temporal support, generates candidate rules of the frequent itemset F_i using a $F_{i-1} \times F_{i-1}$ strategy (see [6]). It is more efficient than the previous version, because only the frequent sets in the previous step are considered and the candidate is generated only if the two sets share exactly $i - 2$ items.

As for characterizing the complexity of the algorithm, we will consider three main parameters: the FoI set size k, the number n of episodes corresponding to temporal facts in the FoI, the cost $S(i, n)$ of computing the temporal support for TARs with cardinality i. The new algorithm has complexity in time $O(k \sum_{i=1}^{k-1} (|F_{i-1}|^2 + i \cdot |F_i| + S(k, n) \cdot |F_i|))$, which is exponential in the size k of the set FoI. In particular, the worst case scenario is the one where all TARs are frequent: the cost $S(i, n)$ for computing the temporal support is in general exponential because the procedure needs to consider all the possible combinations of facts. This happens also during the identification of antecedents, by considering $F_{i-1} \times F_{i-1}$, which is exponential in the size k of FoI. Supposing that $|F_i| = k$, meaning that the frequent rules are about k^2, the algorithm complexity is $(S(k, n)k^3)$, an order of magnitude less than that of the original algorithm (which complexity is $O(k \cdot s(k, n) \cdot \sum_{i=2}^{k-1} (|F_1||F_{i-1}|))$, thus $(S(k, n)k^4)$). The main limitation of the new algorithm lies in the fact that the adopted definition of temporal support is less easily interpreted by the user. Furthermore, we may consider this version as complementary to the previous one in [5], as it can still be used by the user as a *tool for pre-processing*, in order to choose the more suitable parameter values for the original algorithm.

4 An OLAP-Based Approach to Analyse and Visualize Clinical TARs

In this section we present a methodology, and the related design and implementation, for the mining, the OLAP-based analysis and visualization of TARs.

4.1 Deriving TARs for the Hemodialysis Domain

Hemodialysis is the widely used treatment for patients with acute or chronic endstage renal failure. During an hemodialysis session, the blood passes through an extracorporeal circuit where metabolites (e.g., urea) are eliminated, the acid-base equilibrium is re-established, and water in excess is removed. In general, hemodialysis patients are treated 3 times a week and each session lasts about 4 hours. Hemodialysis treatment is very costly and extremely demanding both from an organizational viewpoint and from the point of view of the patient quality-of-life. Indeed, the daily accumulation of huge amounts of data prompts the need for suitable techniques to detect, analyze, and visualize relevant patterns, allowing the physician to take decisions related to different important aspects such as personalizing the treatment of specific patients, and improving the quality of the care delivered. Temporal data mining applications can thus play a crucial role in this context. Modern hemodialyzers are able to acquire up to 50 different parameters from the patient (e.g., heart rate, blood pressure, weight loss due to lost liquids) and from the process (e.g., pressures in the extra-corporeal circuit, incoming blood flow), with configurable sampling time.

The hemodialysis-related database, we considered for evaluating and testing the proposed methodology, contains temporal facts referring to different kinds of trends of vital signs for 6 patients undergoing hemodialysis treatments. More precisely, set FoI contains the 9 available trends in the database: increase, decrease, and stationarity of systolic, diastolic pressure, and heart rate (shortened as Inc_{PS}, Dec_{PS}, Sta_{PS}, Inc_{PD}, Dec_{PD}, Sta_{PD}, Inc_{FC}, Dec_{FC}, Sta_{FC}, respectively). The overall time span of considered temporal facts is of about 2 months.

We first designed and implemented a software tool for the extraction of TARs according to the new proposed approach. Thanks to the proposed extension of the algorithm, the user has also the possibility to carry out an exploratory analysis of the data set using the restricted model, for detecting the optimal values for the parameters LS, RS, GAP for the classical algorithm. As an example, we executed it using $LS = 30$ and $GAP = 15$ as parameter values (in minutes). Since the vital signs are monitored every 15 minutes, assigning 30 minutes to LS value means that an episode of the antecedent may participate in a rule only if it begins at most two samplings earlier than the start of the consequent episode; fixing the value 15 minutes to GAP means that we consider only instances in which the antecedent of rules shall not end earlier than the subsequent sampling. Resulting TARs may be represented in different ways, as discussed in the following sections.

4.2   Multidimensional Analysis of Clinical TARs

The resulting TARs are saved in an OLAP cube as multidimensional facts. According to the usual representation model for data warehouses, a *fact* is an analyzed concept/object; *measures* are quantitative features of the considered fact, while *dimensions*, possibly containing hierarchies, are categorical attributes, according which we may aggregate measures. A *Fact* is represented through a multidimensional cube, where each dimension of the cube corresponds to a fact dimension, and a cell of the cube contains the measure corresponding to the suitable dimension values. *Hemodialysis* is the considered fact, while *Fact measures* are: 1. NAT (total number of antecedent occurrence in the episode set); 2. NARTS (number of antecedent occurrence that occur in a rule instance);

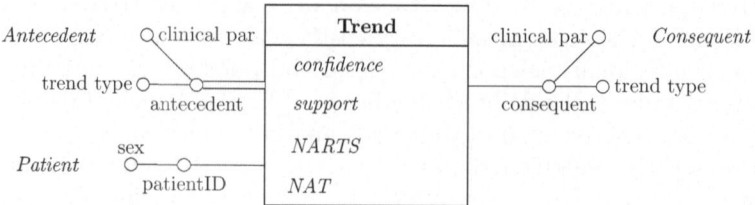

Fig. 2. DFM Schema of the OLAP cube representing the extracted TARs related to hemodialysis patients

3. temporal support; 4. confidence; 5. global support. *Analysis dimensions* are: 1. Antecedent; 2. Consequent; 3. Patient. All the considered dimensions are structured according to given hierarchies: for example, both the Antecedent and the Consequent dimensions specify that we can perform the analysis by aggregating TARs according to the kind of trend (e.g., grouping all TARs dealing with an increase trend) or according to the considered clinical parameter (e.g., grouping all TARs dealing with diastolic pressure). Figure 2 depicts the conceptual schema of cubes related to fact *Hemodialysis* according to the DFM model [3].

We can now proceed with the analysis using OLAP tools, and in particular with the visualization of TARs. Methods for displaying association rules can be divided into three groups, according to the structure adopted for visualization: table, graph, or matrix [7]. Although there are several techniques for displaying association rules, most of them represent the entire set of mined rules in a single screen. In our approach the visualization and analysis of TARs extracted by the algorithm will be done using traditional tools in the context of data warehouses like the OLAP ones.

Such an analysis has been done by the Business Intelligence platform Pentaho[1]. By the *Slicer*, the tool that allows the user to do the typical OLAP operations (*slice, dice, roll-up,* and *drill-down*), it is possible to set the value of one or more dimensions. For example, one may want to consider a TAR set, formed by all TARs, related to a single patient, with the same consequent (e.g., the consequent is either an increase, decrease or stationarity of the *diastolic pressure* i.e. *PD*, for the patient *patient_id* $= 1$). As the consequents and the patient are fixed, the user may decide to hide them and visualize only the antecedent dimension, as depicted in Figure 3. Moreover, it is possible to associate various types of chart to the result: as an example, Figure 3 depicts a bar chart, where the first two bars are the confidence and the temporal support of $Dec_{FC} \rightarrow (Inc_{PD}|Dec_{PD}|Sta_{PD})$, respectively.

4.3   Visualizing Clinical TARs

The analysis tool should display TARs, derived from temporal facts of the modeled clinical domain, providing the usual statistical data, such as support and

---

[1] http://sourceforge.net/projects/pentaho/

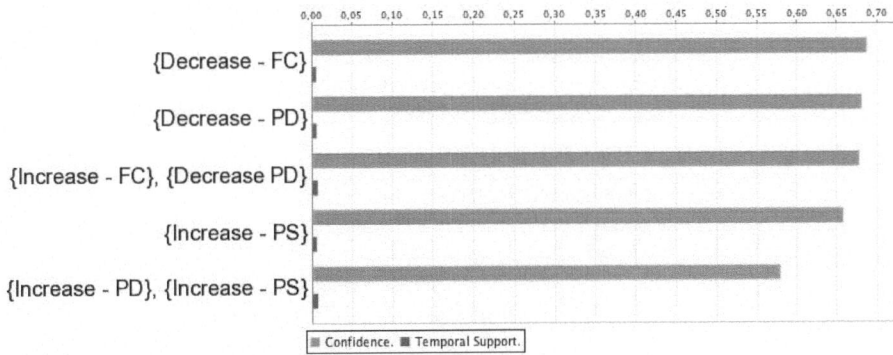

Fig. 3. Bar chart representing the antecedents of TARs obtained from the analysis where the consequent is either an increase, decrease or stationarity of the *diastolic pressure* i.e. *PD*, and the patient is *patient_id* = 1

confidence, as well as hints on how these events temporally relate with each other; moreover, it should show both aggregate information, typical in OLAP systems, and a representation of the raw data (i.e. the episodes of temporal facts). The visualization of temporal features of TARs should give both information about the entire set of the extracted TARs and also information about subsets of TARs, by explicitly considering individual patients/facts. To face this issue, we designed and developed a prototype, to integrate with the existing OLAP tools, focusing on TAR temporal features, by proposing a new visual representation of TARs, depicted in Figure 4. It displays a TAR through *bars*: each bar represents a temporal fact involved in the considered TAR. Using different tones of colors, we can express the *minimum* and the *maximum* duration of episodes of temporal facts, being part of a TAR occurrence. The considered TAR is thus formed by the composition of all its temporal facts. The relative position of bars gives also information about temporal relationships among temporal facts that compose a TAR, such as the relative average start of the corresponding episodes. Furthermore, the smaller bar before facts in the antecedent represents the earliest start with respect to the consequent start. When this bar is associated to the consequent fact, it represents the earliest start with respect to the core start of the given TAR, i.e., when all the episodes composing the antecedent are concurrent. Likewise, the smaller bar after facts in the antecedent represents the latest end with respect to the consequent end; in the case of the consequent, it represents the latest end with respect to the end of the antecedent occurrence. The antecedent and the consequent are separated by an arrow. The interface consists of three main parts as highlighted in Figure 5: (A) *General View* provides a visualization of the aggregate data using the visual representation previously introduced. In addition to numerical values such as *NAT, NARTS* and *temporal support*, all TARs are visually displayed, to emphasize their temporal features; (B) *Temporal View* is closely linked with the general view and shows on a time line the episodes of TARs, in order to allow the user to focus on specific episodes

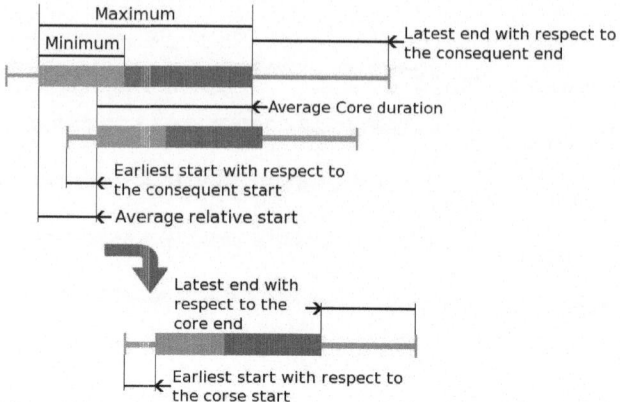

Fig. 4. The visual representation of TARs and of the considered temporal facts

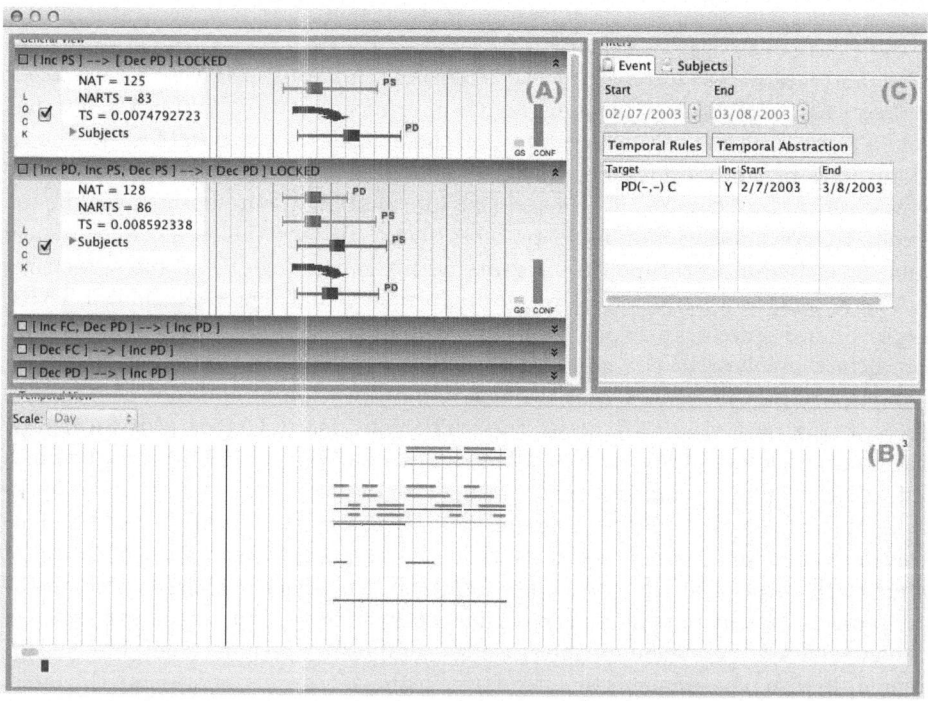

Fig. 5. Result analysis through the interface. (A) General View, (B) Temporal View, and (C) Filters.

or TAR occurrences. TAR occurrences are displayed as bars and their color corresponds to the color of the TAR assigned in the General View. The user can easily interact by clicking on TARs for expanding or collapsing their visual representation; (C) *Filters* consists of all the functions available to users for selection and navigation of the data. We designed it, to maintain a correspondence with the typical OLAP operations analysis (i.e. *roll-up, drill-down, slice* and *dice*).

We also exploit the capacity of human beings to recognize classes of elements based on a color coding [2]. There are two coexisting coloring systems: the first one, in the general view, is used to distinguish different temporal facts within the visualization of TARs, using a coloring system that resembles a street light: *green* for increase, *yellow* for the stationarity and *red* for the decrease; the second one is used for the classification of temporal rules: the coloring is done by the user, allowing one to create a link between the general and the temporal view. As shown in Figure 5, *purple* is used to highlight the rule $\{Inc_{PD}, Inc_{PS}, Dec_{PS}\} \rightarrow Dec_{PD}$. It is worth noting that in the shown TAR there is the presence of increasing and decreasing episodes of the same parameter: it represents up and down patterns, where the two episodes share only one time point (i.e., they intersect only at the beginning/ending point, respectively).

5   Conclusions

In this paper, we revised the specification of *temporal association rules*, by restricting the model proposed in [5] and providing a more efficient algorithm. We have investigated the possibility of using BI and OLAP analysis methodologies and tools for visually exploring the resulting temporal association rules. We also introduced a new visualization technique for TARs. We plan as future work to study the issue of aggregation for TARs in a deep way and to conduct usability test of the developed visualization solutions with medical users.

References

1. Concaro, S., Sacchi, L., Cerra, C., Fratino, P., Bellazzi, R.: Mining healthcare data with temporal association rules: Improvements and assessment for a practical use. In: Combi, C., Shahar, Y., Abu-Hanna, A. (eds.) AIME 2009. LNCS, vol. 5651, pp. 16–25. Springer, Heidelberg (2009)
2. Flatla, D.R., Gutwin, C.: Individual models of color differentiation to improve interpretability of information visualization. In: SIGCHI, pp. 2563–2572 (2010)
3. Golfarelli, M., Maio, D., Rizzi, S.: The dimensional fact model: A conceptual model for data warehouses. Int. J. Cooperative Inf. Syst. 7(2-3), 215–247 (1998)
4. Lin, W., Orgun, M.A., Williams, G.: An overview of temporal data mining. In: Proceedings of the 1st Australian Data Mining Workshop (AusDM 2002), pp. 83–90. University of Technology, Sydney (2002)
5. Sacchi, L., Larizza, C., Combi, C., Bellazzi, R.: Data mining with temporal abstractions: learning rules from time series. Data Mining Knowledge Discovery 15(2), 217–247 (2007)
6. Tan, P., Steinbach, M., Kumar, V.: Introduction to Data Mining. Pearson Addison–Wesley (2005)
7. Techapichetvanich, K., Datta, A.: VisAR: A new technique for visualizing mined association rules. In: Li, X., Wang, S., Dong, Z.Y. (eds.) ADMA 2005. LNCS (LNAI), vol. 3584, pp. 88–95. Springer, Heidelberg (2005)

Learning to Identify Inappropriate Antimicrobial Prescriptions

Mathieu Beaudoin[1], Froduald Kabanza[1], Vincent Nault[2],
and Louis Valiquette[2]

[1] Dept. of Computer Science, Université de Sherbrooke, Canada
{mathieu.beaudoin,froduald.kabanza}@usherbrooke.ca
[2] Dept. of Microbiology and Infectiology, Université de Sherbrooke, Canada
{vincent.nault,louis.valiquette}@usherbrooke.ca

Abstract. Inappropriate antimicrobial prescribing is a major clinical problem and health concern. Several hospitals rely on automated surveillance to achieve hospital-wide antimicrobial optimization. The main challenge in implementing these systems lies in acquiring and updating their knowledge. In this paper, we discuss a surveillance system which can acquire new rules and improve its knowledge base. Our system uses an algorithm based on instance-based learning and rule induction to discover rules for inappropriate prescriptions. The algorithm uses temporal abstraction to extract a meaningful time interval representation from raw clinical data, and applies nearest neighbor classification with a distance function on both temporal and non-temporal parameters. The algorithm is able to discover new rules for early switch from intravenous to oral antimicrobial therapy from real clinical data.

Keywords: Classification, temporal data mining, interval sequence, instance-based learning, nearest-neighbor, antimicrobial optimization.

1 Introduction

Inappropriate antimicrobial (ATM) prescribing is a major clinical problem and health concern, with as many as 50% of ATM prescriptions being unnecessary or inappropriate [1]. ATM stewardship programs have been shown to reduce avoidable adverse effects (toxicity, ATM resistance, *Clostridium difficile*, etc. [1,2]) and length of stay, improve patient health, and reduce unnecessary costs. ATM optimization requires the revision of an overwhelming amount of clinical data by dedicated experts, which proves to be an obstacle in the current context of limited healthcare resources. Therefore, several hospitals rely on automated decision support systems to revise hospital-wide ATM prescriptions.

Over the past five years, we have implemented, deployed, and evaluated an automated system called APSS – antimicrobial prescription surveillance system. It is currently deployed at the *Centre Hospitalier Universitaire de Sherbrooke* (CHUS), a Canadian academic centre of 713 beds. It uses expert rules to identify mismatches between prescribed ATMs and published and local guidelines.

N. Peek, R. Marín Morales, and M. Peleg (Eds.): AIME 2013, LNAI 7885, pp. 248–257, 2013.

A clinical pharmacist first reviews the documented alerts and then contacts the prescribing physician to recommend a prescription modification or discontinuation if deemed appropriate. Over the last two years, pharmacists have rejected as many as 50% of false alerts. On the other hand, 91% of the alerts retained (3 156 total) were accepted by the prescribing physicians. This has contributed to decrease intravenous ATM consumption by 22% and ATM expenses by 688 000 CAD. APSS enabled us to extend our surveillance from high-risk wards (e.g., intensive-care) to every bed of the CHUS' two physical sites.

The high proportion of false alerts generated by APSS is mainly explained by a number of prescription parameters that require fine-tuning, changes in prescription guidelines that are not accurately updated, and other factors that affect the appropriateness of a prescription that are not explicitly accounted for in the guidelines and hence not encoded in the knowledge base. The pharmacists' revision process is impeded by this high rate of false alerts.

In order to reduce the proportion of false alerts generated by APSS, we have been investigating the use of a machine learning algorithm that discovers new rules for classifying inappropriate prescriptions, supervised by user feedback such as the rejection of false alerts by the pharmacist or physician, or the identification of unflagged inappropriate prescriptions. The objective is to automatically improve the knowledge base of APSS based on experience. Given that prescriptions are temporal data by nature, we use a supervised learning algorithm for discovering rules that classify temporal data – this is a binary classification into good and bad temporal data (i.e., prescriptions). The algorithm we use is a combination of rule induction and instance-based learning methods. The application of machine learning to clinical temporal data is not new. We review some applications below. However, to the best of our knowledge this is the first application to the monitoring of ATM prescribing.

To illustrate the temporal nature of ATM prescribing, consider this example. A physician chooses a treatment after the first assessment of a patient. As new information becomes available, he will modify the initial treatment to account for clinical and laboratory test results and variations in the patient's state of health. A key intervention in ATM prescribing is *early switch therapy* where an intravenous ATM is replaced by an oral ATM providing a less costly alternative and allowing the patient to be discharged earlier. An early switch typically occurs after 72 hours of intravenous ATM treatment, if the patient is able to take oral medications and his condition has been stable over the last 48 hours.

In the rest of this paper, we first give an overview of related work. We then describe the supervised learning algorithm that we have integrated into APSS and discuss preliminary experimental results. We conclude with future work.

2   Related Work

There are various applications of data mining and machine learning algorithms to clinical temporal data, including temporal abstraction which is commonly used to extract a meaningful representation of the raw data using qualitative time intervals [3]. Association rule discovery has been used to gain insight into causes of clinical events of interest (e.g.,[4,5]); however it is geared towards discovering rules for frequent patterns and performs poorly when addressing infrequent patterns [6] such as inappropriate prescriptions. It uses an *Apriori*-like strategy [7] with breadth-first search and candidate pruning based on *support* and *confidence*. A problem with this strategy when looking at infrequent patterns is the necessity to lower support thresholds. It inefficiently prunes the candidate space and potentially leads to an intractable search space. Furthermore, it produces an overwhelming quantity of uninteresting patterns from which it is difficult to distinguish interesting ones [6].

Another method used to identify clinical events of interest is case-based reasoning. For example, case-based reasoning has been used to identify potential adverse drug events [8] and hemodialysis treatment failures [9] by looking for similar past cases. While case-based reasoning and instance-based learning are known to perform well with few instances, they are burdened with irrelevant attributes [10] and accumulate large quantities of cases. This is a problem when looking for a small set of highly accurate, concise and intelligible rules aimed at a human user.

A complementary approach to instance-based learning is rule induction. Rule induction is known for its ability to dispose easily of irrelevant features, separate classes with good accuracy, and extract a small set of rules that can lead to better predictions [10]. However, it tends to be affected by a skewed distribution of classes and produce rules that favor the overrepresented classes [11]. Combining instance-based learning and rule induction has been known to address their respective limits with their complementary strengths with traditional non-temporal feature-value data [10].

Our machine learning algorithm also combines instance-based learning and rule induction. However, unlike the approach in [10], which learns classification rules for a labeled set of non-temporal feature-value data, our algorithm learns classification rules for a labeled set of qualitative time interval sequences in addition to non-temporal feature-value data. Before describing the algorithm, we first explain the context of application more precisely and state the problem solved by our algorithm more formally.

3   Application Context and Formal Problem Statement

APSS communicates with the CHUS' electronic health record system and receives administrative and clinical data for every adult inpatient under ATM therapy. For the experiments discussed later in this paper, we selected every adult patient admitted between January 1st 2012 and June 30th 2012. We considered the following attributes: *gender*, *age*, Body Mass Index (*BMI*), patient location (*ward*), temperature (*temp*), white cell count (*WCC*), neutrophil count (*neut*), creatinine clearance (*CrCl*), respiratory rate (*resp*), *pulse*, and blood pressure (*BP*). An attribute was also created for each medication. Prescriptions were described using their *name*, *dose*, *frequency*, and *route* of administration.

We pre-processed this heterogeneous data using simple temporal abstraction mechanisms to extract a uniform and meaningful representation. Figure 1 illustrates the process of state abstractions for the raw *temp* time series where quantitative thresholds were used to identify qualitative states, which we call *episodes*, that hold over a period of time. A temporal granularity of 1 hour was defined. We extracted a single sequence for each hospitalization. Our observation period was restricted to the ongoing ATM of interest, where we considered only data between the first ($t_{\min}$) and last ($t_{\max}$) administered dose. It ensures a common time zero ($t_{\min}$) between sequences.

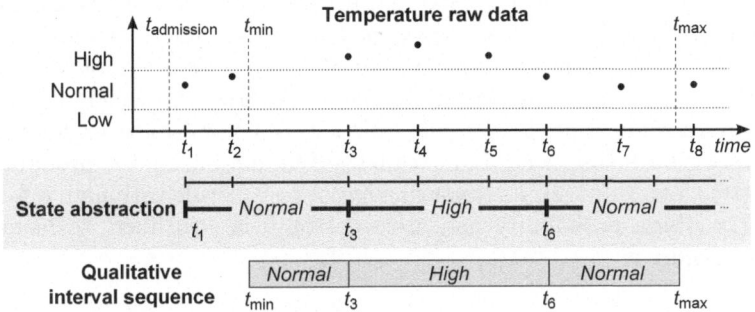

Fig. 1. Example of state abstractions for the *temp* attribute

Let us consider the attribute space A as the finite set of attributes for our domain and the feature space F as the finite set of qualitative states observed for these attributes. An *episode* e is defined as $< a, f, ts, te >$, where $(a = f)$ describes a symbolic state with $a \in A$ and $f \in F$ holding over the time interval $[ts, te[$. We refer to the attribute, feature, start, and end times of an episode as $e.a$, $e.f$, $e.ts$, and $e.te$ respectively. An example of episode from Fig. 1 is $< temp, normal, t_{\min}, t_3 >$.

A *sequence* s is defined by $\{e_1, \ldots, e_n | \forall i = 1, \ldots, n - 1 : e_i.ts \leq e_{i+1}.ts\}$, where $n = |s|$, the size of the sequence. We refer to the subsequence of s for the ith attribute $a_i \in A$ as $att_i(s)$ defined by $\{e_1, \ldots, e_m | \forall e \in att_i(s) : e \in s; e.a = a_i; \forall j = 1, \ldots, m - 1 : e_j.te \leq e_{j+1}.ts\}$, where $m = |att_i(s)|$. A hospitalization is described as a *labeled sequence* ls defined as $\{id, s, l\}$, where id is a unique identifier, s is a sequence, and l is a class label that belongs to the finite set of class labels L. We focus on a binary-class problem where $L = \{negative, positive\}$. We used APSS' revised alerts to label every sequence, where *positive* indicates a true positive and *negative* indicates a negative or false positive.

We can now formally state the supervised machine learning problem that concerns us. Given the finite training set TS of labeled sequences, discover a rule set R for classifying positive sequences. We only have two classes (positive and negative). Learned classification rules identify positive instances. The antecedent of a learned rule is a conjunction of propositions over time intervals whose satisfaction implies membership to the *positive* class; the consequent is *true*.

4   Temporal Induction of Classification Models

Our supervised learning algorithm, called *Temporal Induction of classification Models* (TIM) combines instance-based learning and rule induction. Its main operations are the following: at first, the rule set R is initialized using positive sequences of the training set as maximally specific rules. Distances between rules and sequences of the training set are computed and stored in a multidimensional distance matrix to reduce computation times. These distances are used for nearest neighbor classification. Rules are modified in parallel to increase interclass distance. At each iteration, the most promising local modifications are selected according to the rule's most similar negative sequences. Conditions are eliminated or their time intervals are shortened. Local modifications are performed according to similar negative sequences until they no longer improve a rule.

The rules are evaluated according to the *J-measure* [12], which quantifies the average information content of a rule. We selected the *J-measure* for its ability to account for both simplicity and *goodness-of-fit*, measuring the probability and *cross-entropy* of a rule [12]. As a working hypothesis, a rule with high information content (i.e., high probability and cross-entropy) is also likely to have a high predictive accuracy.

4.1   Classification

The distance function measures the similarity between rules and sequences, where rules classify sequences that involve temporal and non-temporal data. Accordingly, we use a distance function that considers both temporal and non-temporal parameters. A non-symmetric distance function is used where similarity is proportional to the number of conditions that a sequence shares with a rule, i.e., a sequence is perfectly similar to a rule it subsumes.

Given a rule $r \in R$ with N_r attributes and a sequence $s \in TS$, the global *distance*(r, s) function is defined by Equation (1). Normalizing *distance*(r, s) by N_r creates a coefficient between $[0, 1]$, where 0 denotes perfect similarity, that does not arbitrarily favor shorter rules. To ensure that irrelevant sequences are not labeled as positive by the nearest, yet dissimilar, rule we enforce a minimal distance threshold $D_{\min}$ under which a rule is said to **cover** a sequence. In such case, the sequence is labeled as positive by the rule.

$$distance(r, s) = \frac{\sum_{i=1}^{N_r} D_a(att_i(r), att_i(s))}{N_r} \tag{1}$$

The D_a function measures the distance between subsequences $att_i(r)$ and $att_i(s)$ for the ith attribute of r. If $att_i(s) = null$, $D_a = 1$, otherwise we use Equation (2) which measures the distance between the conditions $c_j \in att_i(r)$ and episodes $e_k \in att_i(s)$. An indexing mechanism retrieves attribute-specific subsequences in $O(1)$. We normalize the distance $D_a \in [0, 1]$ to avoid arbitrarily increasing the weight of the ith attribute in the global coefficient.

$$D_{\mathrm{a}}(att_i(r), att_i(s)) = \frac{|att_i(r)| - \left(\sum_{j=1}^{|att_i(r)|} \sum_{k=1}^{|att_i(s)|}(S_{\mathrm{F}}(c_j, e_k) \times S_{\mathrm{T}}(c_j, e_k))\right)}{|att_i(r)|} \tag{2}$$

Feature Similarity. The feature similarity function S_{F} measures the similarity between the symbolic features of c_j and e_k using the *overlap metric* where $S_{\mathrm{F}}(c_j, e_k) = 1$ if $(c_j.f = e_k.f)$ and 0 otherwise.

Temporal Similarity. Temporal similarity is proportional to the temporal overlapping of e_k over c_j, as measured by Equation (3). S_{T} returns a coefficient between $[0, 1]$, where 1 implies $[c_j.ts, c_j.te[\subseteq [e_k.ts, e_k.te[$.

$$S_{\mathrm{T}}(c_j, e_k) = \frac{[c_j.ts, c_j.te[\cap [e_k.ts, e_k.te[}{[c_j.ts, c_j.te[} \tag{3}$$

Consider the attribute-specific subsequences of Fig. 2. A rule's antecedent $att_i(r)$ with conditions c_1 and c_2 overlaps a sequence's $att_i(s)$ with episodes e_1, e_2 and e_3. The distance between these subsequences is 0.2, which is computed as follows:

$$D_{\mathrm{a}}(att_i(r), att_i(s)) = \frac{2 - \left(\sum_{j=1}^{2} \sum_{k=1}^{3}(S_{\mathrm{F}}(c_j, e_k) \times S_{\mathrm{T}}(c_j, e_k))\right)}{2}$$

$$= \frac{2 - ((1 \times 0.6) + (0 \times 0.4) + (1 \times 0) + (0 \times 0) + (1 \times 1) + (0 \times 0))}{2}$$

$$= 0.2$$

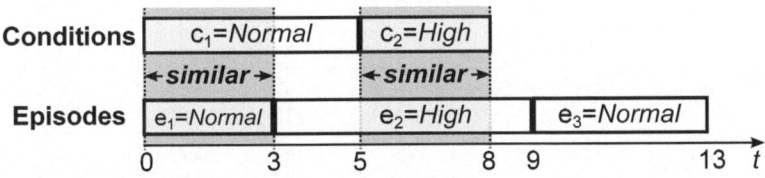

Fig. 2. Example of a rule's conditions and a sequence's episodes

4.2   Refinement of the Rule Set

The intuition behind this rule refinement process is that increasing interclass distance creates more accurate rules. Rules are modified in parallel, where each iteration provides a set of locally promising modifications. Promising modifications are selected by comparing a rule and its most similar negative sequence. Rules are modified by removing the temporal overlapping between a condition *c* and an episode *e*, resulting in a modified condition *c′* being either entirely removed or subsumed by *c*.

Since a new rule is subsumed by the original, it will only be similar to sequences that were already (partially) similar to the original rule. Thus, distances must only be updated for these sequences. TIM uses a multidimensional *distance matrix* to keep track of the partially similar sequences of a rule.

5 Results

As a preliminary experiment for our algorithm, we have tested TIM with learning rules that identify *"early switch therapy"*. A clinically valid recommendation for early switch from intravenous to oral ATM therapy requires the following three indications: 72 consecutive hours of intravenous therapy, 48 hours of stabilized state of health (e.g., normal levels of white cell count and temperature), and 24 hours of concurrent oral therapy. This rule involves non trivial temporal constraints, making it a good test case for the learning algorithm. In this experiment, this rule is not specified. The dataset only contains positive and negative labels specifying if a hospitalization contains or not a recommendation for early switch therapy. The objective is to demonstrate that the rule is eventually learned from these alerts.

We created two datasets of different sizes and ratios of positive sequences. We created the first dataset with patients who received piperacillin-tazobactam (TAZO), our centre's most prescribed intravenous antibiotic. We created another smaller dataset with patients who received metronidazole (METRO), an ATM predominantly prescribed orally. They were partitioned into *training* and *test* datasets, as described in Table 1.

Table 1. Description of the two datasets used in our experiments

	Dataset	Episodes	Sequence	Positive	Attribute
METRO	Training	9,176	132	12	1206
	Test	19,182	278	46	
TAZO	Training	37,428	485	190	1581
	Test	68,188	947	413	

TIM extracted an accurate and sensitive set of 35 rules. While specificity was lower, it remained above APSS without TIM. A microbiology-infectiology expert evaluated their clinical relevance using a five-point Likert scale ranging from 1-no relevance to 5-excellent relevance. Excellent relevance required the presence of all three indications for early switch therapy. Missing or indirect indications decreased the score. Rules with more than 40 conditions were also penalized. Table 2 presents the scores; 63% of the rules were found to be clinically relevant (score ≥ 3). Interestingly, rules with high relevance scores also had the highest

Table 2. Relevance score of 35 extracted rules (1-no relevance to 5-excellent relevance)

Relevance score	1	2	3	4	5
#rules	8 (23%)	5 (14%)	8 (23%)	8 (23%)	6 (17%)

information content (*J-measure*). On the other hand, rules with relevance score of 1 were very specific and covered less than 1% of the test set.

Consider the rule in Example 1 with a relevance score of 5. Clear indications for early switch therapy are respected with normalized white cell count (WCC), extended intravenous (IV) treatment, and concurrent oral treatment. This rule also contains complementary information that was used by our expert to extract profiles of patients associated with early switch recommendations. Prolonged stay at the emergency room (ER), old age, *salbutamol*, and additional ATM coverage with *ciprofloxacin* may indicate suspicion of pneumonia caused by resistant pathogens. Ten rules targeted patients under post-operative ATM prophylaxis, a practice not supported by medical evidence that will be addressed by our ATM stewardship team. Another finding was that eight rules targeted patients with $BMI \geq 40$. It could suggest that extended intravenous treatments are prescribed for very severely obese patients to ensure targeted concentrations are achieved. This new information provides insight into our centre's prescribing practices. These patient profiles are of high interest for further investigation as they identify subgroups of patients that could require closer monitoring or wards that could benefit from targeted in-service training.

Example 1. $\{<$ *gender*, $F, 0, 70 >, <$ *age*, $83, 0, 70 >, <$ *ward*, $ER, 0, 70 >,$
$< WCC, normal, 0, 70 >, <$ *neut*, $high, 0, 70 >, \{tazocin < dose, 3000, 0, 70 >,$
$< freq, 6, 0, 70 >, <$ *route*, $IV, 0, 70 >\}, \{ciprofloxacin < dose, 400, 0, 23 >,$
$< freq, 12, 0, 23 >, <$ *route*, $IV, 0, 23 >\}, \{acetaminophen < dose, 650, 0, 70 >,$
$< freq, 12, 0, 70 >, <$ *route*, $oral, 0, 70 >\}, \{salbutamol < dose, 0.5, 0, 70 >,$
$< freq, 24, 0, 70 >, <$ *route*, $inhaled, 0, 70 >\}\} \implies true$

We also compared TIM to three other algorithms (see Table 3) to evaluate its relative recall, accuracy and computation times. The first was an instance-based learning (IBL) algorithm that performs nearest neighbor classification with every positive sequence of the training set. The second was a classification rule learner (CRL) using a specialization approach with the *J-measure*, removing positive sequences covered by newly created rules. The third algorithm used an association rule mining (ARM) approach. Various strategies were used in CRL and ARM to focus on highly predictive rules for the positive class. For example, ARM used candidate pruning on both support (METRO: ≥ 0.015; TAZO: ≥ 0.02) and confidence ($conf \geq 0.75$), and eliminated dominated patterns [6]. We restricted ARM to a maximum rule size of 4 for the TAZO test.

Overall, TIM achieved relatively similar or better recall and accuracy than CRL and IBL, except for the recall metrics in METRO, where TIM is outperformed by IBL. TIM achieved superior accuracy than IBL with fewer rules, and

Table 3. Compared results of TIM, IBL, CRL, and ARM on two datasets

Dataset	Method	#rules	Time (s)	Precision	Recall	Accuracy
METRO	TIM	5	0.4	53.8	76.1	85.3
	IBL	12	0.2	30.1	95.7	62.6
	CRL	1	46.0	56.5	76.1	86.3
	ARM	8 074	15.2	44.1	32.6	82.0
TAZO	TIM	30	73.5	62.5	99.0	73.7
	IBL	190	9.5	59.3	99.3	70.0
	CRL	6	583.1	71.4	88.1	79.4
	ARM	614 652	17 864.5	66.0	81.4	73.6

80% and 30% less conditions per rule for METRO and TAZO, respectively. TIM was 7 to 100 times faster than CRL. As can be seen in Table 3, ARM demonstrated the worst results and required heavy post-processing to identify a subset of accurate rules.

6   Conclusion and Future Work

The main motivation of this work is to automatically improve the knowledge base of an antimicrobial prescription monitoring system (APSS) by using supervised machine learning. The system analyzes prescriptions and produces alerts on seemingly inappropriate prescriptions. The rejections of alerts by the pharmacist and the physician provide feedback for a supervised machine learning algorithm (TIM) that learns new rules for the knowledge base.

TIM is still in the experimental stage. It combines instance-based learning and rule induction to learn prescription classification rules from feedback. We have discussed preliminary results showing TIM's capability of learning rules for appropriate early switch from intravenous to oral antimicrobial therapy. The majority of learned rules were found to be clinically relevant because they succeeded in identifying the clinical indications for early switch therapy. A clinician identified from these rules patient profiles associated with early switch recommendations providing further insight into our center's prescribing practices and a potential for targeted interventions (e.g., unsupported use of post-operative antimicrobial prophylaxis). TIM's learning capability aims to extract rules for evaluating treatments that must be adjusted to the patient's evolving clinical condition; we believe it could be extended to many other treatments.

We find these preliminary results very promising. The next steps are pursued experimentation of TIM before its release with the currently deployed version of APSS. The release version will require tools for assisting physicians in revising the rules learnt by TIM before they are incorporated in the knowledge base.

Acknowledgements. This project was partially funded by the *Fonds de recherche du Québec – Santé*, the *Fonds de recherche du Québec – Nature et technologies*, and the *Natural Sciences and Engineering Research Council of Canada*.

References

1. Dellit, T.H., Owens, R.C., McGowan, J.E., Gerding, D.N., Weinstein, R.A., Burke, J.P., Huskins, W.C., Paterson, D.L., Fishman, N.O., Carpenter, C.F., Brennan, P.J., Billeter, M., Hooton, T.M.: Infectious Diseases Society of America and the Society for Healthcare Epidemiology of America guidelines for developing an institutional program to enhance antimicrobial stewardship. Clin. Infect. Dis. 44(2), 159–177 (2007)

2. Valiquette, L., Cossette, B., Garant, M.P., Diab, H., Pepin, J.: Impact of a reduction in the use of high-risk antibiotics on the course of an epidemic of clostridium difficile-associated disease caused by the hypervirulent nap1/027 strain. Clin. Infect. Dis. 45(suppl. 2), 112–121 (2007)

3. Shahar, Y.: A framework for knowledge-based temporal abstraction. Artif. Intell. 90(1-2), 79–133 (1997)

4. Bellazzi, R., Larizza, C., Magni, P., Bellazzi, R.: Temporal data mining for the quality assessment of a hemodialysis service. Artif. Intell. Med. 34(1), 25–39 (2005)

5. Concaro, S., Sacchi, L., Cerra, C., Fratino, P., Bellazzi, R.: Mining healthcare data with temporal association rules: Improvements and assessment for a practical use. In: Combi, C., Shahar, Y., Abu-Hanna, A. (eds.) AIME 2009. LNCS, vol. 5651, pp. 16–25. Springer, Heidelberg (2009)

6. Zaki, M., Lesh, N., Ogihara, M.: Planmine: Predicting plan failures using sequence mining. Artif. Intell. Rev. 14(6), 421–446 (2000)

7. Agrawal, R., Srikant, R.: Fast algorithms for mining association rules in large databases. In: Proceedings of the 20th Int. Conf. on Very Large Data Bases, VLDB 1994, pp. 487–499. Morgan Kaufmann Publishers Inc., San Francisco (1994)

8. Hartge, F., Wetter, T., Haefeli, W.E.: A similarity measure for case based reasoning modeling with temporal abstraction based on cross-correlation. Comput. Methods Programs Biomed. 81(1), 41–48 (2006)

9. Montani, S., Portinale, L., Leonardi, G.: Case-based retrieval to support the treatment of end stage renal failure patients. Artif. Intell. Med. 37(1), 31–42 (2006)

10. Domingos, P.: Unifying instance-based and rule-based induction. Machine Learning 24(2), 141–168 (1996)

11. Chawla, N., Japkowicz, N., Kotcz, A.: Editorial: Special issue on learning from imbalanced data sets. ACM SIGKDD Explorations Newsletter 6(1), 1–6 (2004)

12. Smyth, P., Goodman, R.M.: Rule induction using information theory. In: Piatetsky-Shapiro, G., Frawley, W.J. (eds.) Knowledge Discovery in Databases, pp. 159–176. AAAI/MIT Press (1991)

An Approach for Mining Care Trajectories for Chronic Diseases

Elias Egho[1], Nicolas Jay[1], Chedy Raïssi[2], Gilles Nuemi[3], Catherine Quantin[3], and Amedeo Napoli[1]

[1] Orpailleur Team, LORIA, Vandoeuvre-les-Nancy, France
{firstname.lastname}@loria.fr
[2] INRIA, Nancy Grand Est, France
{firstname.lastname}@inria.fr
[3] Service de Biostatistique et d'Information Médicale, CHU de Dijon, Dijon, France
{firstname.lastname}@chu-dijon.fr

Abstract. With the increasing burden of chronic illnesses, administrative health care databases hold valuable information that could be used to monitor and assess the processes shaping the trajectory of care of chronic patients. In this context, temporal data mining methods are promising tools, though lacking flexibility in addressing the complex nature of medical events. Here, we present a new algorithm able to extract patient trajectory patterns with different levels of granularity by relying on external taxonomies. We show the interest of our approach with the analysis of trajectories of care for colorectal cancer using data from the French casemix information system.

Keywords: datamining, chronic illness, claim data, sequential pattern mining, trajectory of care.

1 Introduction

Chronic illnesses are a major burden in both developed and developing countries [5]. Patients with chronic conditions use more services and a greater array of services than other consumers. Multiple encounters of chronic patients with the healthcare system define a so-called "trajectory" of care . Lack of coordination along the trajectory of care, bad implementation of guidelines or inappropriate organization of the healthcare system may have a negative impact on quality and costs of care.

Due to the fragmentation of clinical information systems, little knowledge is readily available to describe and assess the actual processes involved in long-term care, especially in the scope of a cross-institutional analysis. However, in many countries, health information systems routinely collect medical and administrative data at regional or national scale. Among them, case-mix information systems were originally built for hospital activity report and billing purpose[2]. They hold valuable information that could help health care managers and professionals to develop inter-organizational knowledge and bring deeper insights

N. Peek, R. Marín Morales, and M. Peleg (Eds.): AIME 2013, LNAI 7885, pp. 258–267, 2013.

into inpatient care trajectories. In order to produce the expected knowledge and support decision making, case-mix systems have to be turned into longitudinal and patient-centered information systems. This requires the linkage of different stays of a same patient into a sequence that will be further processed. Because of the complex nature and extreme diversity of medical problems, patient care trajectories must be summarized and categorized for allowing meaningful inference about outcomes of particular interest.

Data-mining methods are especially adapted to the analysis of sequences and successfully used in biomedical domain [3,4,7,1]. case-mix systems capture medical problems, procedures, demographic and administrative data using controlled vocabularies and standardized records. In that context, sequences of hospitalizations can be analyzed with sequential pattern mining algorithms[9]. Meanwhile, case-mix records have a multidimensional structure that traditional sequential patterns can not fully reflect. Moreover, the granularity of the initial data may be too fine to generate interesting patterns. The availability of classifications and ontologies used to code information in case-mix systems is an opportunity to integrate additional knowledge into the mining process and achieve better results. Although a few approaches have been developed to tackle the problems of granularity and multidimensionality in sequential pattern mining[8], they are still not adapted to the problem of mining care trajectories.

In this paper, we present an new algorithm, MMISP (Mining Multidimensional Itemsets Sequential Patterns). MMISP is able to extract patterns from care trajectories in a multidimensional temporal database, using external taxonomic knowledge at appropriate levels of granularity. We illustrate this approach in analysing care trajectories for colorectal cancer using data from the french case-mix information system.

2   Problem Statement

The PMSI[1] is the french adaptation of the Diagnoses Related Groups[2]. In the PMSI database, each stay is a standardized record of administrative and clinical data, especially about the institution, the patient's principal diagnosis and the realized medical procedures. In order to formalize the problem, we accordingly model each hospitalization along three dimensions: (i) healthcare institution, (ii) diagnosis and (iii) medical procedure. Two dimensions, i.e. healthcare institutions and diagnosis, are considered as ordered sets with an associated subsumption relation (i.e. a partial ordering). The set of healthcare institutions H, the set of diagnosis DG and the set of medical procedures MP, are given:

- H=$\{t_h, uh, gh, uh_p, uh_n, gh_p, gh_l\}$.
- DG=$\{t_d, c, r, c_1, c_2, r_1, r_2\}$.
- MP=$\{mp_1, mp_2, mp_3, mp_4\}$.

The subsumption relation for H and DG is defined as below (Figure 1).

---

[1] Programme de Médicalisation des Sytèmes d'Information.

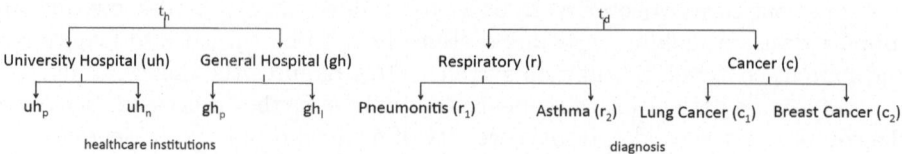

Fig. 1. The subsumption relation for the healthcare institutions set H and the diagnosis set DG

Definition 1. *A **partially ordered set (poset)** is a pair $(D, \leqslant)$, where D is a set and $\leqslant$ is a partial order relation on D. For $x \in D$ the **down set** of x, denoted by $\downarrow x$, is a set of all specializations of x; $\downarrow x = \{y \in D | y \leqslant x\}$. The **up-set** of x is $\uparrow x = \{y \in D | x \leqslant y\}$.*

Among the three basic dimension, H and DG are posets. The hospitalization of a patient is then considered as a vector with 3 components, (H, DG, MP).

Example 1. $(uh_p, c_1, \{mp_1, mp_2\})$ is an hospitalisation for a patient. It is a vector with three components $uh_p \in H, c_1 \in DG$ and $\{mp_1, mp_2\} \subseteq MP$.

Definition 2. *(Elementary vector) An elementary vector $v = (v_1, v_2, v_3)$ is a vector with 3 elements. Given two vectors $v = (v_1, v_2, v_3)$ and $v' = (v'_1, v'_2, v'_3)$, v is more general than v', denoted by $v' \leq_v v$, for every $i = 1...3$*
$$v'_i \leqslant v_i \quad \text{if } v_i, v'_i \text{ are elements in a poset}$$
$$v_i \subseteq v'_i \quad \text{if } v_i, v'_i \text{ are sets}$$

Example 2. $v = (uh_p, c_1, \{mp_1, mp_2\})$ is a vector with 3 elements uh_p, c_1 and $\{mp_1, mp_2\}$. The vector $v' = (uh, t_d, \{mp_1\})$ is more general than v, $v \leq_v v'$, because of:

- $uh_p \leqslant uh$; $uh_p, uh \in H$
- $c_1 \leqslant t_d$; $c_1, t_d \in DG$.
- $\{mp_1\} \subseteq \{mp_1, mp_2\}$; $\{mp_1\}, \{mp_1, mp_2\} \subseteq MP$.

Definition 3. *(Patient Trajectory) A patient trajectory is a pair $(V, <_t)$, where V is a set of elementary vectors and $<_t$ is a temporal order relation on V. The patient trajectory represents like $P = \langle P_1 P_2 ... P_l \rangle$, where $P_1, P_2, ..., P_l \in V$ and $P_1 <_t P_2 <_t P_3... <_t P_l$. Given two trajectories $P = \langle P_1 P_2 ... P_l \rangle$ and $T = \langle T_1 T_2 ... T_{l'} \rangle$, P is more general than T, denoted by $T \leq_p P$, if there exist indices $1 \leq i_1 < i_2 < ... < i_l \leq l'$ such that $T_j \leq_v P_{i_j}$ for all $j = 1 ... l$ and $l \leqslant l'$. We say that T is more specific than P.*

Example 3. $\langle (uh_p, c_1, \{mp_1, mp_2\})(gh_l, r_1, \{mp_2\}) \rangle$ represents a patient trajectory with two hospitalizations. It expresses the fact that a patient was admitted to the hospital uh_p for a lung cancer c_1, and underwent procedures mp_1 and mp_2. Then he went to the hospital gh_l for pneumonitis r_1 where he underwent procedure mp_2.

Table 1. An example of a database of patient trajectories

Patients	Trajectories
$patient_1$	$\langle (uh_p, c_1, \{mp_1, mp_2\})(uh_p, c_1, \{mp_1\})(gh_l, r_1, \{mp_3\}) \rangle$
$patient_2$	$\langle (uh_n, c_1, \{mp_4\})(uh_p, c_2, \{mp_1, mp_2\})(gh_l, r_1, \{mp_2\}) \rangle$
$patient_3$	$\langle (uh_p, c_1, \{mp_4\})(gh_l, r_2, \{mp_3\}) \rangle$
$patient_4$	$\langle (uh_p, c_2, \{mp_1, mp_2\})(gh_p, r_2, \{mp_3\})(gh_l, r_2, \{mp_2\}) \rangle$

Let P_{DB} be the patient trajectories for four patients $patient_1$, $patient_2$, $patient_3$ and $patient_4$, Table 1.

Let supp(P) be the number of trajectories that are more specific than P in P_{DB} and σ be a minimum support threshold specified by the end-user. Let P be a trajectory, P is a frequent trajectory pattern in P_{DB} if and only if $supp(P) \geq \sigma$.

Using the poset for some dimensions, we can extract a large number of frequent trajectory patterns. To avoid the patterns overfloading, our approach only extracts the set of all most specific frequent trajectory patterns in P_{DB}. Actually, frequency is anti-monotonic (i.e if $P = \langle (uh_p, c1, \{mp_1, mp_2\}) \rangle$ is a frequent then $T = \langle (uh, c, \{mp_1\}) \rangle$ which is more general than P is also frequent). So, all the most specific frequent trajectory patterns can lead to some general frequent trajectory patterns.

Definition 4. *(Most Specific Frequent Trajectory) Let P be a trajectory. P is a most specific frequent trajectory, if and only if: $supp(P) \geq \sigma$ and for all T such that $T \leq_p S$; $supp(T) \leqslant \sigma$*

Example 4. Let $\sigma = 0.75$ (i.e. a trajectory is frequent if it appears at least three times in P_{DB}). The trajectory $P = \langle (uh_p, c, \{mp_1, mp_2\}) \rangle$ is frequent. $T = \langle (uh, c, \{mp_1\}) \rangle$ is also frequent. Nevertheless, T is not a most specific frequent trajectory pattern while P is one.

3   Mining Patient Trajectory Patterns

In this section, we present an approach for extracting all the most specific frequent trajectory patterns from patients trajectories. Our approach is called **MMISP** (*Mining Multidimensional Itemsets Sequential Patterns*). The basic idea of MMISP is finding a way to transfer the multidimensional itemsets sequential database into a classical sequential database (i.e. sequence of itemsets). So, MMISP is based on three steps:

1. Extract all the frequent elementary vector v without taking into account the temporal relation between them in each trajectory.
2. Map the frequent elementary vectors which extracted in the first step to an alternate representation. Then, the patient trajectories are encoded by using the new representation of frequent elementary vectors.
3. Apply a standard sequential mining algorithm to enumerate frequent patient trajectories.

3.1 Generating Frequent Elementary Vectors

MMISP starts by searching for the frequent elementary vectors in the trajectories. MMISP firstly studies the patient's trajectory like a set of elementary vectors without taking into account the temporal relation order between them. The support of elementary vector v is defined as follows,

Definition 5. *(Support of elementary vector v, $supp(v)$) Let P_{DB} be a database of patient trajectories with m patients and let $P =< P_1P_2...P_l >$ be a patient trajectory in P_{DB}. The support of elementary vector v is defined as follows*

$$supp(v) = \frac{|\{P \in P_{DB}; \exists j \in [1,..,l];\ P_j \leq_v v\}|}{m}$$

Example 5. In our example, the support of $(gh, r, \{mp_3\})$ is $\frac{3}{4}$, because of:

- $(gh_l, r_1, \{mp_3\}) \in patient_1$ where $(gh_l, r_1, \{mp_3\}) \leq_v (gh, r, \{mp_3\})$.
- $(gh_l, r_2, \{mp_3\}) \in patient_3$ where $(gh_l, r_2, \{mp_3\}) \leq_v (gh, r, \{mp_3\})$.
- $(gh_p, r_2, \{mp_3\}) \in patient_4$ where $(gh_p, r_2, \{mp_3\}) \leq_v (gh, r, \{mp_3\})$.

MMISP generates all the frequent elementary vectors by building a poset $(L, \leq_v)$. Building $(L, \leq_v)$ is done as follows:

- Firstly, we generate the most general elementary vector. In our running example, we have two dimensions with posets H and DG and one dimension with a set MP, so the most general elementary vector is $(t_h, t_d, \{\})$.
- Then, the recursive generation of the new elementary vectors continues by using each previously generated frequent elementary vector (v). For each element $v_1, v_2, v_3 \in v$, we replace v_k, where $k \in [1,3]$ with each of its specialization from the set $special(v_k)$. At each step, we take only the frequent elementary vector which has support greater than σ.

We define the set $special(v_i)$ as follows:

Definition 6. *Let v_i be the ith-element in the vector $v = (v_1, v_2, v_3)$ and let D be the ground set of the component v_i*

$$special(v_i) = \begin{cases} \{a \in D; a \leq v_i \text{ and } \nexists b \in D;\ a \leq b \text{ and } b \leq v_i\} & \text{if } D \text{ is a poset} \\ \{v_i \cup \{a\}; a \in D \setminus v_i\} & \text{if } D \text{ is a set} \end{cases}$$

Example 6. In our example, $special(t_h)=\{uh, gh\}$, $special(t_d)=\{r, c\}$ and $special(\{\}) =\{\{mp_1\}, \{mp_2\}, \{mp_3\}, \{mp_4\}\}$. With $\sigma = \frac{3}{4}$ we can generate new seven frequent elementary vectors from $(t_h, t_d, \{\})$. They are $(uh, t_d, \{\}), (gh, t_d, \{\})$, $(t_h, r, \{\})$, $(t_h, c, \{\})$, $(t_h, t_d, \{mp_1\})$,$(t_h, t_d, \{mp_2\})$ and $(t_h, t_d, \{mp_3\})$. The first and the second are generated by replacing t_h by $child(t_h)$, the third and the forth are generated by replacing t_d by $special(t_d)$, and the rest are generated by replacing $\{\}$ by $special(\{\})$.

The objective of MMISP is to generate all the most specific frequent patient trajectories, thus it retains only the most specific frequent elementary vectors from $(L, \leq_v)$.

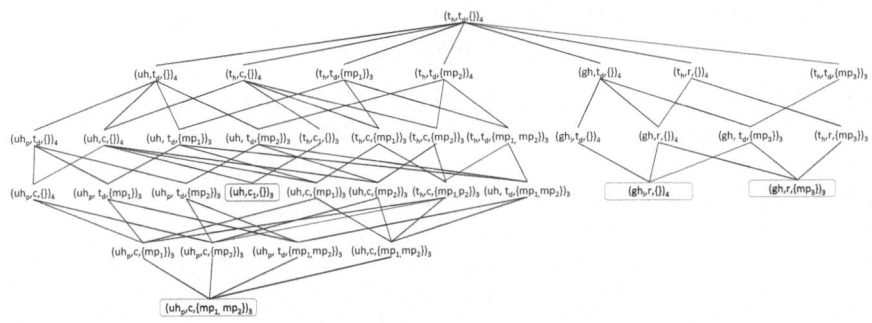

Fig. 2. The poset $(L, \leq_v)$ is generated by taking into account the two posets H and DG in Figure 1 and the set $MP = \{mp_1, mp_2, mp_3, mp_4\}$ with minsup$= \frac{3}{4}$

Definition 7. *(Most specific frequent elementary vector, MSFV) Let v be an elementary vector, v is a most specific frequent elementary vector, if and only if $supp(v) \geq \sigma$ and $\nexists \, v'$ an elementary vector, where $supp(v) = supp(v')$ and $v' \leq_v v$.*

Table 2. The most specific frequent elementary vectors extracted from $(L, \leq_v)$ in Figure 2

id	MSFV
1	$(uh_p, c, \{mp_1, mp_2\})$
2	$(uh, c_1, \{\})$
3	$(gh_l, r, \{\})$
4	$(gh, r, \{mp_3\})$

Example 7. Figure 2 illustrates the generation of all frequent elementary vectors on our example with $\sigma = \frac{3}{4}$. Table 2 shows the hash table of all *MSFV* extracted from $(L, \leq_v)$.

3.2 Mining Patient Trajectory

The next step of MMISP is studying the temporal relation between the most specific frequent elementary vectors extracted in previously step. This is done by taking each patient trajectory $P = \langle P_1 P_2, ..., P_l \rangle$ from the database of patient trajectories P_{DB}, then replacing each elementary vector $P_i \in P$; $i \in [1..l]$ with all elementary vectors $v \in MSFV$ where $P_i \leq_v v$.

Example 8. In our example, the trajectory of $patient_3, \langle (uh_p, c_1, \{mp_4\})(gh_l, r_2, \{mp_3\}) \rangle$, is transformed into $\langle \{(uh, c_1, \{\})\} \{(gh_l, r, \{\}), (gh, r, \{mp_3\})\} \rangle$ because the first elementary vector of $patient_3$, $(uh_p, c_1, \{p_4\})$, can only be replaced with $(uh, c_1, \{\})$ from the *MSFV* set where $(uh_P, c_1, \{p_4\}) \leq_v (uh, c_1, \{\})$ and the second elementary vector of $patient_3$, $(gh_l, r_2, \{mp_3\})$, can be replaced by $(gh_l, r, \{\})$ and $(gh, r, \{mp_3\})$ from the $MSFV$ set.

Table 3 shows the transformation of patient trajectories in P_{DB} by using the set of all most specific frequent elementary vector $MSFV$ in Table 2.

Table 3. Transforming a patient trajectories in Table 1 by using the set of all most specific frequent elementary vector in Table 2

Patients	Trajectories
$patient_1$	$\langle\{(uh_p, c, \{mp_1, mp_2\}), (uh, c_1, \{\})\}\{(uh, c_1, \{\})\}\{(gh_l, r, \{\}), (gh, r, \{mp_3\})\}\rangle$
$patient_2$	$\langle\{(uh, c_1, \{\})\}\{(uh_p, c, \{mp_1, mp_2\})\}\{(gh_l, r, \{\})\}\rangle$
$patient_3$	$\langle\{(uh, c_1, \{\})\}\{(gh_l, r, \{\}), (gh, r, \{mp_3\})\}\rangle$
$patient_4$	$\langle\{(uh_p, c, \{mp_1, mp_2\})\}\{(gh, r, \{mp_3\})\}\{(gh_l, r, \{\})\}\rangle$

We apply a classical sequential pattern mining algorithm (e.g. [6,11,10]) to extract the frequent sequential patterns. This extraction has be done as follows: firstly we transform each patient trajectory into a sequence simple (i.e sequence of itemset like $< \{a, b\}\{a, d\} >$) and then we apply a CloSpan [10] on the transformation patient trajectories. The transformation has be done as follows:

- Each elementary vector in the $MSFV$ set is assigned a unique id which will be used during the mining operation. This is illustrated in Table 2 .
- For each elementary vector v in a patient trajectory in Table 3, we replace v with its id in Table 2.

Example 9. In our example, the patient trajectory $patient_3 = \langle\{(uh, c_1, \{\})\} \{(gh_l, r, \{\}), (gh, r, \{mp_3\})\}\rangle$ in Table 3 is transformed into $\langle\{2\}, \{3, 4\}\rangle$, because $(uh, c_1, \{\})$ has an id 2, $(gh_l, r, \{\})$ has an id 3 and $(gh, r, \{mp_3\})$ has an id 4.

Table 4. Transformed database in Table 3

Patients	Trajectories
$patient_1$	$\langle\{1, 2\}\{2\}\{3, 4\}\rangle$
$patient_2$	$\langle\{2\}\{1\}\{3\}\rangle$
$patient_3$	$\langle\{2\}\{3, 4\}\rangle$
$patient_4$	$\langle\{1\}\{4\}\{3\}\rangle$

Table 5 displays all frequent sequences in their transformed format and the frequent patient trajectories in which identifiers are replaced with their actual values with minsup=$\frac{3}{4}$.

Table 5. Frequent patient trajectory patterns with minsup=$\frac{3}{4}$

Frequent sequential patterns	Frequent patient trajectory patterns	Support
$\langle\{3\}\rangle$	$\langle(gh_l, c)\rangle$	1
$\langle\{2\}\{3\}\rangle$	$\langle(uh, c_1)(gh_l, c)\rangle$	0.75
$\langle\{4\}\rangle$	$\langle(gh, r, \{mp_3\})\rangle$	0.75
$\langle\{1\}\{3\}\rangle$	$\langle(uh_p, c, \{mp_1, mp_2\})(gh_l, c)\rangle$	0.75

4   Results

This section describes the results obtained with MMISP on a set of 2618 trajectories of care of patients from the Burgundy region in France. Using data from
the PMSI, the so-called french case mix system, we reconstituted the sequence
of hospitalizations of patients having undergone surgery for colorectal cancer
between 2006 and 2008, with a one year follow-up. Each event in a sequence was
characterized by the following dimensions : hospital, principal diagnosis, procedures delivered during the stay. The hospital dimension was associated with a
geographical taxonomy of 4 levels : root (France), administrative region, administrative department, hospital. Principal Diagnosis could be described at 5 levels
of the 10th International classification of Diseases (ICD10): root , chapter, block,
3-character, 4-character, terminal nodes. Procedures were represented by their
first CCAM[2] code.

Figure 3 shows the number of discovered patterns at different thresholds according to their length. The total number of patterns grows exponentially for
support below 34%. However, the increase is extremely variable considering the
length of patterns and the number of short patterns (length<6) is still manageable. The high number of length 7 patterns can probably be explained by a
combinatorial effect resulting from a high number of sequences of length 14-15
in the database. They correspond to the patients who underwent chemotherapy
and usually had around 14 and 15 stays for 1 cycle.

Table 6 shows the items appearing in the Principal Diagnoses dimension of
patterns for which support is over 32%. It can be noticed that the ICD10 tree has
been mined at different levels. In the neoplasm branch, the most specific observed
item is of depth 3, Malignant neoplasm of colon. In the branch of "Factors
influencing . . . ", items of depth 4 (chemotherapy session for neoplasm) have been
extracted. Children of "Malignant neoplasms of colon" are not frequent enough
to be extracted, but "chemotherapy session" appears in a sufficient proportion of
trajectories to be seen. Such results could not have been obtained by representing
items at an arbitrary pre-determined level.

Multidimensional sequential patterns can be analysed per se. For example,
the pattern $\langle(\text{Root,C15-C26}, \{\text{Colectomy}\}), (\text{Burgundy,Z00-Z99},\{\})\rangle$ shows that
69% of patients had a colectomy for a digestive cancer and a subsequent stay

---

[2] Classification Commune des Actes Médicaux : the french classification of medical
and surgical procedures.

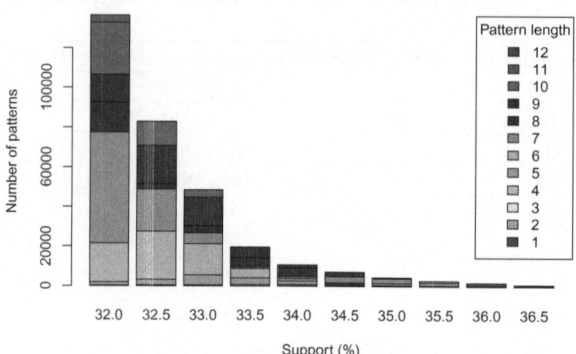

Fig. 3. Number of sequential patterns by support and length (stacked bars)

Table 6. Items extracted in the Principal Diagnosis dimension, (minsupp=32%)

ICD10 level – Item
0– Root
1– Neoplasms
2– Malignant neoplasms of digestive organs
3– Malignant neoplasm of colon
1– Factors influencing health status and contact with health services
2– Persons encountering health services for specific procedures and health care
3– Other medical care
4– Chemotherapy session for neoplasm

in the Burgundy region for complementary treatments and follow-up. This kind of information can help healthcare managers and deciders in planning and organizing healthcare resources at a regional level. Besides, sequential patterns can be seen as condensed representations of the care trajectories. As such, they can be reused as new variables to distinguish subgroups of patients in subsequent analysis. As an illustrative example, we selected a subset of frequent patterns to analyze the relationship between accessibility of care facilities and trajectories of care, as it has been shown that geographical disparities might be related to less favourable outcome in terms of survival. The cumulative driving distance travelled by patients to access facilities along their care trajectory was used to fit a classification tree with patterns as predictors. As expected, longer distances were associated to trajectories involving chemotherapy sessions. However differences were observed according to the occurrence of hospitalizations in specific places. In particular, patients initially treated outside of the burgundy region travelled longer distances. Theses findings can bring experts to investigate specific hypothesis regarding the links between organization of care and health outcomes.

5   Conclusion

Care trajectories of chronic patients can be analysed using administrative databases and sequential pattern mining. The MMISP algorithm relies on external knowledge to enrich the mining process and produces results with appropriate levels of granularity. Experiments on data from the french case-mix information system show that MMISP is flexible enough to reflect both the relational and temporal structure of the care trajectories.

References

1. Batal, I., Sacchi, L., Bellazzi, R., Hauskrecht, M.: A temporal abstraction framework for classifying clinical temporal data. In: AMIA Annu. Symp. Proc., pp. 29–33 (2009)
2. Fetter, R.B., Shin, Y., Freeman, J.L., Averill, R.F., Thompson, J.D.: Case mix definition by diagnosis-related groups. Med. Care 18(2), 1–53 (1980)
3. Huang, Z., Lu, X., Duan, H.: On mining clinical pathway patterns from medical behaviors. Artif. Intell. Med. 56(1), 35–50 (2012)
4. Kim, M., Shin, H., Su Chung, T., Joung, J.-G., Kim, J.H.: Extracting regulatory modules from gene expression data by sequential pattern mining. BMC Genomics 12(suppl. 3), S5 (2011)
5. Nolte, E., McKee, M. (eds.): Caring for people with chronic conditions: A health system perspective. Open University Press (2008)
6. Pei, J., Han, J., Mortazavi-Asl, B., Pinto, H., Chen, Q., Dayal, U., Hsu, M.: Prefixspan: Mining sequential patterns by prefix-projected growth. In: ICDE, pp. 215–224 (2001)
7. Petitjean, F., Masseglia, F., Gançarski, P., Forestier, G.: Discovering significant evolution patterns from satellite image time series. Int. J. Neural. Syst. 21(6), 475–489 (2011)
8. Plantevit, M., Laurent, A., Laurent, D., Teisseire, M., Choong, Y.W.: Mining multidimensional and multilevel sequential patterns. ACM Trans. Knowl. Discov. Data 4, 4:1–4:37 (2010)
9. Srikant, R., Agrawal, R.: Mining sequential patterns: Generalizations and performance improvements. In: Apers, P.M.G., Bouzeghoub, M., Gardarin, G. (eds.) EDBT 1996. LNCS, vol. 1057, pp. 3–17. Springer, Heidelberg (1996)
10. Yan, X., Han, J., Afshar, R.: Clospan: Mining closed sequential patterns in large datasets. In: SDM, pp. 166–177 (2003)
11. Zaki, M.J.: Spade: An efficient algorithm for mining frequent sequences. Mach. Learn. 42(1-2), 31–60 (2001)

Similarity Measuring between Patient Traces for Clinical Pathway Analysis

Zhengxing Huang, Xudong Lu, and Huilong Duan*

College of Biomedical Engineering and Instrument Science of Zhejiang University,
The Key Laboratory of Biomedical Engineering, Ministry of Education, China
duanhl@zju.edu.cn

Abstract. Clinical pathways leave traces, described as activity sequences with regard to a mixture of various latent treatment behaviors. Measuring similarities between patient traces can profitably be exploited further as a basis for providing insights into the pathways, and complementing existing techniques of clinical pathway analysis, which mainly focus on looking at aggregated data seen from an external perspective. In this paper, a probabilistic graphical model, i.e., Latent Dirichlet Allocation, is employed to discover latent treatment behaviors of patient traces for clinical pathways such that similarities of pairwise patient traces can be measured based on their underlying behavioral topical features. The presented method, as a basis for further tasks in clinical pathway analysis, are evaluated via a real-world data-set collected from a Chinese hospital.

1 Introduction

Clinical pathway analysis (CPA) has experienced increased attention over the years due to its importance to health-care management in general and to its usefulness for capturing the actionable knowledge and interesting insights to administrate, automate, and schedule the best practice for individual patients in clinical pathways [1]. A carefully inspection of patient traces can support health-care organizations to analyze and improve clinical pathways. By measuring similarities between patient traces, it can be useful to health-care organizations for a number of reasons including better overall clinical pathway management and maintenance [2].

In order to measure similarities between patient traces, it is a common technique to provide a measure of distance in the features' space, e.g., to compute similarity primarily by using activity sequences of patient traces. Traditional techniques of sequence similarity measures are focused on direct matching between sequences applying commonly the classical distance concepts. They may not be appropriate to measure similarities between patient traces for clinical pathways.

In this study, we employ a probabilistic graphical model, i.e., Latent Dirichlet Allocation (LDA) [3], to measure similarities between patient traces for clinical

---

* Corresponding author.

N. Peek, R. Marín Morales, and M. Peleg (Eds.): AIME 2013, LNAI 7885, pp. 268–272, 2013.

pathways. The assumption made is that the possibly treatment behaviors of patient traces in clinical pathways may be represented by a relatively small number of simple and common behavioral topics, which can be combined with the original patient traces to measure similarities between traces. We use real-life data from Zhejiang Huzhou Central Hospital of China to evaluate the proposed method.

2 Method

In this study, we assume that it is possible to sequentially record various kinds of clinical activities in clinical pathways. In general, hospital information systems record such information. To introduce the patient trace representation model and our similarity measure method, we first define the following concept.

Definition 1. *Let $\mathcal{A}$ be the set of clinical activities. A patient trace is a non-empty sequence of clinical activities performed on a particular patient, i.e., $c = \langle a_1, a_2, \ldots, a_n \rangle$, where $a_i \in \mathcal{A}$ $(1 \leq i \leq n)$ is a particular clinical activity. For convenience, let $c(i)$ be the ith clinical activity in the trace. A patient trace repository R is a multi-set of patient traces.*

In general, LDA helps to explain the behavioral similarity of patient traces by grouping clinical activities into unobserved sets. A mixture of these sets then constitutes the observable patient trace. The generative process of LDA is as follows. For each patient trace c, a mixture of topic proportion $\theta_c \sim Dir(\alpha)$ is sampled from a Dirichlet distribution parameterized by the hyperparameter α. Each clinical activity a in a trace is generated by first sampling a topic t from a multinomial distribution $t \sim Mult(\theta)$, and then sampling $a \sim Mult(\phi_t)$ also from a multinomial distribution. Given a treatment behavioral topic t, each $\phi_t \sim Dir(\beta)$ is sampled from a Dirichlet distribution parameterized by β. In LDA, each patient trace c is a mixture of topics represented by θ_c and each topic t is a distribution over all activities represented by $\phi_{t,a} = Pr(a|t)$.

Using this generative model, the treatment behavioral topic assignments for clinical activities can be calculated based on the current topic assignment of all the other clinical activity positions. More specifically, the topic assignment is sampled from:

$$Pr(t_i = t | t_{\neg i}, c) = \frac{n_{t,\neg i}^a + \beta}{\sum_{b \in A} n_t^b + \beta |A|} \frac{n_{c,\neg i}^t + \alpha}{\sum_{j \in K} n_c^{t_j} + \alpha K} \tag{1}$$

where $t_i = t$ represents the assignment of the ith occurrence to topic t, $t_{\neg i}$ represents all treatment behavioral topics assignments not including the ith occurrence, K is the number of topics, $|A|$ is the number of clinical activities, $n_{t,\neg i}^a$ is the number of times activity a is assigned to topic t, not including the current instance, and $n_{c,\neg i}^t$ is the number of times topic t is assigned to the patient trace c, not including the current instance.

From these count matrices, we can estimate the topic-activity distribution θ and trace-topic distribution ϕ by,

$$\theta_{t,a} = \frac{n_t^a + \beta}{\sum_{b \in A} n_t^b + \beta|A|}, \quad \phi_{c,t} = \frac{n_c^t + \alpha}{\sum_{t \in T} n_c^t + \alpha K} \tag{2}$$

Exact inference in LDA is generally intractable. In particular, we use Gibbs sampling to estimate the parameters of the LDA model. Once we have learned the model parameters, we can measure the similarity between patient traces. In particular, for a specific trace c in the repository R, we obtain the topic distribution $\overrightarrow{\theta_c} = \{\hat{\theta}_{c,t_1}, \hat{\theta}_{c,t_2}, \cdots, \hat{\theta}_{c,t_K}\}$, where each $\hat{\theta}_{c,t_i}$ is the posterior estimate of θ_{c,t_i} for the treatment behavioral topic t_i $(1 \leq i \leq K)$. Upon this, we are able to calculate the similarity between two traces c and c^* $(c, c^* \in R)$ as follows:

$$sim(c, c^*) = \frac{\sum_{t \in T} \hat{\theta}_{c,t} \times \hat{\theta}_{c^*,t}}{\sqrt{\sum_{t \in T} \hat{\theta}_{c,t}^2} \sqrt{\sum_{t \in T} \hat{\theta}_{c^*,t}^2}} \tag{3}$$

To illustrate the feasibility of the proposed approach, we present a specific application, i.e., patient trace clustering, based on similarities between patient traces. Patient trace clustering helps reveal the underlying characteristics and commonalities among a large collection of traces. The information extracted by clustering can also facilitate subsequent analysis, for instance, to extract common treatment patterns of execution in the traces, or speed up trace indexing and anomaly detection. A reasonable similarity measure $sim(c, c')$ is critical for the patient trace clustering. The objective of the clustering methods that work on similarity measure function is to maximize the intra cluster similarities and minimize the inter cluster similarity. In this study, we adopted a hierarchical micro-clustering algorithm to generate partitions of patient traces in the repository.

3   Case Study

The experimental data set was extracted from Zhejiang Huzhou Central hospital of China. In the experiments, we build a specific patient trace repository of clinical pathways of several specific types of cancer, i.e., branchial lung cancer, colon cancer, rectal cancer, breast cancer, and gastric cancer, from the system. The collected data is from 2007/08 to 2009/09. In detail, there are 258 traces, 11028 clinical activities with 266 activity types. In the experiments, we conducted topic analysis for the experimental repository using LDA with the different number of treatment behavioral topics ($K = 1, 2, \cdots, 20$). The Dirichlet prior α and β of LDA are set to 0.2 and 0.1. The number of iterations of Gibbs sampling is set to 10000. In addition, to expand the number of trials when we construct the LDA model, we adopt a fivefold cross-validation strategy.

As shown below, the presented method is evaluated by a specific application, i.e., patient trace clustering. In particular, we compare the presented LDA-based similarity measure with the traditional edit-distance-based similarity measure

[4]. In the following experiments, we refer to LDA-based similarity measure with K-topic model ($K = 1, 2, \cdots, 20$) as LDA-K, and edit-distance-based similarity measure as ED.

The benchmark clusters are identified from the experimental repository. In particular, we use the first diagnosis code to category patient traces. As mentioned above, 5 categories, i.e., bronchial lung cancer, colon cancer, rectal cancer, breast cancer, and gastric cancer, are extracted from the repository, which can be used as benchmark clusters for evaluating the overall performance of clustering. For evaluation on patient trace clustering, we measure "$F_{0.5}$" to calculate the accuracy of the system on a per-trace basis and then build a global score for all patient traces in the repository.

Using the benchmark clusters, we can evaluate clustering performance on $F_{0.5}$. In particular, by taking the maximum value of $F_{0.5}$ (among different merging thresholds ε from 0.0 to 0.4), we compare the performance of ED and LDA-K ($K = 1, 2, 3, \cdots, 20$). As shown in Figure 1, when the number of topics is larger than a particular value ($K \geq 8$), the $F_{0.5}$ is quite stable. Certainly, $k \approx 8$ is probably the suitable number of topics for the experimental patient trace repository.

Now we study the impact of the parameter ε on both the experimental results, where ε is the merging threshold in the clustering step. We vary the value of ε from 0.0 to 0.4. Figure 2 shows the results of ED and LDA-8 (using the 8-topic model). From Figure 2, we can see that LDA-8 can provide significant improvement over ED. The maximum value of $F_{0.5}$ of LDA-8 is 0.6422, which is nearly 56% better than ED (0.1044). Note that when margining threshold is zero, each patient trace is classified into a specific cluster. That explains why both curves have the same starting value of $F_{0.5}$ shown in Figure 2. In addition, the inclusion of latent topics increases similarity among patient traces. As a result, when merging threshold is small, LDA-8 does not show an advantage over ED. When merging threshold increases, LDA-8 obtains better results on $F_{0.5}$ than ED, while the latter remains stable regardless of the value of ε. In particular, LDA-8 provides the most significant improvements when ε is 0.15. Note that we can always obtain better results with LDA-8 except $\varepsilon = 0$ in comparison with

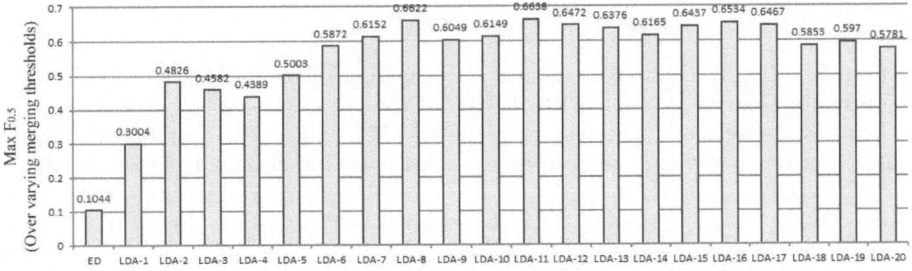

Fig. 1. Performance of clustering using ED and LDA with different latent treatment behavioral topic models on the experiment repository

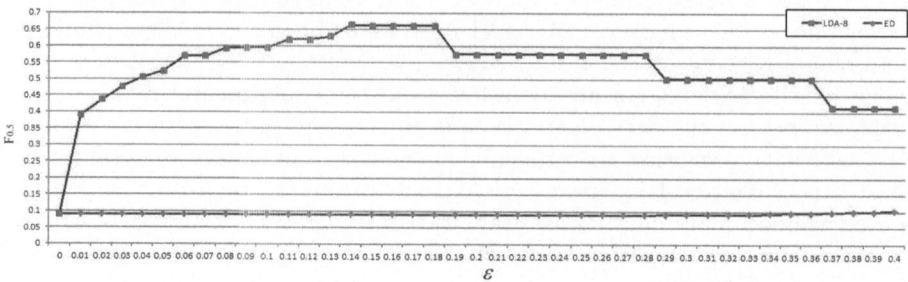

Fig. 2. The comparison between ED and LDA-8 on patient trace clustering

ED. It indicates that the treatment behavioral features have more influences on the similarity measure and subsequent analysis (e.g., patient trace clustering) than the sequential order of clinical activities of the traces.

4   Conclusion

In this paper, we have introduced a new method of measuring the similarities between patient traces for clinical pathways, which can profitably be exploited as a basis for further tasks of CPA, e.g., critical/essential treatment behaviors can be detected, analyzed, and optimized based on the topic analysis presented in this study, association rules between recognized anomalies and patient states can be derived, etc. We will address these tasks by exploiting the potential of the proposed similarity measure between patient traces and its applications, as a crucial advantage over traditional techniques for clinical pathway analysis and optimization.

Acknowledgment. This work was supported by the National Nature Science Foundation of China under Grant No 81101126.

References

1. Huang, Z., Lu, X., Duan, H.: Latent treatment topic discovery for clinical pathways. Journal of Medical Systems 37(2), 1–10 (2013)
2. Combi, C., Gozzi, M., Oliboni, B., Juarez, J.M., Marin, R.: Temporal similarity measures for querying clinical workflows. Artificial Intelligence in Medicine 46(1), 37–54 (2009)
3. Blei, D.M., Ng, A.Y., Jordan, M.I.: Latent dirichlet allocation. Joural of Machine Learning Research 3, 993–1022 (2003)
4. Gusfield, D.: Algorithms on strings, trees and sequences, Computer Science and Computational Biology. Cambridge University (1997)

Instantiating Interactive Narratives from Patient Education Documents

Fred Charles[1], Marc Cavazza[1], Cameron Smith[1], Gersende Georg[2],
and Julie Porteous[1]

[1] School of Computing, Teesside University, Middlesbrough, United Kingdom
[2] Haute Autorité de Santé, 2 Avenue du Stade de France, Saint-Denis, France
{f.charles,m.o.cavazza,c.g.smith,j.porteous}@tees.ac.uk,
g.georg@has-sante.fr

Abstract. In this paper, we present a proof-of-concept demonstrator of an Interactive Narrative for patient education. Traditionally, patient education documents are produced by health agencies, yet these documents can be challenging to understand for a large fraction of the population. In contrast, an Interactive Narrative supports a game-like exploration of the situations described in patient education documents, which should facilitate understanding, whilst also familiarising patients with real-world situations. A specific feature of our prototype is that its plan-based narrative representations can be instantiated in part from the original patient education document, using NLP techniques. In the paper we introduce our interactive narrative techniques and follow this with a discussion of specific issues in text interpretation related to the occurrence of clinical actions. We then suggest mechanisms to generate direct or indirect representations of such actions in the virtual world as part of Interactive Narrative generation.

Keywords: Interactive Narratives, Natural Language Processing, Patient Education.

1   Introduction and Objectives

Patient information and education are major challenges for public health. The main medium for patient education is currently constituted by documents produced by health agencies, which are not unlike clinical guidelines, albeit simplified ones. Yet these documents may still be challenging for many patients to understand. The constraints governing completeness and accuracy of the content of these documents are not always compatible with readability and memorisation, and what is considered simplified by health professionals may still look complex to some patient populations. For all these reasons, there has been an increasing interest in the use of new media, in particular interactive ones to promote patient education. The use of technologies traditionally associated with interactive entertainment for this type of application is often referred to as "serious games". The development of these interactive systems is

N. Peek, R. Marín Morales, and M. Peleg (Eds.): AIME 2013, LNAI 7885, pp. 273–283, 2013.
© Springer-Verlag Berlin Heidelberg 2013

time consuming, and not always principled: it is important, particularly in a medical context, that the underlying knowledge model should properly capture the causal structure of clinical situations and of patient's actions and decisions, so as to allow the exploration of appropriate behaviour. The recent development of interactive narrative technologies precisely supports such knowledge models by ordering relevant situations dynamically, taking into account user interaction with the world objects and characters. These technologies are predominantly based on Planning, which supports action representation and causal propagation; actions can be associated with animations in the virtual world, with the plan execution generating a real-time 3D animation.

In this paper, we describe a proof-of-concept, yet fully-implemented, prototype of an interactive narrative for patient education. The narrative features the main stages of bariatric surgery (surgical therapy for obese patients) which requires accurate patient information and education. One specific aspect of our work is that the instantiation of the underlying narrative actions can use information directly extracted from the original patient education documents using NLP techniques. This should in the long term enable to speed up the development of interactive narratives using a set of default actions and representations, to be later instantiated to the specific knowledge content of individual patient documents. The next section gives an overview of the system through its interactive 3D visual presentation. We then describe in more detail our interactive narrative engine, based on state-of-the-art planning techniques. We show how individual action representations can be parameterised from the original text of the patient document using off-the-shelf dependency parsing; in the process we identify specific issues on the nature of reference actions described in the text. Throughout the paper the discussion is illustrated by examples from our prototype.

2   Previous and Related Work

In recent years, there has been significant interest in serious games for health applications, including patient education, with too many applications being developed to be listed here [1]. These were based on bespoke development without significant use of AI techniques. In [2], Bers et al. explored storytelling techniques for cardiac care in children, again, however, not using recent AI-based interactive storytelling techniques. Previous research in the analysis of documents to construct virtual worlds has concentrated on the creation of virtual scenes [3], or the analysis of procedural instructions to be executed by a virtual agent [4]. The latter project has also proposed methods to parameterise action representations from natural language [5]. In comparison to previous work, our research aims at developing state-of-the-art interactive narratives capturing as much domain knowledge as possible. This is not simply about staging the events described in a narrative text but giving the most appropriate representation of the underlying situations. Further, in contrast to previous work on understanding instructions, our application defines default knowledge not conveyed by the text, and seeks to contextualise it from the document's statements. The knowledge instantiation from text that we propose, although more attainable than complete understanding, still constitutes a form of deep understanding. Deep natural language understanding in Medicine [6], which aims at connecting semantic representations of linguistic input to domain knowledge, has not attracted much attention in recent years, as the emphasis has been on large coverage systems that are often shallow in knowledge terms.

3 System Overview

Our prototype application can be described as a serious game for patient education about obesity surgery[1] such as gastric reduction or bypass techniques Developed in partnership with the French Health Agency (HAS, Haute Autorité de Santé) it is meant to facilitate the understanding of the various stages of therapy including eligibility, preparation, decision making and post-operative care. The interactive narrative is driven by user exploration of the virtual environment, and uses cinematic principles to blend phases of active user exploration and the staging of visual explanations (for instance for surgery). Its principles and underpinning techniques will be described in more detail in the next sections.

System development was based on UDK, a state-of-the-art professional game engine with its inherent layout, interaction and navigation procedures, which supports high-quality visualisation of environments and characters' animations, including emotional expressions. The graphic database, which references all the objects of the environment as well as providing a basic navigational mechanism, is interfaced with the knowledge layer. This makes it possible to gain direct access to an object location and to plan characters' motion accordingly. The game operates in third-person mode, with the user controlling an avatar representing an overweight patient (male or female). Interaction takes place through various means including navigation through the environment, the avatar's physical interaction with objects and the user responding to prompts. When some actions take place that explain specific situations (e.g. the patient undergoing certain investigations or surgery), the avatar becomes part of the action without being constantly under the control of the user, not unlike "quicktime events" in recent computer games.

In contrast to traditional serious games, which rely on scripted behaviour of characters, our system features an interactive storytelling engine, embedding the main actions and situations of bariatric surgery. The main difference with ad hoc scripted rules is that it constitutes a consistent driver for all actions in the environment. This firmly places the unfolding of the narrative under the control of user interaction which allows an exploration of the underlying knowledge by the user. Another difference is the enhanced modularity of behaviour description that derives from using an AI technique such as Planning, which avoids tedious encoding of procedural behaviour.

---

[1] http://www.has-sante.fr/portail/jcms/c_765529/
obesite-prise-en-charge-chirurgicale-chez-l-adulte

The action takes place in a virtual hospital whose full-scale surface would be equivalent to 3500 m², and contains most of the features (reception, waiting area, doctor's office, examination rooms) and equipment of a hospital (MRI, X-Ray, Operating theatre). Navigation through this space is correlated to the patient education data/knowledge, as the various stages of the patient's care are naturally associated with specialised areas of the hospital. As such, it constitutes a natural way of exploring the domain as well as rehearsing real-world actions that the patient will perform such as hospital visits. Because part of the education of patients refers to their daily activities, we have also extended the virtual environment to incorporate the patient's kitchen and living area in their home: this makes it possible to stage and rehearse actions, e.g. those related to eating habits, as part of the overall narrative. For example, these eating habits form a condition for the level of preparation of the patient for bariatric surgery. At this stage the simulation of eating habits is essentially centred on the choice of healthy foods. The user is presented with a clear choice between low and high-calorie meals in the virtual kitchen.

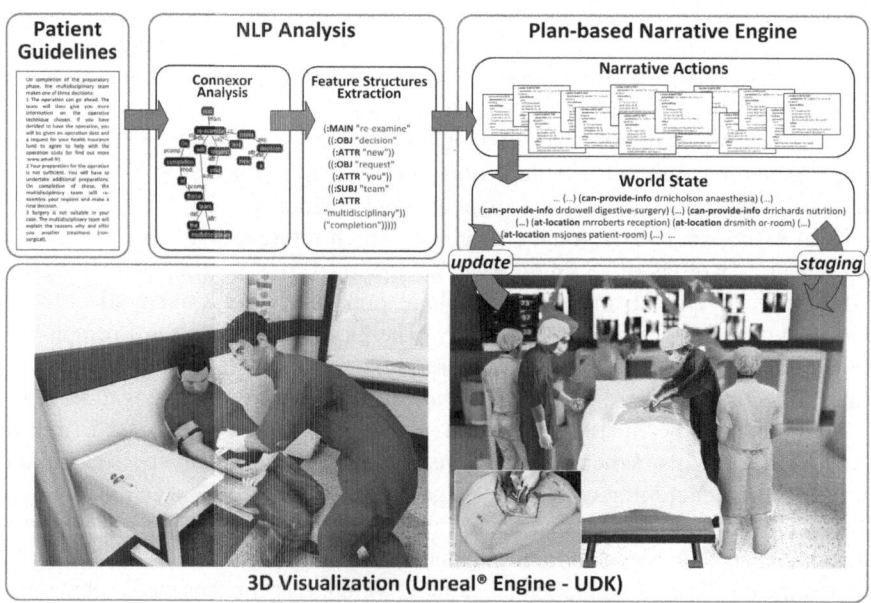

Fig. 1. System Architecture: the Interactive Narrative is generated by a Planning system whose actions, corresponding to the clinical domain, are staged in real-time in the virtual environment

Figure 1 describes the system architecture and its main mode of operation. The end-system consists of the interactive narrative, in which a fully interactive virtual world is under the control of a dynamic plan representing the various possible stages of bariatric surgery, whose execution responds to real-time user interactions. The left-side of the figure shows the instantiation procedure from the original patient education document. The initial representation contains planning operators representing typical domain actions such as `consultation-with-specialist`, `blood-test`, `gastro-endoscopy-test`, `laparoscopy-procedure`, `complications-post-op`, `prompt-interaction-surgery-decision`, ..., which form the basis for an interactive narrative based on these actions. They constitute the domain knowledge, including significant default and specialised knowledge, not part of the patient education documents. The objective of the instantiation module is to customise the baseline planning representation, centred on standard domain actions, to capture the actual text intentions and stage appropriately the actions mentioned. This is exploring how to tune interactive narratives endowed with baseline domain knowledge in one medical specialism to the specific contents of medical documents (patient education, clinical guidelines). Our implementation uses standard rather than temporal planning, which is not a limitation as most actions are centred on the user, without any real need for synchronisation or scheduling. Action duration is based on implicit time although it is possible to define mandatory duration for actions (e.g. waiting time, examinations).

4   Interactive Narrative Techniques

The rationale for using interactive narrative in simulation and training, since early work such as [7] [8], is to support a better integration of knowledge access within user experience. On one hand, the dramatization of situations improves their realism, allowing the user to better relate to them. On the other hand, interactive aspects provide a unique mechanism with which to test the appropriateness of the user behaviour throughout the application itself, without having to stage *ad-hoc* tests.

Interactive storytelling has developed significantly over the past ten years with Planning emerging as one of the most popular AI techniques supporting it. Our system capitalises on our previous research in the area [9], and consists of a plan-based interactive narrative describing the various phases of bariatric surgery from the patient's perspective. In essence, an interactive narrative assembles a coherent story by selecting a subset of all possible actions consistent with the context and the user actions: it is this combinatorial aspect that truly distinguishes it from any sort of pre-scripted narrative (even with optional actions or explicit branching points). From a dynamic perspective, the story actions are continuously generated to take into account the evolution of context, including the user's actions. User influence takes various forms:

- the presence of the user at a given location is a condition for some actions to be possible (it is obviously the case for most actions involving the user, but the order of actions is also important, so visiting an exam room before going through admissions will not trigger an examination action)
- the user can be prompted to accept or refuse a course of action (the user would need to accept surgical intervention if offered this possibility during consultation)
- previous actions may have an influence on a later situation (e.g. eating habits may disqualify the user for surgery while incorrect preparation may make certain investigations, or even make surgery on that day, impossible)

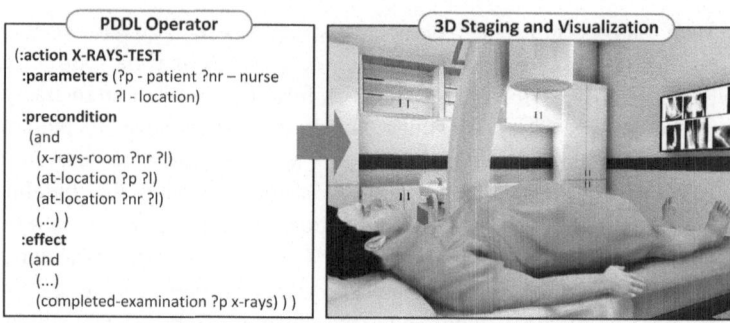

Fig. 2. Actions as the basis for the Interactive Narrative. Each elementary action, represented as a Planning operator, has associated 3D animations that enable the action's visualisation in the virtual world.

The interactive narrative system is based on the state-of-the-art Metric-FF planner [10]. Action representation follows the PDDL standard [11], whose format is well-suited to describe the occurrence conditions of an action and its immediate consequences. For instance, Figure 2 shows the PDDL operator for the action x-rays-test corresponding to the x-ray examination of the patient, which is presented staged on the right of the figure. A typical PDDL operator is composed of a set of parameters (here: a patient, a nurse, and a location), a set of pre-conditions which must be validated (here: the patient and the nurse must be located in the x-ray examination room) and a set of effects which are a description of the domain updates that this specific action will engender (here: this action specifies that the examination has been successfully undertaken by the patient; which may become a pre-condition for subsequent actions). Since this planner can produce a complete solution for this domain complexity in less than 300ms on average, rather than developing a bespoke real-time version of the planner, we have modified its activation so that, at each world state update, it can be invoked to recompute the remainder of the narrative.

To support an Interactive Narrative in the virtual environment, the Planner (including its domain) is integrated into the visualisation environment at two levels: action visualisation and domain update. Planning actions (x-rays-test, check-preparatory-phase, patient-ready-for-surgery, anaesthesia) are visualised through associated UDK actions: these provide high-level control of virtual actors relieving the planner of low-level motion control (i.e. path planning when navigating to a target destination), and can concentrate on the high-level narrative actions. All aspects of low-level motion are associated with a library of appropriate animations. A high-level action can be parameterised with its constituent actors, objects and execution modalities so as to limit the overhead in knowledge elicitation: this parameterisation can also be performed using NLP analysis of the patient documents, as described in the next section. While the baseline knowledge representation is elaborated manually (in the form of a planning domain enhanced with default knowledge on actions' roles), the parameterisation of actions and situations from the patient education document is ultimately meant to take place with no further human intervention. To compensate for the partial recognition of some events by the NLP module, the system should rely on its default knowledge.

As well as executing high-level actions in the virtual world, UDK's embedded event system can detect changes resulting from the user's avatar's physical interaction with the virtual world. Through this mechanism the planning domain can be updated in real-time; e.g. the location of the user's avatar can be passed to the planning domain, as can the location of other relevant objects (e.g. patient files, admin documents), or the user's response to prompts in certain situations (acknowledgement of information or approval during pre-op consultations).

5   NLP Tuning of Baseline Knowledge Representation

Our objective is not to merely visualise explicit actions or instructions described in the document. We also want to demonstrate the possibility of tuning a baseline knowledge representation to the actual text contents and thereby capturing some of the document's true intention of conveying knowledge about specific situations. The first step is to devise a baseline set of actions for the bariatric surgery domain, many actually quite generic (admissions, consultations…), as described above.

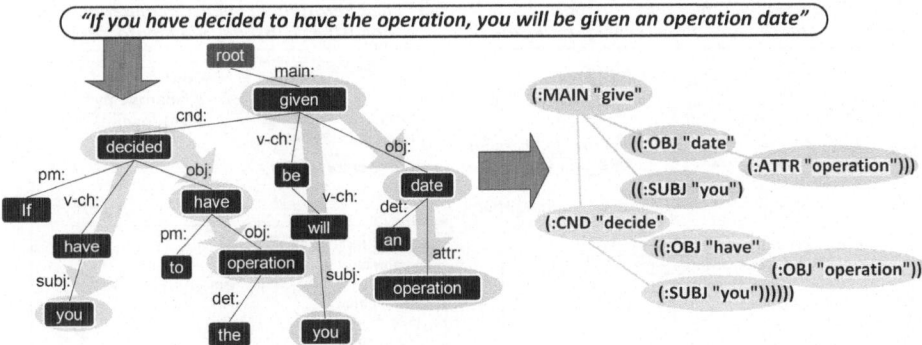

Fig. 3. Extracting feature structures (right) from the Connexor dependency parse (left) of a sentence (top). Features are nested with the main action "give" having various dependents including the condition "decide" which has dependents of its own.

A second step is to perform an NLP analysis on individual text sentences in order to extract the information relevant to the instantiation of these planning operators. NLP analysis is based on the off-the-shelf Connexor (http://www.connexor.com/nlplib/) parser for English: we have developed a dedicated module to extract feature structures from the Connexor dependency parse (Figure 3). This step operates on a sentential basis, not making use of discourse markers or phenomena: part of this is covered by the consistency properties of the virtual world, although on an empirical basis only. For instance, coreference to surgical interventions is assumed to refer to the same operation, unless there are specific adverbial markers.

Many actions represented as PDDL operators cover both generic and specific situations. Generic actions such as appointments, admissions, or certain examinations can be reused across applications. The specific nature of an action derives from either its potential for instantiation (in which case it can share a common base with other actions in related domains), or its unique nature (e.g. domain-dependant surgical interventions). This is the case for instances of consultations (between various physicians and patients, in different settings, for different purposes such as diagnosis, assessment, eligibility, etc). The instantiation of PDDL operators is a two-step process comprising recognition and parameterisation. Recognition proceeds top-down from the list of available actions, which are associated with a set of lexical units behaving like a *Synset* that are compared to the contents of the latest output of the NLP step. Once a PDDL action is recognised, parameterisation proceeds in a similar way but processes the case structure using a set of ad-hoc procedures extracting case values (up to a list depth of two) and looking for patterns to be matched to predefined PDDL structures. The simplest form of parameterisation is to actually set the type of actors (e.g. various medical professional such as mapped in PDDL to: anaesthetist, endocrinologist, dietician, psychiatrist, psychologist) as they are mentioned, by recognising lexical entries for actors in the case structure, associated with a compatible case. More complex parameterisation is required for the phenomena described next.

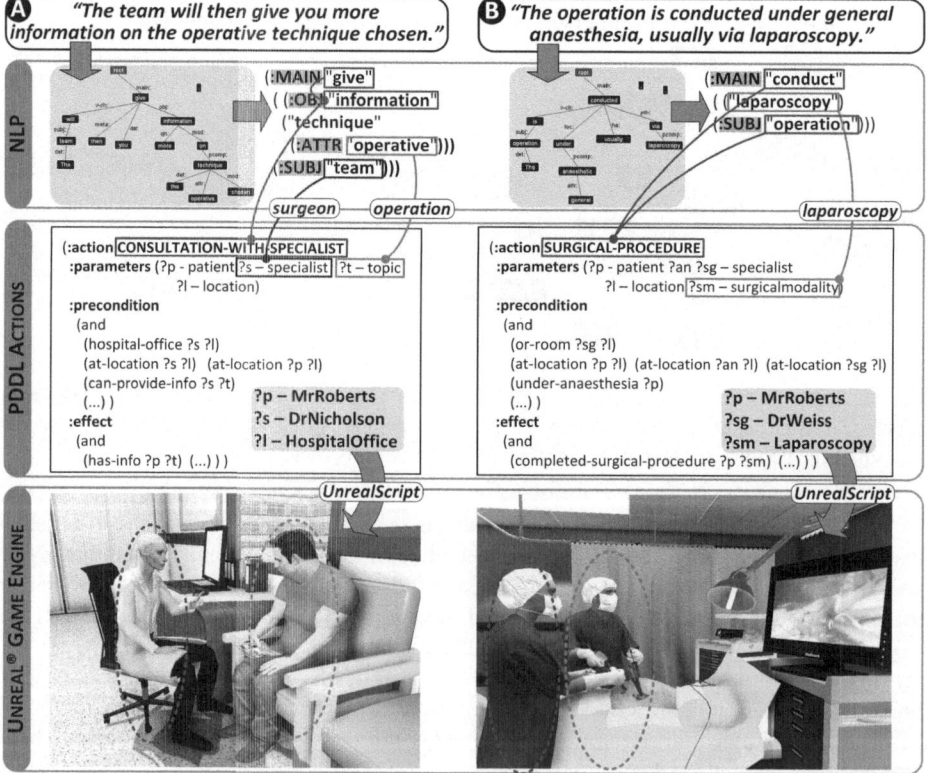

Fig. 4. Indirect or direct reference to a similar action depending on text contents. On the left, the main action staged in the virtual world is a consultation whose topic is surgery (this is parameterised using an appropriate leaflet). On the right, the text actually describes the surgical intervention itself and results in the instantiation of the corresponding scene.

One of the specific phenomena encountered at the interface of natural language understanding and visualisation is one of indirect reference: in other terms, when is an action mentioned in the text the subject of a discussion and when is the text actually describing the course of action itself. Figure 4 illustrates examples of both: the indirect references (A) include the provision of information about an operation ("*The team will then give you more information on the operative technique chosen.*") while the direct references (B) correspond to all actual descriptions of surgery ("*The operation is conducted under general anaesthesia, usually via laparoscopy.*"). One of the first steps is to devise a heuristic that could determine the type of reference at hand, and the simplest heuristic is to consider the case (ergative versus accusative) of the word referring to the surgical intervention. To be applicable, this heuristic should take into account various sorts of negation when terms denoting surgery are the subject of a sentence (as in "*Surgery is not suitable in your case.*").

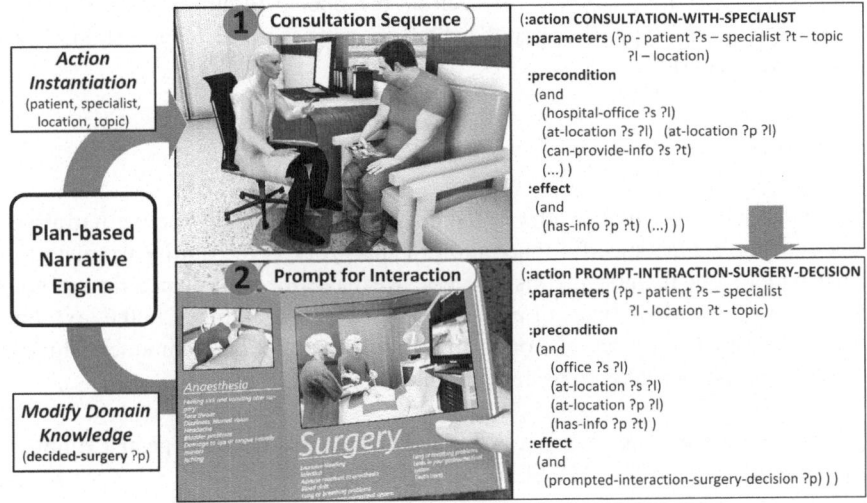

Fig. 5. An action sequence including a user prompt: in specific situations the user is prompted for a response, such as in the case of informed consent represented here

We have incorporated such heuristics as part of the mapping functions. The difference in instantiation, and later in the execution of the interactive narrative is that two very different actions would be instantiated, one being an information action whose object is the surgical intervention, and the other being an action corresponding to surgery itself, which can be further parameterised with any available details of the surgical technique itself.

The recognition of conditional statements is of particular relevance to properly stage corresponding actions in the virtual world. The significance of conditional statements has to be analysed from the specific perspective of the staging of the interactive narrative, considering the entire course of action rather than simply on a sentential basis. Conditional statements are related to the reference issue discussed above, in that they may affect whether to stage the resulting action or not. However, in many cases they describe conditions that are very much part of the default course of action. In that sense, the mapping process can be used to inform the completion of certain high-level pre-conditions. More interestingly, the same mechanism can also support the long-term consequences of user actions, which are an essential part of a proper exploration of the document knowledge. The interactive narrative contains a kitchen and living area, which makes it possible to simulate the eating habits of the patient through user control. The outcome of any such interactions are passed back to the system, which in turns registers eating habits, to be used later as a pre-condition for those conditional actions requiring it (related to surgery eligibility).Another interpretation is to convert conditional statements into interactive scenes requiring user input. Conditional statements in which the user is a subject (valid for active voice only) form such a basis. For instance, any conditional statement about user acceptance of a therapy, including bariatric surgery itself, will have to instantiate a `Prompt-Interaction-Surgery-Decision` such as the one in Figure 5. This is achieved through a specialised type of operator, which prompts the user for a response during an interactive scenario.

6   Conclusions

We have described the first results in the development of an interactive narrative for patient education. One specific innovation of this work is the ability to relate to the original patient documents: in this process, we have identified specific integration issues such as the various types of reference to an action mentioned in the text. Future work will benefit from more elaborate Information Extraction techniques which will increase the proportion of actions actually instantiated from text.

Acknowledgements. This work was funded in part by the European Commission through the FP7 Open FET "MUSE" Project (ICT-296703).

References

1. Graafland, M., Schraagen, J.M., Schijven, M.P.: Systematic review of serious games for medical education and surgical skills training. British Journal of Surgery 99(10), 1322–1330 (2012)
2. Bers, M.U., Ackermann, E., Cassell, J., Donegan, B., Gonzalez-Heydrich, J., DeMaso, D.R., et al.: Interactive storytelling environments: Coping with cardiac illness at Boston's Children's Hospital. In: SIGCHI Conference on Human Factors in Computing Systems, pp. 603–610. ACM Press/Addison-Wesley Publishing Co. (1998)
3. Coyne, B., Sproat, R.: WordsEye: An automatic text-to-scene conversion system. In: 28th Annual Conference on Computer Graphics and Interactive Techniques (SIGGRAPH 2001), pp. 487–496. ACM, New York (2001)
4. Badler, N., Webber, B.L., Steedman, M., Achorn, B., Becket, W., Di Eugenio, B., et al.: The AnimNL Project. Research in the Language, Information and Computation Laboratory of the University of Pennsylvania. Technical Report MS-CIS-95-07, pp. 94–95 (1995)

5. Badler, N., Allbeck, J., Zhao, L., Byun, M.: Representing and parameterizing agent behaviours. In: Computer Animation, Geneva, Switzerland, pp. 133–143. IEEE Computer Society (2002)
6. Cavazza, M., Doré, L., Zweigenbaum, P.: Model-based natural language understanding in medicine. In: Lun, K.C., Degoulet, P., Piemme, T., Rienhoff, O. (eds.) Medical Informatics (MedInfo 1992), pp. 1356–1361 (1992)
7. Kenny, P., Parsons, T.D., Gratch, J., Leuski, A., Rizzo, A.A.: Virtual Patients for Clinical Therapist Skills Training. In: Pelachaud, C., Martin, J.-C., André, E., Chollet, G., Karpouzis, K., Pelé, D. (eds.) IVA 2007. LNCS (LNAI), vol. 4722, pp. 197–210. Springer, Heidelberg (2007)
8. Swartout, W.R., Gratch, J., Hill Jr, R.W., Hovy, E., Marsella, S., Rickel, J., Traum, D.: Toward virtual humans. AI Magazine 27(2), 96–108 (2006)
9. Porteous, J., Cavazza, M., Charles, F.: Applying planning to interactive storytelling: Narrative control using state constraints. ACM Trans. Intell. Syst. Technol. 1(2), article 10, 21 pages (2010)
10. Hoffmann, J.: The Metric-FF Planning System: Translating "Ignoring Delete Lists" to Numeric State Variables. Journal of Artificial Intell. Research. 20, 291–341 (2003)
11. Gerevini, A., Long, D.: BNF Description of PDDL3.0 (2005), http://zeus.ing.unibs.it/ipc-5/

Added-Value of Automatic Multilingual Text Analysis for Epidemic Surveillance

Gaël Lejeune, Romain Brixtel, Charlotte Lecluze, Antoine Doucet,
and Nadine Lucas

Normandy University – UNICAEN, GREYC CNRS UMR-6072
Boulevard du Maréchal Juin, CS 14032 Caen Cedex France
firstname.lastname@unicaen.fr

Abstract. The early detection of disease outbursts is an important objective of epidemic surveillance. The web news are one of the information bases for detecting epidemic events as soon as possible, but to analyze tens of thousands articles published daily is costly. Recently, automatic systems have been devoted to epidemiological surveillance. The main issue for these systems is to process more languages at a limited cost. However, existing systems mainly process major languages (English, French, Russian, Spanish...). Thus, when the first news reporting a disease is in a minor language, the timeliness of event detection is worsened. In this paper, we test an automatic style-based method, designed to fill the gaps of existing automatic systems. It is parsimonious in resources and specially designed for multilingual issues. The events detected by the human-moderated ProMED mail between November 2011 and January 2012 are used as a reference dataset and compared to events detected in 17 languages by the system DAnIEL2 from web articles of this time-window. We show how being able to process press articles in languages less-spoken allows quicker detection of epidemic events in some regions of the world.

1 Introduction

The early detection of disease outbursts is critical for epidemic surveillance. One of the main sources of information is the press articles written all over the world, since diseases erupt anywhere. With the increasing amount of newspapers accessible on the Internet, tens of thousands of articles are available online daily. It has become one of the main lead to improve the early detection of epidemic events using computer driven information filtering and extraction.

Many projects use press articles for extracting epidemic events. ProMED [8] or GPHIN [9] rely on human intervention to extract epidemic events from press articles. Other systems are fully automated like BioCaster [13], EpiSpider [15], PULS [16] or DAnIEL [6]. Another approach is to propose an aggregation of events already collected by other systems, it is the choice of the researchers working on HealthMap [3].

One of the limitation encountered in classical natural language processing is the number of languages covered by any single system [14]. Table 1 shows the

N. Peek, R. Marín Morales, and M. Peleg (Eds.): AIME 2013, LNAI 7885, pp. 284–294, 2013.
© Springer-Verlag Berlin Heidelberg 2013

different languages[1] processed by the previously cited systems and an estimation of the number of speakers for each language [4]. English (en) and Russian (ru) are handled by all the systems previously mentioned. Arabic (ar), Chinese (zh), French (fr), Portuguese (pt) and Spanish (es) are also well represented with 4 to 5 systems able to process them. The Japanese BioCaster system covers three Asian languages in addition: Korean (ko), Thai (th) and Vietnamese (vi). The DAnIEL system processes five European languages, including two, Polish (pl) and Greek (el), not available in other systems.

Table 1. Languages processed by existing epidemic surveillance systems and an estimation of their number of speakers (10^6)

	ar	cz	de	el	en	es	fi	fr	it	ko	nl	no	pl	pt	ru	sv	th	tr	vi	zh
#Speakers	255	10	166	13	1,000	500	5	200	62	78	21	5	46	240	277	8	60	75	86	1,151
GPHIN	✓				✓	✓		✓							✓					✓
HealthMap	✓				✓	✓		✓						✓	✓					✓
PULS					✓										✓					
Biocaster	✓				✓	✓		✓	✓	✓				✓	✓		✓		✓	
DAnIEL				✓	✓			✓					✓		✓					✓
DAnIEL2	✓	✓	✓	✓	✓	✓	✓	✓	✓		✓	✓	✓	✓	✓	✓		✓		✓

Twenty languages are covered by at least one system, having a total of four billions of speakers. However, this number is over-estimated since people speaking two languages are counted twice. That means that the dropped-out languages represent more than 40% of the world's population. It is true that many events are eventually reported in English or another major language appearing in Table 1. However, two problems arise. First, it is extremely difficult to judge silence: some diseases can be ignored. Second, even in the case of delayed report, the problem is the time elapsed for response to be effective [10]. While medical reports use major languages for diffusion, press articles may report an epidemic event in a local language, but this valuable information is often by-passed.

Work has already been carried out on the impact of covering multiple languages on the informations extracted in different domains. Piskorski *et al.* [12] showed a significant improvement of the quality of the information extracted when more languages were processed. Lyon *et al.* [7] studied specifically this impact for epidemic surveillance by comparing BioCaster, EpiSPIDER and Health-Map. But, the number of languages involved (five) was quite small with respect to the number of languages for which press articles are published online (more than 20 languages on Google News for instance).

An important issue is to check to which extent the number of processed languages will give an added-value to the early detection of diseases and thus epidemic events. To this purpose, this study proposes a comparison between human-produced ProMED-mail, taken as a reference, and an extended implementation called DAnIEL2, based on the multilingual system DAnIEL [6,5].

---

[1] ISO 639-1 codes : http://www.loc.gov/standards/iso639-2/php/code_list.php

ProMED approach is efficient, with many experts employed, but it is costly and slow. ProMED is an expert-based relevance gold standard. To the contrary, DAnIEL (Data Analysis for Information Extraction in any Language) claims to minimize the marginal cost for the analysis of new languages but handles only six languages, French, English, Russian, Greek and Polish (fr, en, ru, el, pl), plus Chinese (zh).It was used to process up to a total of 17 languages, allowing comparison of both geographic coverage and timeliness of event detection with ProMED.

The DAnIEL2 system processes 11 more languages than DAnIEL and 9 European languages not available yet in other systems. This study will focus on the impact of extended multilingual analysis for timeliness. Epidemic events detected through both ProMED and DAnIEL2 will be compared. The impact of multilingual automatic coverage will be measured on the timeliness of event detection and the coverage of different regions of the world.

ProMED and DAnIEL2 are presented in Section 2. The datasets for each approach are described in Section 3. The results obtained for both approaches are presented in Section 4. The conclusions and perspectives of this study are detailed in Section 5.

2   Multilingual Surveillance with ProMED and DAnIEL2

This section presents the characteristics of the two compared information systems: Section 2.1 for ProMED and Section 2.2 for DAnIEL2.

2.1   The ProMED System

ProMED-mail publishes daily reports disseminating information on disease outbreaks worldwide [8,2]. ProMED moderators, with the help of ProMED subscribers, screen different sources of information to produce their reports. The main sources exploited are local media reports, official reports and information from local observers. The number of different languages used on the field is not known. ProMED published reports in English since the beginning of the project in 1994. Reports are now also available in French, Portuguese, Russian and Spanish. ProMED relies on the accuracy of its human experts analysis to produce highly reliable reports [11]. It is therefore used as a source in automatic information processing [1]. The question raised is whether the complexity of the reporting chain has a bad impact on the timeliness of public reporting.

2.2   The DAnIEL2 System

DAnIEL2 takes advantage of genre-based analysis, requiring little expert knowledge in medicine and making it easier to use for various languages [6]. A quick presentation of the approach used by DAnIEL is made here, more details can be found in a previous article [5]. DAnIEL uses the collective style of journalists in order to build one multilingual core analysis, relying on expert knowledge on news discourse rather than on specific languages syntax. Decisions are taken at text-level. DAnIEL relies on a character-level analysis, so it can handle languages where graphical words do not exist (for instance Chinese).

DAnIEL2 compares the text and the disease names found in its database extracted from Wikipedia. Repetitions of substrings of disease names occurring at key positions are used to check if the document is relevant for epidemic surveillance and which disease is involved. The same algorithm is used for detecting the location. If no location is found *implicit location* heuristic is used: the location of the reported event is the same as the location of the source. DAnIEL2 extracts disease-location pairs in 17 languages, as given in Table 2. They include 7 European languages not yet reported to our knowledge, for automatic news filtering: Czech (cz), German (de), Finnish (fi), Norwegian (no) and Swedish (sv). The datasets used for this evaluation are described in the next section.

3   Datasets for ProMED and DAnIEL2

The ProMED reference dataset has been built with reports presented in Section 3.1. For DAnIEL2 a corpus of press articles was constituted using available data processed by DAnIEL and extra material presented in Section 3.2.

3.1   ProMED Dataset

The reports produced by ProMED-mail from October 2011 to February 2012 have been automatically harvested on the ProMED website[2]. The data hereby obtained includes 2,558 structured reports in 5 main languages (English, Russian, Portuguese, Spanish and French). In this period, a few reports are also available in Thai and Vietnamese but for these particular languages, no reports were available after the 4th of November.

Each report from ProMED contains a triplet describing the event: the disease name, the location of the event and the date of the report. For each unique disease-location pair, the earliest report date in the period was kept to get *first reports*. The events appearing only in October were excluded from the dataset since the objective was to measure the delay between first reports of DAnIEL2 and ProMED, for the same disease-location pair. It was therefore necessary to extend the time-window to feed DAnIEL2 with press articles that give hints for the November 2011 events. In the same way, events reported by ProMED in February 2012 were kept, to check if they were connected to events reported by DAnIEL2 in January.

Details about the data collected are presented in Table 2. Reports in English represent more than 50% of the total number of reports published by ProMED. Most of these reports come from the analysis of a newswire in English. The importance of English in this corpus is due to the fact that is used as a *lingua franca* for many reports and news. Table 3 shows that English sources allow

---

[2] http://www.promedmail.org/

ProMED to cover a high number of different locations (153) and a great number of disease-location pairs. For English three locations (USA, Australia and United Kingdom) are involved in 40% of the reports.

Table 2. ProMED reports repartition by language and by month

	English	French	Portuguese	Russian	Spanish	Thai	Vietnamese
#Reports	**819**	148	129	127	220	25	78
#November 2011	285	3	26	49	68	25	78
#December 2011	291	33	15	28	78	0	0
#January 2012	193	62	48	37	37	0	0
#February 2012	54	50	40	33	38	0	0

Table 3. ProMED reports details: number of diseases, locations and disease-location pairs per language

	English	French	Portuguese	Russian	Spanish	Thai	Vietnamese
#Reports	819	148	129	127	220	25	78
#Diseases	**183**	33	34	47	58	10	31
#Locations	**151**	37	23	15	46	8	26
#Disease-location pairs	**366**	63	40	55	46	12	26

3.2   Corpus for DAnIEL2

The corpus used by DAnIEL2 in this study was constituted by downloadable data processed by DAnIEL, plus extra press articles belonging to the same time-window collected from Google News health category for Arabic (ar), Chinese (zh), Czech (cz), English (en), French (fr), German (de), Italian (it), Norwegian (no), Portuguese (pt), Russian (ru), Spanish (es), Swedish (sv) and Turkish (tr). For Finnish (fi), Greek (el) and Polish (pl), articles have been collected in health categories of national newspapers and health-related RSS feeds.

The DAnIEL2 corpus contains documents from the 1st of October 2011 to the 31th of January 2012. The repartition by language and by date are shown in Table 4. 40% of these documents are written in languages probably not covered by ProMED. Since DAnIEL2 does not process original html files, a phase of pre-processing was needed to allow the system to process the documents. For this purpose, an in house unpublished scrapping tool was used to clean non relevant content of original html pages. The scrapping quality differed according to the source/language of the documents. This could worsen results as compared with the original system.

DAnIEL2 needs a list of disease names and countries for each language to perform its analysis. These lists were obtained by translations provided by Wikipedia of a list of most common disease names in English. From the corpus mentioned above, DAnIEL2 extracted 1,571 epidemic events. They are detailed in Table 5 and Table 6. 32% of these events were extracted from documents in

Table 4. Number of articles by language and by month for the DAnIEL2 dataset

	ar	cz	de	el	en	es	fi	fr	it	nl	no	pl	pt	ru	sv	tr	zh
Articles	3,093	208	2,509	1,380	4,742	4,389	132	2,132	703	876	311	801	1,362	1,896	196	239	1,122
10.2011	780	42	631	220	1,301	952	23	412	173	197	52	182	343	240	41	74	243
11.2011	819	99	809	289	1,181	1,020	37	506	100	172	61	199	205	312	72	79	174
12.2011	735	37	712	400	1,082	1,517	32	832	224	253	111	122	485	487	37	52	303
01.2012	759	30	357	471	1,178	900	40	382	206	254	87	298	329	857	46	34	402

Table 5. Number of epidemic events extracted by DAnIEL2 by language and by month

	ar	cz	de	el	en	es	fi	fr	it	nl	no	pl	pt	ru	sv	tr	zh
#Reports	30	15	63	83	285	230	7	142	54	24	11	140	92	296	26	0	73
October 2011	3	2	7	17	63	42	2	17	12	2	0	15	30	49	2	0	12
November 2011	5	7	13	25	75	62	0	50	27	4	4	37	22	84	10	0	25
December 2011	12	3	24	18	67	71	3	48	15	12	4	36	25	54	9	0	14
January 2012	10	3	19	23	80	55	2	27	8	6	3	52	15	109	5	0	22

Table 6. Details for epidemic events extracted by DAnIEL2: number of diseases, locations and disease-location pairs per language.

	ar	cz	de	el	en	es	fi	fr	it	nl	no	pl	pt	ru	sv	tr	zh
#Reports	30	15	63	83	285	230	7	142	54	24	11	140	92	296	26	0	73
#Diseases	7	6	12	13	33	29	6	32	22	9	6	19	23	21	7	0	16
#Locations	3	2	19	7	55	35	2	39	9	7	1	45	14	70	2	0	6
#Disease-location pairs	12	9	32	25	161	115	4	85	28	11	6	83	50	141	10	0	23

languages probably not covered by ProMED. Few events were found in Arabic, despite the high number of documents in this language reported in Table 4. Turkish was the only language in which the system extracted no event.

Table 6 exhibits the different diseases and locations involved in the events extracted. Major languages permitted to extract events in many countries, e.g. the 285 events signaled in English cover 55 different locations. Less common languages like Finnish or Swedish seem to be more specific to their country.

4   Evaluation

This evaluation aims to assess the benefit, if any, of the parsimonious scheme of DAnIEL for multilingual epidemic surveillance reproduced by DAnIEL2. The main hypothesis is that a local disease outburst is first reported in a local language. Consequently, there may be a delay between this very first report and the report in main languages processed by existing systems. The geographic repartition of the time elapsed between the publication of the event by ProMED and DAnIEL2 will also be studied.

From the datasets presented in Section 3, 167 events were in common between ProMED and DAnIEL2, which amounts to 15% (over 1,082). This figure is consistent with the study made by Lyon *et al.* [7]: the intersection between different epidemic surveillance systems is quite small. Table 7 shows a sample of events first reported by ProMED and by DAnIEL2.

Table 7. Examples of events detected by both systems with the differences in timeliness in number of days. A positive (resp. negative) value indicates that ProMED (resp. DAnIEL2) reported earlier. Language of detection and date of publication for ProMED and DAnIEL2 are indicated.

Pair		Timeliness	ProMED		DAnIEL2	
Disease	Location	(days)	Lang.	Date	Lang.	Date
Cholera	Zimbabwe	+43	en	2011-12-18	en	2012-01-30
Influenza	Canada	+27	en	2011-11-04	en	2011-12-01
Scabies	Spain	+18	en	2011-12-25	es	2012-01-12
Hepatitis	Russia	+14	en	2011-11-22	ru	2011-12-06
Botulism	Finland	-11	en	2011-11-01	fi	2011-10-21
Rabies	Russia	-12	ru	2011-12-21	fr	2011-12-09
Jap. Encephalitis	India	-22	en	2011-11-02	en	2011-10-11
Norovirus	Russia	-29	ru	2011-12-27	ru	2011-11-28

From the 167 events extracted by both approaches, 37% were first reported by DAnIEL2 (Table 8). DAnIEL2 gives better results than ProMED for regions where it processed more documents in local languages. Most examples are found in European countries, for instance Czech Republic, Finland or Greece. To the contrary, in America, ProMED is clearly better. Table 9 exhibits the comparison between the two systems. When DAnIEL2 shows a better timeliness it is frequently due to the fact its coverage in languages is complementary. However, the impact of this coverage was difficult to assess for some languages and some countries, such as Turkey and Norway, for lack of common data.

Table 8 shows that the result of the comparison between the two systems is mainly affected by the locations. ProMED clearly outperforms DAnIEL2 in English-speaking and Spanish-speaking regions, specially North and Central America. ProMED also has a better timeliness in Portuguese-speaking and French-speaking regions in America and Africa. DAnIEL2 reports sooner on local events in African regions where news are published in Arabic.

ProMED is rarely slower than DAnIEL2 when reports are coming from articles in major languages (with the exception of Russian), confirming the idea that in major languages human analysis remains the reference [1]. Table 9 shows that the repartition of languages allowing DAnIEL2 to outperform ProMED is quite large. The hypothesis that a local language conveys information on its country of origin is valid, but not sufficient. It is also common that a neighbor country signals a disease when it spreads, thus becoming an epidemic event. This fact is correlated with the accuracy by zone presented in Table 8.

Table 8. Locations of events first reported by ProMED and DAnIEL2

	ProMED		DAnIEL2	
	Languages	#First reports	Languages	#First reports
France,Portugal,Spain,UK	en,es,fr,pt	31	en,es,fr,nl,pt	12 (28%)
Rest of Europe	en,fr	7	cz,de,el,fi,fr,it,sv	12 (63%)
Russia,Ukraine	en,ru	4	pl,ru	6 (60%)
North Africa	en,fr	5	ar,fr	3 (38%)
Rest of Africa	en,fr,pt	10	fr	3 (23%)
China,India	en	5	cn,en	3 (38%)
Rest of Asia	en	6	cn,ru	9 (60%)
North America	en,es	22	en,es	4 (15%)
Central,South America	en,es,pt	16	en,es,pt	9 (36%)
All locations	5	106	15	61 (37%)

Table 9. Repartition by language of events first reported by ProMED and DAnIEL2,
"-" means a non-covered language

	ar	cn	cz	de	el	en	es	fi	fr	it	nl	no	pl	pt	ru	sv	tr
ProMED	-	-	-	-	-	54	27	-	5	-	-	-	-	15	6	-	-
DAnIEL2	1	3	2	3	4	8	8	2	8	3	3	0	2	4	9	1	0

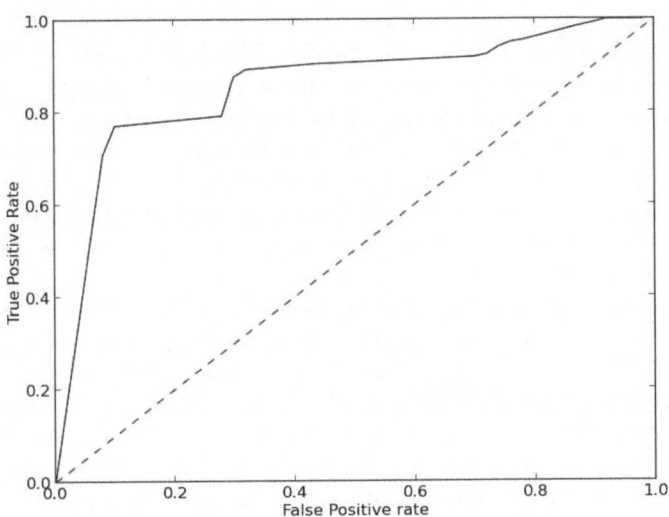

Fig. 1. ROC curve for DAnIEL2 (plain black). Results for a manually annotated subset
of 2,089 documents. The Area Under the Curve is 0.86.

DAnIEL2 shows better results in Europe, in countries where it is the only system to analyze reports in the local languages, whereas it is outperformed by ProMED in other countries. The influence of Russian is difficult to assess since few events are reported by both systems. Their results are comparable in Russia and Ukraine. DAnIEL2, however, reported events occurring in Asia earlier than ProMED, thanks to documents in Russian.

We ran an evaluation on a manually annotated subset containing 2,089 documents in five languages (el, en, pl, ru and zh). Figure 1 presents the ROC curve of DAnIEL2 results. The area under the curve for this experiment is 0.86. One can see that DAnIEL2 achieves a good equilibrium between True Positive (TP) rates and False Positive (FP) rates. For instance, for a 0.91 TP rate the system shows a 0.31 FP rate.

5   Conclusion

This paper proposed a comparative study of ProMED-mail, the reference human-based analysis for epidemic surveillance, and a multilingual automatic surveillance system, DAnIEL2, checked for 17 languages including little-studied ones. It was derived from an existing system called DAnIEL intended to process multiple languages at a limited cost. ProMED proposes highly reliable human-produced reports and seems to mostly use sources in the five major languages used to disseminate reports (English, French, Portuguese, Russian and Spanish). DAnIEL2, on the other hand, is a light automatic system using only parsimonious resources. It was indeed possible to extend the previous DAnIEL coverage by eleven languages in a very short time, each addition taking a couple hours once the crawling was done. This is a major breakthrough in disease monitoring.

From the events signaled by ProMED in a three-month time period, around 15% (167 over 1,082) were also extracted by DAnIEL2 and thus allowed comparison on a common set. The overlap between the two systems is quite small but the figures are comparable to those presented in previous studies [7]. The two characteristics studied here were the timeliness of the first description of events and their geographic repartition. Among the 167 epidemic events, roughly two out of three was first extracted by ProMED, leaving one third first detected automatically. DAnIEL2 gave worst results than ProMED for regions where English, French, Portuguese and Spanish are the main languages. The timeliness of the two approaches was comparable in Russian.

However, DAnIEL2 offers an important improvement for countries where it takes advantage of the local language news, mainly in Europe in the experiment related here. The human-based approach and the style-based automatic approach are complementary. When human analysts for one language are available, DAnIEL2 is outperformed. To the contrary, ProMED gives a great importance to English and Spanish. It is noteworthy that ProMED also relies on automatic surveillance systems, heavily if not exclusively based on English. This causes a bias in geographic coverage.

DAnIEL2 offers an interesting added-value for parts of the world where minor languages are used. It would clearly be worthwhile to test more languages for Africa and Asia, all the more so since the cost is low. The parsimonious approach behind this system seems to be well adapted for covering these regions. Therefore, the complementarity between opposite approaches seems to be important in terms of massive multilingual coverage. To complete this study, relevance tests to compare DAnIEL2 with reference data are needed to assess its sensitivity. This study shows that an automatic system does not replace manual systems, but could well assist experts to filter the web news and help detect epidemic events early.

References

1. Collier, N.: Towards cross-lingual alerting for bursty epidemic events. Journal of Biomedical Semantics 2(supp. 5), 1–11 (2011)
2. Cowen, P., Garland, T., Hugh-Jones, M.E., Shimshony, A., Handysides, S., Kaye, D., Madoff, L.C., Pollack, M.P., Woodall, J.: ProMED-mail as an electronic early warning system for emerging animal diseases: 1996 to 2004. JAVMA 229(7), 1090–1099 (2006)
3. Freifeld, C.C., Mandl, K.D., Reis, B.Y., Brownstein, J.S.: Healthmap: Global infectious disease monitoring through automated classification and visualization of internet media reports. Journal of the American Medical Informatics Association 15(2), 150–157 (2008)
4. Katsiavriades, K., Qureshi, T.: The 30 most spoken languages of the world (2007), http://www.krysstal.com/spoken.html
5. Lejeune, G., Brixtel, R., Doucet, A., Lucas, N.: DAnIEL: Language Independent Character-Based News Surveillance. In: Isahara, H., Kanzaki, K. (eds.) JapTAL 2012. LNCS, vol. 7614, pp. 64–75. Springer, Heidelberg (2012)
6. Lejeune, G., Doucet, A., Yangarber, R., Lucas, N.: Filtering news for epidemic surveillance: Towards processing more languages with fewer resources. In: 4th Workshop on Cross Lingual Information Access, pp. 3–10 (2010)
7. Lyon, A., Nunn, M., Grossel, G., Burgman, M.: Comparison of Web-Based Biosecurity Intelligence Systems: BioCaster, EpiSPIDER and HealthMap. Transboundary and Emerging Diseases 59(3), 223–232 (2011), http://dx.doi.org/10.1111/j.1865-1682.2011.01258.x
8. Madoff, L., Freedman, D.: Detection of Infectious Diseases Using Unofficial Sources. In: Infectious Diseases: A Geographic Guide, pp. 11–21. Wiley-Blackwell (2011)
9. Mawudeku, A., Blench, M.: Global Public Health Intelligence Network (GPHIN). In: 7th Conference of the Association for Machine Translation in the Americas (AMTA), pp. 7–11 (2006)
10. Mondor, L., Brownstein, J.S., Chan, E., Madoff, L.C., Pollack, M.P., Buckeridge, D.L., Brewer, T.: Timeliness of nongovernmental versus governmental global outbreak communications. Emerging Infectious Diseases 18(7), 1184–1187 (2012)
11. Morse, S.S.: Public health surveillance and infectious disease detection. Biosecurity and Bioterrorism: Biodefense Strategy, Practice, and Science 10(1), 6–16 (2012)
12. Piskorski, J., Belyaeva, J., Atkinson, M.: Exploring the usefulness of cross-lingual information fusion for refining real-time news event extraction: A preliminary study. In: Proceedings of Recent Advances in Natural Language Processing, pp. 210–217 (2011)

13. Son, D., Quoc, H.N., Ai, K., Collier, N.: Global Health Monitor - A Web-based system for detecting and mapping infectious diseases. In: Proc. International Joint Conference on Natural Language Processing (IJCNLP), pp. 951–956 (2008)
14. Steinberger, R.: A survey of methods to ease the development of highly multilingual text mining applications. Language Resources and Evaluation, 1–22 (2011)
15. Tolentino, H., Kamadjeu, R., Fontelo, P., Liu, F., Matters, M., Pollack, M.P., Madoff, L.: Scanning the Emerging Infectious Diseases Horizon - Visualizing ProMED Emails Using EpiSPIDER. Advances in Disease Surveillance 2, 169 (2007)
16. Yangarber, R., von Etter, P., Steinberger, R.: Content collection and analysis in the domain of epidemiology. In: Proceedings of DrMED-2008: International Workshop on Describing Medical Web Resources (2008), http://www.mendeley.com/research/content-collection-analysis-domain-epidemiology/

An Approach for Query-Focused Text Summarisation for Evidence Based Medicine

Abeed Sarker[1], Diego Mollá[1], and Cécile Paris[2]

[1] Centre for Language Technology,
Department of Computing, Macquarie University,
Sydney, NSW 2109, Australia
{abeed.sarker,diego.molla-aliod}@mq.edu.au
http://www.clt.mq.edu.au
[2] CSIRO – ICT Centre,
Locked Bag 17, North Ryde, Sydney, NSW 1670, Australia
cecile.paris@csiro.au
http://www.csiro.au

Abstract. We present an approach for extractive, query-focused, single-document summarisation of medical text. Our approach utilises a combination of target-sentence-specific and target-sentence-independent statistics derived from a corpus specialised for summarisation in the medical domain. We incorporate domain knowledge via the application of multiple domain-specific features, and we customise the answer extraction process for different question types. The use of carefully selected domain-specific features enables our summariser to generate content-rich extractive summaries, and an automatic evaluation of our system reveals that it outperforms other baseline and benchmark summarisation systems with a percentile rank of 96.8%.

Keywords: Automatic Text Summarisation, Medical Natural Language Processing, Evidence Based Medicine, Query-focused Summarisation.

1 Introduction

Evidence Based Medicine (EBM) is a practice that requires practitioners to incorporate the best evidence from published research, when answering clinical queries. Due to the plethora of electronically available medical publications (e.g., PubMed[1] indexes over 22 million articles), practitioners generally face the problem of information overload. Research has shown that practitioners often fail to comply with EBM guidelines because of time constraints, particularly at point-of-care [7]. As such, there is a strong motivation in this domain for systems that can summarise text, according to the information needs expressed by practitioners. In this paper, we present an extractive, query-focused, single document summarisation system that relies on statistics generated from a specialised corpus. In particular, our system incorporates novel, domain-specific statistical

---

[1] http://www.ncbi.nlm.nih.gov/pubmed/ (Accessed on: 5th March, 2013).

N. Peek, R. Marín Morales, and M. Peleg (Eds.): AIME 2013, LNAI 7885, pp. 295–304, 2013.

features involving query types, medical semantic types, and associations between semantic types. We show that our approach outperforms other summarisation systems, with a percentile rank of 96.8%, in this challenging domain.

2   Related Work

While automatic text summarisation research has made significant progress in various domains (e.g., news), the medical domain still lacks complete end-to-end summarisation systems. This domain is particularly challenging because of a number of reasons including the complex nature of medical text and the large volume of domain-specific terminologies, concepts, and relationships that must be taken into account [1]. Some of the work on summarisation for this domain has been carried out under the broader research area of Question Answering (QA). [10] present a QA system whose summarisation component relies on the classification of information present in medical abstracts into PICO (**P**opulation, **I**ntervention, **C**omparison and **O**utcome) elements [14]. Text segments classified as *Outcome* are presented as the final summary. [13] perform polarity identification of medical sentences and show that summarisation can be improved with the use of this information. More recently, [2] proposed the AskHermes[2] system that performs multi-document summarisation via key-word identification and clustering of information. Our recent pilot study on query-focused summaristion [15] revealed that the content of extracted summaries can be improved via the use of target-sentence-specific statistics and specialised corpora.

In terms of automatic evaluation of summarisation systems, the most popular tool is perhaps ROUGE (Recall-Oriented Understudy for Gisting Evaluation) [9], which provides several evaluation metrics that have been shown to have strong correlation with human judgements. Recently, [4] have shown that ROUGE scores for extractive summaries within a domain follow a normal distribution with most combinations of sentences giving a ROUGE score that is very close to the mean. The relative performance of a system can be measured by computing its percentile rank from the score distribution.

3   Data and Methods

We used a publicly available corpus that is specialised for the task of summarisation for EBM [11]. The corpus is collected from the Journal of Family Practice[3]. The corpus consists of a set of records, $R = \{r_1 \ldots r_m\}$. Each record, r_i, contains one clinical query, q_i, so that we have a set of questions $Q = \{q_1 \ldots q_m\}$. Each r_i has associated with it a set of one or more bottom-line answers to the query, $A_i = \{a_{i1} \ldots a_{in}\}$. For each bottom-line answer of r_i, a_{ij}, there exists a set of detailed justifications (single-document summaries) $L_{ij} = \{l_{ij1} \ldots l_{ijo}\}$.

---

[2] http://www.askhermes.org
[3] http://www.jfponline.com

Each detailed justification l_{ijk} is in turn associated with at least one source document d_{ijk}. Thus, our corpus has a set of source documents, which we denote as $D = \{d_{ij1} \dots d_{ijo}\}$, each d_i consisting of a set of n sentences $S_i = \{s_{i0} \dots s_{in}\}$ and a title t_i. In the research work described in this paper, we use the set of questions from our corpus (Q), the set of human authored summaries (L), and the set of referenced documents (D); and divide the corpus into two sets: training $(R_{TRAIN}: 1388$ documents$)$ and evaluation $(R_{EVAL}: 1319$ documents$)$.

3.1 Generation of Ideal Summaries

Our intent is to generate a query-focused summary from each d_i by extracting three sentences from it which most closely resemble the associated human authored summary (l_i). We define the ideal extractive summary of d_i to be a set of three sentences, $S_{BEST,i} \subseteq S_i$, from d_i, that produce the highest ROUGE-L f-score when compared with l_i. We choose three as our target number of sentences in line with past research in this area [10]. To identify $S_{BEST,i}$ for d_i, we generate all possible three sentence combinations for d_i, $S_{combs,i}$, and then perform an exhaustive search to select the combination that has the best ROUGE-L f-score. We thus have a set of ideal summaries from each d_i, $S_{BEST} = \{S_{BEST,0} \dots S_{BEST,1388}\}$, and we use this set to derive much of the required statistics. The target of our summarisation task is therefore to use statistics derived from S_{BEST} to attempt to select a set of sentences, S_{sel}, from an unseen document d, such that S_{sel} has the highest scoring ROUGE-L f-score among all the three-sentence combinations in d. We select a summary containing a set of three sentences, $S_{summary,i} = \{s_{first}, s_{second}, s_{third}\}$, from document d_i, using separate statistics, wherever appropriate, for each of s_{first}, s_{second} and s_{third}. We now discuss the features for which we derive statistics.

3.2 Generation of *Question Type* Independent Statistics

We apply two broad categories of statistics for the summarisation process. The first category involves features that are independent of the *types* of the questions:

Relative Sentence Position. Given a document d_i, we want to assign three scores to each sentence in S_i. Each score assigned to a sentence is an estimate of a probability measure, and depends on which target summary sentence $(tn = 1, 2,$ or $3)$ we are attempting to select. The score for a sentence with relative position j is:

$$RP_{s_{ij}} = P(s_{ij}|tn) \tag{1}$$

i.e., the probability estimate of a sentence with relative position j to be chosen as the target sentence, tn. We first create normalised histograms of each of the three relative sentence position distributions for S_{BEST}. Then, for a sentence in a document with a relative position j, the score assigned is equal to the normalised frequency of the jth bin of the histogram. Since we have a separate distribution for each target sentence position, the same sentence gets a different score based on which distribution is used for scoring (e.g., when selecting the first target summary sentence, sentences earlier in the documents get high scores, because of higher likelihood). Thus, the scoring is not biased towards a predetermined region of text, but is determined by probability distributions from seen data.

Sentence Length. We use the equation in [15] and reward longer sentences:

$$LEN_{s_{ij}} = \frac{len(s_{ij}) - avg(len(all))}{len(d_i)} \qquad (2)$$

where $len(s_{ij})$ is the length of sentence s_{ij}, $avg(len(all))$ is the average sentence length over the whole training set, and $len(d_i)$ is the length of the document.

Sentence-Query Similarity. We assign a score to each sentence based on its similarity with the question, since our analyses suggest that answers tend to contain similar contents as the associated questions. We use Maximal Marginal Relevance (MMR), which has been used for summarisation in the past [3]:

$$MMR_{s_{ij}} = \lambda(CosSim(s_{ij}, q_i)) - (1 - \lambda)max_{s_k \in S_s}(CosSim(s_{ij}, s_k)) \qquad (3)$$

where $CosSim()$ is a *cosine similarity* function that returns a score ranging from $1 - 0$ (1 = complete match; 0 = no match). Our cosine similarity metric represents the two sets as vectors of word and the UMLS medical semantic type *tf.idf* features. Incorporation of the medical semantic types ensures that we don't only consider word-level similarity, but also concept level similarity.

Sentence Type Statistics. We use two probabilistic measures involving the *type* of each sentence. We use the system proposed by [8] to classify all the sentences of the abstracts in our corpus into PIBOSO (population, intervention, background, other, study, outcome) elements. We generate frequency distributions of the PIBOSO elements in R_{TRAIN} and S_{BEST} and use the normalised frequency distributions for making probability estimates. The first score, which we call the Position Independent PIBOSO Score (PIPS) is computed as:

$$PIPS_{s_{it}} = \frac{P(s_t|S_{BEST})}{P(s_t|R_{TRAIN})} \qquad (4)$$

where $P(s_t|S_{BEST})$ is estimated as the proportion for PIBOSO element t among the sentences in S_{BEST}, and $P(s_t|R_{TRAIN})$ is estimated as the proportion of that PIBOSO element among the sentences in R_{TRAIN}. Thus, this score is higher for sentences belonging to PIBOSO categories that have a higher proportion among the best sentences compared to all sentences. The second score is computed as follows:

$$PDPS_{s_{it}} = \frac{P(s_t|tn = x)}{P(s_t|S_{BEST})} \qquad (5)$$

where $P(s_t|S_{BEST})$ is as before, and $P(s_t|tn = x)$ is the proportion for PIBOSO element t in a target sentence-specific distribution. We call this the Position Dependent PIBOSO Score (PDPS). For example, when selecting the first sentence (i.e., $tn = 1$), a sentence classified as Background is given a much higher score compared to a sentence classified as Outcome, because of the greater frequency.

There can be six possible *PIPS* scores as there are six types of sentences. We normalise these scores by dividing each score by the sum of all six scores. Similarly, for each target sentence, there can be six possible *PDPS* scores, giving a total of 18 possible scores (six for each tn). We normalise these scores in the same way. The intuitions behind these scores have been explained in [15].

3.3   Generation of *Question Type* Dependent Statistics

Our preliminary analyses suggest that the content of a summary is influenced by the type of question. For example, the content of the answer to a question that asks about the treatment of a disease is generally different from that of a question that asks about a diagnostic procedure. Our intent is to categorise the questions in our corpus into *types*, analyse the medical concepts that are prevalent in the answers to each of the question types, and devise techniques that reward sentences by taking into account the question types and the domain-specific concepts present in the sentences. We define two scores: $SEMTYPE_{s_{ij}}$ and $ASSOC_{s_{ij}}$. We classify the questions in our corpus using the same categories, training data, and approach as [17]. There are 12 possible classes, and each question can have multiple categories or none. In our corpus, 216 questions have a single category, 167 have 2 categories, 61 have 3, 9 have 4, and 3 have no categories. *Treatment and Prevention, Pharmacological, Diagnosis*, and *Management* are the four most frequent question types in the data set.

Semantic Types for Sentence Scoring. We use the categorised questions of our corpus to identify the UMLS semantic types that are important for each question type. Similar to some of our previous scoring approaches, we rely heavily on probability estimates from frequency distributions. We generate a frequency distribution of all the UMLS semantic types present in the human authored summaries (l_i) of R_{TRAIN}. Next, we generate separate frequency distributions of l_i for each question type. The two sets of distributions illustrate how the UMLS semantic types are distributed over the whole training set and for each type of question. If a semantic type st has a high frequency in the distribution for question type t, but a low frequency in the overall distribution, it indicates that st is an important semantic type for answers to all questions of type t. The score for a semantic type st is calculated as follows:

$$semtype\_score(st, t) = \frac{P(st|t)}{P(st)} \qquad (6)$$

where $P(st)$ is the probability estimate of semantic type st in the complete set of questions and $P(st|t)$ is the probability estimate of st in the questions of type t. Thus, the *semtype_score()* is large for semantic types that are more frequent for question type t than the whole training set and vice versa. When scoring the sentences of an abstract, each sentence receives a score ($ST_{s_{ij}}$) based on the set of UMLS semantic types it contains ($SEMT_{s_{ij}}$). This score is the sum of the normalised $semtype\_score()$ for the UMLS semantic types contained in that sentence, as shown below:

$$ST_{s_{ij}} = \sum_{st \in SEMT_{s_{ij}}} semtype\_score(st, t) \tag{7}$$

Semantic Associations for Sentence Scoring. The intuition behind this score is that medical terms in the questions generally have some relationships with the terms in the summary sentences. For example, if a question has a term representing a disease and the summary contains a term that acts as the cure for a disease, we can assume that there is a *is_treated_by* relationship between the disease term and the cure term. In our domain, the disease and cure terms are represented by the UMLS semantic types. The UMLS semantic network also provides associations between semantic types, and we attempt to use these associations to identify sentences in the source texts that are related to the associated questions.

To identify important associations for each type of question, we first identify: (i) important question semantic types, and (ii) important answer semantic types. (i) is identified from the questions in R_{TRAIN}, while (ii) is identified from the manual summaries (l_i) in R_{TRAIN}. We use an approach identical to the one described in the previous subsection, and remove semantic types that have relative frequencies below a given threshold (we empirically chose 0.01 as the threshold). Once both sets of semantic types are identified, we identify the important associations that exist within a question type by applying yet another frequency distribution. For each question type t, we compute a normalised frequency distribution of all the associations between the important question and answer UMLS semantic types. Given a question q_i of type t, the probability estimate of the answer to that question having an association $assoc_l$ is the relative frequency of $assoc_l$ in the association frequency distribution for t. When scoring a sentence s_{ij}, we first identify the set of all associations s_{ij} has with the question ($AS_{s_{ij}}$), find the relative frequencies of the associations, and sum the relative frequencies. We use the function $assoc\_freq(assoc, t)$, which, given an association type and a question type, computes the relative frequency of $assoc$ for t. The score assigned to the sentence is the sum of the relative frequencies, normalised by dividing the value by the total number of unique semantic types present in the question and the sentence. For questions with multiple types, the association frequency distributions for all the types are combined and normalised before computing sentence scores. The following equation summarises the scoring process:

$$ASSOC_{s_{ij}} = \sum_{assoc \in AS_{s_{ij}}} \frac{assoc\_freq(assoc, t)}{|st_{q_i} \cup st_{s_{ij}}|} \tag{8}$$

where st_{q_i} and $st_{s_{ij}}$ represent the semantic types present in the question and the sentence being scored respectively.

3.4 Combining Statistics for Sentence Extraction

We use the following *Edmundsonian* [6] equation to compute the score for s_{ij}:

$$SCORE_{s_{ijt}} = \alpha RP_{s_{ij}} + \beta LEN_{s_{ij}} + \gamma PIPS_{s_{it}} + \delta PDPS_{s_{it}} \\ + \epsilon MMR_{s_{ij}} + \zeta ST_{s_{ij}} + \eta ASSOC_{s_{ij}} \tag{9}$$

where $SCORE_{s_{ijt}}$ is the score for candidate sentence s_{ijt}; i represents the document number, j represents the sentence position, and t represents the question type. When extracting the first sentence, we replace the MMR score with the cosine similarity score in the equation.

To automatically find good approximations for optimal values of the weights (α, β, γ, δ, ϵ, ζ and η), and the λ parameter in MMR, we perform a grid search through all values from 0.0 to 1.0 using step sizes of 0.1. Our intent is to find a combination of weights that maximises the chances of selecting the sentences, from an abstract, that belong to S_{BEST}. Therefore, for each combination of weights, we compute the recall values for the first, second and last sentences over R_{TRAIN}. The combination producing the best combined recall is chosen. We also apply and alternative regression based approach for comparison. In this approach, separate weights are learned for each target sentence using an SVM regression algorithm [5]. For each sentence, all the above mentioned scores are derived, along with an additional score for the degree of overlap between the sentence and the human summary. Our intuition is that the higher the overlap score, the more likely is the sentence to be in the final summary. We use the *jaccard similarity* measure to compute overlap, and compute values for the weights using the overlap scores as the dependent variables.

4 Evaluation and Results

We are interested in assessing the performance of our system relative to those of other systems, on this data set. We use the ROUGE tool for this, and compare the ROUGE-L f-scores of different systems using the percentile-rank based approach proposed by [4]. Figure 1 shows the probability distribution (pd) obtained using this technique for all abstracts in R_{EVAL}. The pd shows the range of possible scores an extractive summarisation system can have given this data set. The distribution is long-tailed, meaning that the scores for most of the extracts in the summary space are clustered around the mean. This suggests that most systems are likely to produce scores that are around the mean of the pd. The two ends of the distribution are shown on Figure 1 via the short vertical lines. The longer vertical line shows the best score achieved by our system.

Using the pd, the percentile rank for a ROUGE-L f-score, sc, is given by the cumulative distribution funtion for pd evaluated at sc. The baselines we use are: Last three sentences, last three PIBOSO *outcome* sentences (this is comparable to the summarisation component presented in [10]), random, first three sentences, all PIBOSO *outcome* sentences, SumBasic [12], FastSum (modified) [16],

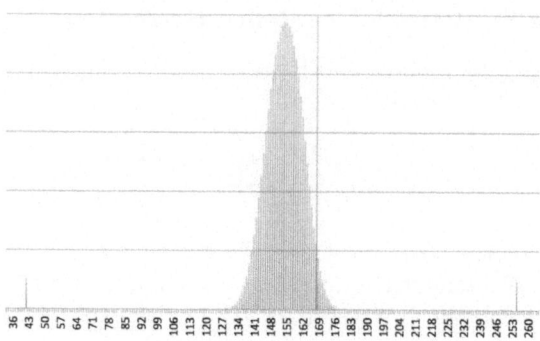

Fig. 1. The normalised histogram for all ROUGE-L f-scores in R_{EVAL}

Sentence Position Independent (SIP), and Naïve Bayes. For the Naïve Bayes summariser, a separate classifier is trained for each target sentence using the abstracts in R_{TRAIN} with the features mentioned in the previous section. For the FastSum system, modifications were made (e.g., no redundancy removal step) to customise it to single document summarisation. The SIP system is our system without any target sentence-specific features. Table 1 presents the ROUGE-L f-scores for our system and the baselines, the 95% confidence intervals for the f-scores as reported by ROUGE, and the percentile rank for each score. In the table, QSpec represents our system, which outperforms all systems with a percentile rank of 96.8%[4]. Learning the weights via regression results in a slight degradation of performance (not statistically significant), but is still better than the other systems. The next best performing baselines are: SIP, and the *Outcome*-based systems, one of which is our implementation of the system proposed by Lin and Demner-Fushman [10]. The poor performances of SumBasic and FastSum indicate that word-frequency based approaches are perhaps not suited for this domain. Figure 2 shows a sample summary produced by the QSpec system.

To assess the contribution of each feature towards the ROUGE scores, we performed two simple experiments: (i) sentence scoring using single features only, and (ii) sentence scoring by leaving out one feature. All the single features scores indicate statistically significant improvements over the score that is obtained using no features (i.e., first three sentence summaries). Importantly, none of the single feature scores are better than the score obtained by the combination of features. The same is true for the leave-one-out scores. None of the scores are statistically significantly lower than the best score, which indicates that the final score is not biased by the influence of a single score. *MMR* and *ST* are shown to be the most important features from this analysis, with score drops of 0.00234 and 0.00295 units respectively in the leave-one-out experiments.

---

[4] The percentile ranks for some systems in this paper are different to the ones presented in our pilot study [15]. This is because a different implementation of the same algorithm for generating the *pd* is used, which gives very slightly different values after the thousands of computations that must be performed. Relative performance comparison among the systems, however, is not different for the different *pds*.

Table 1. ROUGE-L f-scores, 95% confidence intervals and percentile ranks for our system and several baselines

System	F-Score	95% CI	Percentile (%)
Last Three	0.15482	0.151 - 0.158	55.9
Last Three Outcome	0.16050	0.158 - 0.164	78.1
Random	0.15251	0.149 - 0.156	46.1
First Three	0.13994	0.136 - 0.143	36.9
All Outcomes	0.15936	0.155 - 0.164	74.2
SIP	0.16019	0.157 - 0.164	78.1
Naïve Bayes	0.15551	0.152 - 0.159	55.9
SumBasic	0.15818	0.155 - 0.162	69.9
FastSum (modified)	0.15769	0.154 - 0.161	69.9
QSpec (grid search)	0.16780	0.164 - 0.172	96.8
QSpec (regression)	0.16479	0.161 - 0.169	92.5

Question: What medications are effective for treating symptoms of premenstrual syndrome (PMS)?

Summary: Forty women with premenstrual tension received either placebo, 100, 200 or 400 mg danazol daily for 3 months in a pilot study arranged as a double-blind trial. In patients treated with danazol, symptom scores for breast pain during the second and third months and for irritability, anxiety and lethargy during the third month were significantly (P less than 0.05) lower than scores in those given placebo. By the end of the trial more than 75% of patients who were still taking danazol were essentially free of breast pain, lethargy, anxiety and increased appetite, but results for other common symptoms were no better than with placebo.

Fig. 2. A sample 3-sentence, query-focused, extractive summary generated by QSpec

5   Conclusions

In this paper, we have presented an approach for query-focused, automatic, extractive summarisation that utilises target sentence-specific statistics, question type information, and novel domain-specific features. Statistics are derived from a corpus that specialises in summarisation for EBM and the sentence extraction process relies on these derived statistics. We evaluated our system against several baselines using ROUGE and show that our system outperforms all the baselines with a percentile rank of 96.8%. This shows that use of specialised corpora, target sentence-specific statistics, and the customisation of the sentence extraction procedure to query types can significantly improve the performance of such domain specific summaristion systems. The approach is fast, as it does not apply computationally expensive NLP techniques (e.g., parsing), and can therefore be readily used post retrieval. Our future work will focus on using single-document, extractive summaries to generate multi-document, bottom-line summaries.

References

1. Athenikos, S.J., Han, H.: Biomedical question answering: A survey. Computer Methods and Programs in Biomedicine, 1–24 (2009)
2. Cao, Y., Liu, F., Simpson, P., Antieau, L.D., Bennett, A., Cimino, J.J., Ely, J.W., Yu, H.: AskHermes: An Online Question Answering System for Complex Clinical Questions. Journal of Biomedical Informatics 44(2), 277–288 (2011)
3. Carbonell, J., Goldstein, J.: The use of mmr, diversity-based reranking for reordering documents and producing summaries. In: Proceedings of SIGIR, pp. 335–336 (1998)
4. Ceylan, H., Mihalcea, R., Özertem, U., Lloret, E., Palomar, M.: Quantifying the limits and success of extractive summarization systems across domains. In: Proceedings of NAACL, pp. 903–911 (2010)
5. Chang, C.-C., Lin, C.J.: LIBSVM: A library for support vector machines. ACM Transactions on Intelligent Systems and Technology 2, 1–27 (2011)
6. Edmundson, H.P.: New methods in automatic extracting. J. ACM 16(2), 264–285 (1969)
7. Ely, J.W., Osheroff, J.A., Ebell, M.H., Bergus, G.R., Levy, B.T., Chambliss, L.M., Evans, E.R.: Analysis of questions asked by family doctors regarding patient care. BMJ 319(7206), 358–361 (1999)
8. Kim, S.N.N., Martinez, D., Cavedon, L., Yencken, L.: Automatic classification of sentences to support Evidence Based Medicine. BMC Bioinformatics 12(2) (2011)
9. Lin, C.Y., Hovy, E.: Automatic Evaluation of Summaries Using N-gram Co-occurrence Statistics. In: Proceedings of HLT-NAACL 2003, pp. 71–78 (2003)
10. Lin, J.J., Demner-Fushman, D.: Answering clinical questions with knowledge-based and statistical techniques. Computational Linguistics 33(1), 63–103 (2007)
11. Mollá-Aliod, D., Santiago-Martinez, M.E.: Development of a Corpus for Evidence Based Medicine Summarisation. In: Proceedings of ALTW, pp. 86–94 (2011)
12. Nenkova, A., Passonneau, R.: The impact of frequency on summarization. MSR-TR, Microsoft Research, Redmond, Washington (2005)
13. Niu, Y., Zhu, X., Hirst, G.: Using outcome polarity in sentence extraction for medical question-answering. In: Proceedings of the AMIA Annual Symposium, pp. 599–603 (2006)
14. Richardson, S.W., Wilson, M.C., Nishikawa, J., Hayward, R.S.: The well-built clinical question: A key to evidence-based decisions. ACP Journal Club 123(3), A12–A13 (1995)
15. Sarker, A., Mollá, D., Paris, C.: Extractive Evidence Based Medicine Summarisation Based on Sentence-Specific Statistics. In: Proceedings of the 25th IEEE International Symposium on CBMS, pp. 1–4 (2012)
16. Schilder, F., Kondadadi, R.: Fastsum: Fast and accurate query-based multi-document summarization. In: Proceedings of ACL-HLT, Short Papers, pp. 205–208 (2008)
17. Yu, H., Cao, Y.G.: Automatically extracting information needs from ad hoc clinical questions. In: AMIA Annu. Symp. Proc., pp. 96–100 (2008)

Clustering of Medical Publications
for Evidence Based Medicine Summarisation

Sara Faisal Shash and Diego Mollá

Department of Computing,
Macquarie University, Sydney, 2109 NSW, Australia
{sara-faisal.shash,diego.molla-aliod}@mq.edu.au
http://web.science.mq.edu.au/~diego/medicalnlp/

Abstract. We present a study of the clustering properties of medical publications for the aim of Evidence Based Medicine summarisation. Given a dataset of documents that have been manually assigned to groups related to clinical answers, we apply K-Means clustering and verify that the documents can be clustered reasonably well. We advance the implications of such clustering for natural language processing tasks in Evidence Based Medicine.

1 Introduction

Evidence Based Medicine (EBM) is the practice that highlights the use of proven and current medical research and literature, when making clinical decisions. The process of EBM requires physicians to search, read and appraise medical literature in order to obtain recommendations for decisions. However, research has shown that accurate evidence in EBM is retrieved using a time consuming and resource intensive process that is largely manual and does not take advantage of emerging information processing technologies [1].

This paper contributes to solve this problem by outlining the application of document clustering to help identify the clusters of documents relevant to a given question. This will contribute to the eventual construction of an evidence based summary and create clusters of reference documents that will ultimately allow medical practitioners to improve their effective practice of EBM.

2 Clustering for Evidence Based Medicine

The ultimate goal of our research is to build a query-based multi-document summarisation system that takes, as input, a clinical question and a list of relevant documents, and generates a summary of the key relevant information extracted from the original documents that is relevant to the clinical question.

Document clustering is an unsupervised machine learning task that aims to discover natural groupings of data [2]. Document clustering has been used to aid the practice of EBM in various ways. Work done by Pratt and Fagan [3] showed that organising medical search results into meaningful groups that correspond to

N. Peek, R. Marín Morales, and M. Peleg (Eds.): AIME 2013, LNAI 7885, pp. 305–309, 2013.

a given query increases the efficiency of the search experience for users. Lin and Demner-Fushman [4] also show how grouping MEDLINE citations into clusters, based on extracted interventions from document abstract texts, improves the understanding of literature search results. A text mining framework for assisting bio-medical researchers through automatic document clustering and ranking was also developed by Lin et al. [5].

For the present study we use a corpus of clinical questions and evidence-based summaries obtained from the "Clinical Inquiries" section of the Journal of Family Practice (JFP)[1] [6]. The corpus is freely available and comprises 456 questions. Each question is accompanied with the group of documents from which answers are obtained. The answer to a clinical question in the corpus has several parts. Each part has a number of documents associated to it.

It is our goal to determine whether traditional clustering techniques applied to the set of documents relevant to a clinical question can be used to re-create the groups of documents relevant to the answer parts. Thus, we will perform 456 distinct clustering tasks and compare the resulting clusters with the document groupings in our dataset. In this paper, we will name the clusters produced by our method "clusters", and the clusters defined in the annotated data "source clusters". It is anticipated that the clustering criteria used in each question will be different, and therefore separate clustering methods would be required. In this paper, however, we study effect of clustering techniques without using the question information, as a first step towards query-based summarisation.

3 Clustering Experiments

In the original data set, documents were in the PubMed XML format[2] that comprises the article's abstract and metadata such as the title of the article, publication type, author, year of publication, medical subject headings (MeSH),[3] and country. We used MetaMap [7], a program developed to map biomedical terms to concepts in the Unified Medical Language System (UMLS), to select the medical terms from the text. We then conducted preliminary clustering experiments on four representations of the data set: (i) whole XML (original format), (ii) abstracts of articles only, (iii) terms that have an UMLS concept, and (iv) UMLS medical semantic types. Words were lowercased, stopwords removed, and remaining words were weighted based on *tf.idf*.

We used K-means as the clustering approach, using the original numbers of source clusters as the K parameter. This value of K is different for each question. Since this assumes prior knowledge we can take the result as an upper bound.

To determine clustering quality we used the cluster entropy measure. The entropy of cluster i is:

$$Entropy(i) = -\sum_{j} p_{i,j} \log_2 p_{i,j}$$

[1] http://jfponline.com
[2] http://www.nlm.nih.gov/bsd/licensee/data_elements_doc.html
[3] http://www.nlm.nih.gov/mesh/

Where $p_{i,j}$ is the number of documents in cluster i that belong to source cluster j, divided by the number of documents in cluster i.

The entropy measure of the clusters generated in a particular question of our data set is the weighted average of the entropies of all clusters from the question, where the weight is a ratio of the cluster size relative to the total set of documents relevant to the question. We then computed the average entropy across all questions. The results are in Table 1.

Table 1. Average entropy for optimal K clusters. The best result is marked in bold.

Measure	Whole XML	Abstract only	Concepts only	Semantic types
Euclidean	0.260	0.264	0.274	0.310
Correlation	0.348	0.362	0.349	0.347
Cosine	**0.249**	0.266	0.277	0.298
Dice	0.332	0.328	0.324	0.334
Jaccard	0.320	0.330	0.317	0.327
Manhattan	0.288	0.299	0.305	0.296

To interpret the results, note that purely random clustering would give an entropy of $-\log_2(1/K)$. For the average number of clusters in the dataset $K = 2.4$, the resulting entropy would be 1.263. As we can see from Table 1, the resulting clusters have much lower entropy values, indicating good clustering results. We can also observe that the lowest entropy value is obtained when Cosine Distance is used to cluster documents that are represented as whole XML documents. It is important to note that K-means clustering provides disjoint clusters that provide no provisions for clusters that overlap. At this stage, every document is assigned a unique cluster.

In regards to the representation of the data set (Whole XML, Abstract Only, Concept Only, Semantic Type Only), we can observe from Table 1 that there is little disparity between the entropy values obtained from the different representations of the data set. Entropy values for documents represented as Whole XML are, however, producing the best results (lowest entropy) in general. This might be due to the similarity between documents being able to be computed on more information, which in-turn yielded better clustering results. Entropy based on semantic types are the worst, presumably because the semantic types are too general and many words were grouped to the same semantic type. It was interesting to observe that the UMLS concepts did not produce better results than the abstracts only.

To determine the optimal number of clusters we tried the following three methods:

User defined K: This is a constant value of K for each question. We experimented with values of $K = 2, 3$, and 4 which are constant across all questions.

Rule of Thumb: Based on the total number m of documents in a cluster [8]. This provides a value of K that is distinct for each question.

$$K = \sqrt{m/2}$$

Cover Coefficient: Distance to each question and based on the number m of documents, the number n of terms, and the number t of non-zero entries in the matrix of bags of words [9],

$$K = \frac{m \times n}{t}$$

Table 2 shows the values of entropy for all our experiments. We only show the results on full XML documents since these performed best in our previous experiments.

Table 2. Average entropy for different cluster numbers

Measure	$K = 2$	$K = 3$	$K = 4$	RoT	Cover	Original
Euclidean	0.489	0.309	0.205	0.163	0.235	0.260
Correlation	0.604	0.413	0.283	0.238	0.316	0.348
Cosine	0.479	0.298	0.213	0.154	0.224	0.249
Dice	0.572	0.368	0.250	0.204	0.290	0.332
Jaccard	0.562	0.360	0.252	0.191	0.293	0.320
Manhattan	0.522	0.327	0.226	0.174	0.281	0.288

To interpret the above results, note that the entropy values will improve (decrease) as we increase the number of clusters. Therefore one can only compare methods that use (approximately) the same number of clusters. The average number of clusters in the original setting (when the number of clusters is provided) is 2.4. The average numbers of clusters of the rule of thumb and the cover method are 3.8 and 2.8, respectively. The cover method approximates the original number of clusters, and the entropy values are second to the rule of thumb. Thus, the cover method is the best compromise for the number of clusters and the resulting entropy values. This might be because the cover method uses information specific about the words in each document and assigns a higher weighting to documents that have a lot of terms in common.

4   Conclusions and Further Work

We have studied the effect of using K-means clustering for Evidence Based Medicine (EBM). Our system attempts to reproduce the original groupings of documents that provide the clinical evidence to the different components of the answer to a clinical question. The good entropy results demonstrated that K-Means works well in capturing these groupings.

By providing such clusterings we allow the separation of the different components of an EBM answer. This information can be used in future systems to provide the final EBM answers by applying information extraction techniques and redundancy-based approaches on the clusters.

In further work we will explore the use of alternative clustering methods such as Agglomerative Clustering or clustering based on Topic Modelling. More interestingly, we will explore the possibility of using fuzzy clustering methods that will enable a document to be assigned to multiple clusters. This will provide a closer approximation to the real scenario.

The present study considered relevance of the clusters to the question only implicitly in the sense that all documents were relevant to the question to start with. We will study the possibility of integrating supervised clustering techniques and incorporating similarity measures and clustering techniques that tightly incorporate the information of the question.

Further on the ultimate goal to produce the final EBM summaries, we will investigate methods to generate expressions of the cluster topics as means to extract the evidence relevant to the clinical answers.

References

1. Cohen, A.M., Adams, C.E., Davis, J.M., Yu, C., Yu, P.S., Meng, W., Duggan, L., McDonagh, M., Smalheiser, N.R.: Evidence Based Medicine: The essential role of systematic retrieval and the need for automated text mining tools. In: Proceedings of the 1st ACM International Health Informatics Symposium, pp. 376–380 (2010)
2. Andrews, N.O., Fox, E.A.: Recent Developments in Document Clustering. Tech. rep., Virginia Tech. (2007)
3. Pratt, W., Fagan, L.: The Usefulness of Dynamically Categorizing Search Results. Journal of the American Medical Informatics Association 7(6), 605–617 (2000)
4. Lin, J.J., Demner-Fushman, D.: Semantic clustering of answers to clinical questions. In: AMIA Annual Symposium Proceedings (2007)
5. Lin, Y., Li, W., Chen, K., Liu, Y.: A Document Clustering and Ranking System for Exploring {MEDLINE} Citations. Journal of the American Medical Informatics Association 14(5), 651–661 (2007)
6. Mollá, D., Santiago-Martínez, M.E.: Development of a Corpus for Evidence Based Medicine Summarisation. In: Proceedings of the Australasian Language Technology Workshop (2011)
7. Aronson, A.R.: Effective mapping of biomedical text to the UMLS Metathesaurus: the MetaMap program. In: Proceedings of the 2001 AMIA Annual Symposium, pp. 17–21 (January 2001)
8. Mardia, K.V., Kent, J.T., Bibby, J.M.: Multivariate Analysis. Academic Press, London (1979)
9. Can, F., Ozkarahan, E.A.: Concepts and Effectiveness of the Cover-Coefficient-Based Clustering Methodology for Text Databases. ACM Transactions on Database Systems 15(4), 483–517 (1990)

Classifying Measurements
in Dictated, Free-Text Radiology Reports

Merlijn Sevenster

Philips Research North America, Briarcliff Manor, NY 10510, USA
merlijn.sevenster@philips.com

Abstract. Radiological measurements (e.g., '3.2 x 1.4 cm') are the predominant type of quantitative data in free-text radiology reports. We report on the development and evaluation of a classifier that labels measurement descriptors with the exam they refer to: current and/or prior exam. Our classifier aggregates regular expressions as binary features in a maximum entropy model. It has average F-measure 0.942 on 2,000 annotated instances; the rule-based baseline algorithm has F-measure 0.795. Potential applications and routes for future are discussed.

Keywords: Radiology report, natural language processing, measurements.

1 Introduction

Radiology reports of cancer patients, amongst others, address interval change of disease burden both in qualitative and quantitative terms. Radiological measurements are the predominant type of quantitative data. Unlike other numerical, phenotypic evidence, such as lab values, measurements are described in free text, which hampers utilization of such data by automated agents.

In this paper we address the challenge of classifying measurement descriptors by the exam they refer to: current and/or prior exam. This classifier can be integrated in solutions that utilize radiological measurements, with varying application areas, including detection of mismatches between quantitative and qualitative lesion data; transcription support of measurement data for the sake of clinical trial management by highlighting measurement descriptors that refer to the current exam; and, automatically tabulating measurements to allow for clinical knowledge discovery.

Measurement descriptors (e.g., a string of the form '3.2 x 1.4 cm') can be recognized using pattern recognition techniques, such as regular expressions. We divided measurement descriptors in four classes. Let E be a given exam, and let m be a measurement descriptor in the radiology report of E. Then, m belongs to the first class whose definition it satisfies in the following ordered list:

- Relative position — m specifies the location of an image finding relative to another image finding, e.g., the underlined descriptor in *Stable tracheostomy tube, terminating <u>5 cm</u> above the carina.*

N. Peek, R. Marín Morales, and M. Peleg (Eds.): AIME 2013, LNAI 7885, pp. 310–314, 2013.
© Springer-Verlag Berlin Heidelberg 2013

- Comparison — m refers to a measurement made on E and in the sentence that contains m, this measurement is compared to a measurement on an exam predating E, e.g., *There is a 1.6 x 0.9 cm lytic focus in the right iliac wing, unchanged from previous examination.*
- Current — m refers to a measurement made on E, e.g., the first underlined descriptor in *There is an anterior mediastinal lymph node which measures 2.9 x 1.7 cm, previously measured 2.8 x 1.5 cm.*
- Prior — m refers to a measurement made on an exam that predates E, e.g., the second underlined descriptor in the above sentence.

Measurements belonging to the second to fourth class address dimensions of clinical findings, such as tumors.

Other quantitative data points extracted from medical content include medication strength [1] and image dose [2]. An important body in the medical natural language processing literature is dedicated to concept extraction [3] and normalizing narrative content [4]. MedLEE [5] is a general-purpose engine that maps radiology reports into an XML data structure. MedLEE recognizes measurements as special entities and maps them into dedicated <measure .../> XML nodes.

2   Materials and Methods

Corpus — A set of free-text radiology reports was obtained from an academic hospital in the Midwest spanning at least two weeks' worth of production. The radiology department uses Nuance dictation technology. Reports were deidentified and automatically separated in sections, paragraphs and sentences. Using the corpus, a regular expression was developed to recognize measurements of up to three dimensions. A string matching this expression is called a *marked phrase*.
Regular expressions — Per class C, two sets of regular expressions are developed: P_C and R_C. The expressions in P_C give the specific sentence contexts in which marked phrases of C occur. This set aims at high precision: if a marked phrase matches a regular expression from P_C then in all likelihood it belongs to C. For instance, the following expression is in $P_{current}$:

```
"measur(e|es|ing) *" + approx + m,
```

where `approx` matches phrases like 'approximately' and 'up to,' and `m` matches measurement descriptors. Similarly, the following expression is in P_{prior}:

```
"(enlarged|changed|decreased) *(in size *)?from *" + approx + m.
```

Not all sentence–phrase pairs match an expression in any of the sets P_C. To avoid that such pairs would go uncharacterized, a second series of sets R_C is installed that aim at high recall. The regular expressions in the sets R_C are essentially disjunctions of keywords. For instance, the keywords for prior are: 'previous(ly),' 'prior,' 'earlier,' and 'measured.'

Naive rule-based (NR) — A baseline classifier that exploits the strengths of the high-precision regular expressions. It is defined as a set of four rules, one for each class C, inheriting the class ordering: rel-pos > comparison > current > prior. For a given sentence s and marked phrase t, each rule is of the form:

If (s, t) matches at least one regular expression in P_C, then assign C.

The antecedent of each rule contains only one argument, hence the adjective naive.

Maximum entropy (ME) — Every sentence s and marked phrase t is represented as a binary vector. Each set P_C and R_C has an entry in the vector that is 1 if s and t match at least one of its regular expressions. In addition, we have three entries that hold 1 if t is one, two or three dimensional, respectively. Finally, for each n, we have a binary feature that returns 1 if there are n measurement descriptors in s.

A maximum entropy model (SharpEntropy) is trained on the binary vectors of the instances in the training set with default parameters. Maximum entropy models are known to be a "viable and competitives" [6] approach to a variety of natural language processing problems.

Evaluation — Ground truth was created from a randomly selected list of sentences with at least one marked phrase. The first 2,000 proper sentences s containing a measurement descriptor t were manually classified. The ground truth was compared against a control annotation (not discussed in this paper) yielding κ statistics higher than 0.922 for all classes.

The maximum entropy classifier is evaluated in a ten-fold cross-validation protocol: In each fold, nine parts are used for training the model, the remaining part is used for evaluation. The naive rule-based classifier requires no training data, and is thus evaluated in a one-fold protocol. The results are compared against the ground truth using standard metrics.

3   Results

The confusion matrix of the two classifiers is given in Table 1. Accuracy of NR is 0.887 (1,774/2,000); accuracy of ME is 0.960 (1,920/2,000).

In an one-against-all analysis, our four-class problem is reduced to four binary decision problem: for each class C, does an instance belong to C or not? The performance of the classifier on the four one-against-all problems are presented in Table 2. Average F-measure of NR on all classes is 0.795, that of ME is 0.942.

4   Discussion

The strong performance of NR on rel-pos (F-measure 0.992) indicates that the high-precision regular expressions match this class' instances and do not match instances of other classes. The score of ME is comparable to that of NR on this class (F-measure 0.985).

Table 1. Confusion matrix of ground truth (columns) and the classifiers (rows)

	\multicolumn{8}{c}{Ground truth}							
	current		prior		comparison		rel-pos		Sum	
	NR	ME	NR	ME	NR	ME	NR	ME	NR	ME
current	1,399	1,365	93	17	120	19	1	3	1,613	1,404
prior	2	3	182	259	5	1	0	0	189	263
comparison	1	34	3	2	61	166	0	0	65	202
rel-pos	0	0	0	0	1	1	132	130	133	131
Sum	1,402	1,402	278	278	187	187	133	133	2,000	2,000

Table 2. Scores of the classifiers on the four one-against-all problems

| | current | | prior | | comparison | | rel-pos | |
	NR	ME	NR	ME	NR	ME	NR	ME
Precision	0.867	0.972	0.663	0.985	0.910	0.822	0.992	0.992
Recall	0.998	0.974	0.955	0.932	0.326	0.888	0.992	0.977
F-measure	0.928	0.973	0.779	0.957	0.480	0.853	0.992	0.985
Accuracy	0.891	0.962	0.949	0.989	0.934	0.972	0.999	0.998
κ	0.711	0.909	0.751	0.951	0.453	0.838	0.992	0.984

On comparison, NR combines poor recall (0.326) with high precision (0.910), despite the fact that the rule of this class was second in NR's rule order. This shows that the regular expressions in its high-precision set indeed have high precision and apply infrequently. By taking into account the keywords and weighing the high-precision features of the other classes, ME obtains higher precision and recall scores, resulting in increased F-measure: 0.853 versus 0.480.

Confusion between current and comparison is the main source of error for ME: 34 of the 80 misclassified instances are current mistaken for comparison, whereas 19 are misclassified the other way around. None of these instances match any of the high-precision regular expressions of comparison; all match at least one of the comparison keywords in its set of high-recall regular expressions. The number of measurements in the sentence, modeled as a series of binary features, plays a role in the decision making of ME. Of the 34 current instances misclassified as comparison, only four appear in a sentence with one or more other measurements. Possibly, ME relies on a pattern to the effect that a sentence with one measurement descriptor is more likely to compare two measurements on different exams than a sentence with two or more measurement. This makes sense as a rule of thumb, but our data shows that it still causes relatively many errors.

ME has fewer prior/comparisonthan current/comparisonerrors. Since the number of instances of these classes are of the same order of magnitude (187 versus 278), this may signal that the comparison versus current errors are due to skewed class frequency (70.1% of all instances are current).

In our work, the narrative context of measurements is characterized by means of hard-coded patterns. Alternative approaches might use more advanced linguistic features, for instance, by using scopal information of keywords like 'previous,' bearing similarity to the Negex take on negation detection [7].

The class comparison is defined with respect to the sentence in which the measurement descriptor appears. A more liberal definition would involve the entire paragraph in which it appears. Consider for instance the following two sentences: *Hilar lymph node measures 2.1 x 0.8 cm. Grossly unchanged.* By our criteria, the measurement descriptor is current although comparison is consistent with the criteria's spirit. The impact of loosening the definition in this way must be investigated.

Our ME classifier can be leveraged to register measurements across reports. Consider the following sentence: *There is an anterior mediastinal lymph node which measures 2.9 x 1.7 cm, previously measured 2.8 x 1.5 cm.* If the most recent prior report contains a measurement with dimensions 2.8 x 1.5 cm labeled current or comparison, then with high likelihood they measure the same mediastinal lymph node albeit at different points in time.

Limitations of this work are as follows. The ground truth data cannot be shared because of legal restrictions. The classifiers were evaluated on the data set of only one institution. We did not conduct a formal ablation study.

Our work shows that a brute force enumeration of lexical patterns (in the form of regular expressions) combined with a statistical decision-making layer achieves formidable results. The described work can be leveraged in applications that are driven by quantitative clinical data, in the form of workflow support tooling or automated construction of sizeable databases.

References

1. Xu, H., Stenner, S.P., Doan, S., Johnson, K.B., Waitman, L.R., Denny, J.C.: MedEx: A medication information extraction system for clinical narratives. J. Am. Med. Inform. Assoc. 17(1), 19–24 (1996)
2. Cook, T.S., Zimmerman, S., Maidment, A.D., Kim, W., Boonn, W.W.: Automated extraction of radiation dose information for CT examinations. J. Am. Coll. Radiol. 7(11), 871–877 (2010)
3. Aronson, A.R., Lang, F.M.: An overview of MetaMap: Historical perspective and recent advances. J. Am. Med. Inform. Assoc. 17(3), 229–236 (2010)
4. Dreyer, K.J., Kalra, M.K., Maher, M.M., Hurier, A.M., Asfaw, B.A., Schultz, T., Halpern, E.F., Thrall, J.H.: Application of recently developed computer algorithm for automatic classification of unstructured radiology reports: Validation study. Radiology 234(2), 323–329 (2005)
5. Friedman, C., Alderson, P.O., Austin, J.H.M., Cimino, J.J., Johnson, S.B.: A general natural-language text processor for clinical radiology. J. Am. Med. Inform. Assoc. 1, 161–174 (1994)
6. Nigam, K.: Using maximum entropy for text classification. In: IJCAI 1999 Workshop on Machine Learning for Information Filtering, pp. 61–67 (1999)
7. Chapman, W.W., Bridewell, W., Hanbury, P., Cooper, G.F., Buchanan, B.G.: A simple algorithm for identifying negated findings and diseases in discharge summaries. J. Biomed. Inform. 34(5), 301–310 (2001)

Author Index